Paediatric Practice in Developing Countries

Second Edition

G. J. EBRAHIM

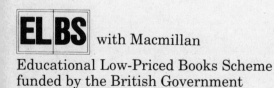

with Macmillan

Educational Low-Priced Books Scheme
funded by the British Government

The Macmillan Press Ltd
London and Basingstoke

*Associated companies and representatives
throughout the world*

© G. J. Ebrahim 1981, 1993

The Educational Low-Priced Books Scheme
is funded by the Overseas Development
Administration as part of the British
Government overseas aid programme.
It makes available low-priced, unabridged
editions of British publishers' textbooks to
students in developing countries.

First published 1981
Second edition 1993

ELBS edition first published 1984
Reprinted in 1987, 1988, 1990, 1991
ELBS edition of second edition 1993

ISBN 0–333–57346–3

Printed in China

Contents

Preface to the Second Edition

The first edition of Paediatric Practice in Developing Countries came out at about the same time as the Alma Ata Declaration on Primary Health Care (PHC). As countries commenced the task of reorienting their health services towards PHC, the book soon became the standard text for in-service training of health workers in several countries, and later for undergraduate and postgraduate teaching. The book's focus on high standards of clinical care with emphasis on prevention, and equal commitment to those who come seeking medical attention as well as to those who do not or cannot has been appreciated by colleagues around the world.

Since the publication of the first edition major changes have taken place. All developing countries have experienced a rise in their populations, even though the growth rate has slowed from 2 per cent annually in the 1970's to the current 1.7 per cent. But the serious and growing demographic challenge of the 1990's is the rise in urban population, with between 45 and 50 per cent of them living below the poverty line. Increase in poverty also means exclusion from the conventional type of services. Hence dealing with diseases of poverty will continue to remain the main concern for this decade and beyond.

In all developing countries PHC for the disadvantaged communities must be organised in a world climate of economic recession, made worse by a heavy burden of external debt. Even in the more affluent countries economic downturn has necessitated the closing down of prestigious institutions and transfer of resources to grass roots level.

And yet remarkable progress has been achieved during the past decade in global health indices. Access to PHC has increased dramatically with 70 per cent of the population in the least developed countries enjoying access to health care. Global programmes like the Expanded Programme of Immunisation, Oral Rehydration Therapy, control of Acute Respiratory Infections, The Child Survival Revolution and several others are helping to establish a strong foundation for child health in the developing world. Immunisation coverage rate is now in excess of 80 per cent compared to less than 20 per cent in the 1970's. More than 40 per cent of children in the world with episodes of diarrhoea are being treated by oral rehydration, and the proportion is increasing annually. There have been a number of beneficial spin-offs from these global programmes. For example, there has been unprecedented growth of relevant health infrastructure, a great deal of managerial experience has been gained, and there has been the social mobilisation of the population to meet health targets.

As the count down to Health For All by the Year 2000 begins, it is time to consolidate the progress made and to build towards the future. This second edition of Paediatric Practice in Developing Countries takes a forward look at the post-PHC era. From that point of view all the chapters have been brought up-to-date, and the majority have been rewritten. A new chapter on HIV infection has been added. Throughout the book the approach remains as before viz. striving for high standards of clinical care in hospital whilst endeavouring to deal with the determinants of disease in the community. Though principally aimed at the district medical officer, the book's target audience also remains the same as before, namely all those concerned with improving the health of children in the developing world.

G.J.E.

Section I

The Background

1 Introduction

Developing countries carry a heavy burden of disease and death. This is seen mainly in vulnerable groups such as children and women in the reproductive phase of life; in these groups inadequate nutrition, physiologic demands and lack of resistance make the effects of disease more serious. The hostile physical environment manifests itself in heavy infant and child mortality and a low expectancy of life, and these two indices taken together give an indication of the health of a community.

Low standards of health affect a society in many different ways. A heavy childhood mortality, where 30 to 40 per cent of the children born do not reach the age of five years, is a strong indicator of the prevalence of ill-health in the community as a whole. This is seen in table 1.1.

In an Inter-American Investigation of Mortality in Childhood (Pan American Health Organisation, 1973) the under-five mortality in El Salvador and Bolivia was found to be as high as 50.5 per 1000 population. As might be expected, a large proportion of this mortality occurred under the age of one year (table 1.2).

A striking feature of all studies in childhood mortality is that most of the morbidity and deaths are caused by only a handful of diseases. The Registrar General's office in India has reported on causes of mortality in rural areas from data recorded in 786 villages with a total population of 2.3 million. More than 80 per cent of deaths were categorised under eight causes or symptoms. Similarly, mortality studies in Iran show that respiratory illnesses account for 30 per cent and infectious and parasitic diseases for another 28 per cent of all attendances at health institutions. Thus 58 per cent of all illnesses were accounted for by two of the 17 major disease groups in that country.

It is not only the children who develop disease and die, but the entire community is exposed to ill-health, and the children succumb easily because they are more vulnerable. Also, not only do 30 or 40 per cent of the children develop disease and die, but the entire child community is at risk and only the fortunate survive. It is also likely that among the survivors, growth potential has been compromised because of illness in early childhood, or that the body's physiological processes may become suboptimal and thus unable to withstand stress. This is especially so in the case of girls who take on responsibilities of parenthood at a very early age.

Widespread ill-health in the community can produce far-reaching effects on the national economy. In most developing countries there are too few people in the productive age-groups supporting a large number of individuals.

Table 1.1 Selected developing countries: per cent who die before fifth birthday

Country	Per cent dying before fifth birthday	Age at which the same per cent die in USA
India	28.1	63
Pakistan	31.0	66
Egypt	24.8	61
Guinea	36.7	68
Cameroon	26.5	62
Guatemala	18.5	57

Sources: *UN Demographic Yearbooks* 1963, 1967, 1969 and 1970. Washington, Population Bureau *1970 World Population Data Sheet.*

Table 1.2 Mortality by age group in the Inter-American Investigation of Childhood Mortality

Age group	Deaths	Per cent
Under 5 years	35 095	100
Under 1 year	27 602	78.6
Neonatal (0–27 days)	12 674	36.1
Post-neonatal (28 days–11 months)	14 928	42.5
1 year	4 361	12.4
2–4 years	3 132	8.9

Certain characteristics of developing countries

Many developing countries share the following characteristics

The demographic pattern

The populations are predominantly young. Approximately 45 per cent consists of individuals under the age of 15 years and up to 20 per cent may be children under the age of five (figure 1.1).

Thus the child health services have to carry a heavy work load. If to the above figures is added the number of women in the reproductive phase of life, the maternal and child health services have the task of looking after 65–70 per cent of the population. The demographic pattern calls for a fundamental reorganisation of services and allocation of resources.

Rurality with urban shift

Rurality with widespread subsistence farming has characterised most African, Asian and Latin American countries for centuries, but the pattern is now changing. Urban migration and expansion is a feature which will dominate the future, with many implications for health services.

At present India's population is 80 per cent rural, distributed among 570 000 or more villages and hamlets, and nine-tenths of East Africa's population is living in scattered homesteads. Such a widely scattered population creates many difficulties in communication and in delivery of health care. Furthermore, physical and social isolation, together with illiteracy, often make peasant societies conservative and suspicious of all outside influences. Hence programmes of health care need careful planning and implementation with community involvement at all stages.

In 1940 only 25 per cent of the world's 2295

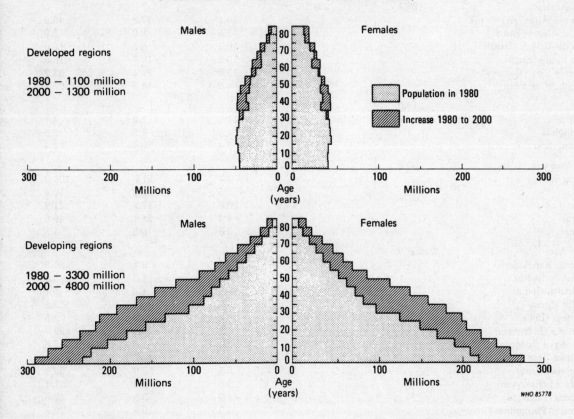

POPULATION BY AGE AND SEX (1980 AND 2000)

Figure 1.1 Population pyramids

million population lived in cities, but by the end of the century 51 per cent of the projected population of 6254 million will live in cities. This represents enormous growth and shifts of people. Even over 25 years (1975 to 2000) the urban population is expected to increase by some 250 per cent in the less developed countries of the world (table 1.3). This uncontrolled urban population explosion is a particular threat to the health of children, because most will live in slums and shanty towns where destitution, environmental degradation and moral disruption are worse than in most impoverished villages. The health problems of the urban poor are a mixture of a heavy burden of malnutrition and infection together with chronic and social diseases of industrial countries. Although the prospects for

Table 1.3   Urban population increase

	Total urban population 1975 (millions)	Total urban population increase 1975–2000 (millions)	Principal city's population in 1980 (millions)	Principal city's population as % of: national population	Principal city's population as % of: total urban population
Northern Africa	38.2	71.6			
Cairo (Egypt)			7.4	17.6	38.6
Sub-Saharan Africa	66.0	185.9			
Addis Ababa (Ethiopia)			1.7	5.2	36.6
Jos (Nigeria)			2.7	3.5	17.0
Kinshasha (Zaire)			3.1	11.0	28.0
Lagos (Nigeria)			1.2	1.6	7.9
Nairobi (Kenya)			1.3	7.9	57.3
Latin America	198.1	230.1			
Buenos Aires (Argentina)			10.1	37.3	45.2
Porto Alegre (Brazil)			2.5	2.0	3.0
Rio de Janeiro (Brazil)			10.7	8.5	13.0
Sao Paulo (Brazil)			13.5	10.7	16.5
Mexico City (Mexico)			15.0	21.4	32.2
Bogota (Colombia)			4.9	18.2	25.8
China	218.0	273.9			
Beijing			11.4	1.2	4.7
Shanghai			14.3	1.5	5.9
Guangzhou			3.4	0.4	1.4
East Asia	30.6	34.0			
Hong Kong			4.4	91.0	100.0
Osaka			9.5	8.2	10.4
Tokyo			20.0	17.2	21.9
Seoul			8.4	22.1	40.6
Taipei			3.3	0.3	1.3
South Asia	265.9	455.8			
Dacca (Bangladesh)			3.0	3.4	30.0
Bombay (India)			8.4	1.2	5.4
Calcutta (India)			8.8	1.3	5.7
Delhi (India)			5.4	0.8	3.5
Madras (India)			5.4	0.8	3.5
Jakarta (Indonesia)			7.2	4.7	23.3
Surabaya (Indonesia)			2.4	1.6	7.8
Tehran (Iran)			5.4	14.2	28.4
Baghdad (Iraq)			5.1	39.0	54.6
Karachi (Pakistan)			5.0	6.1	21.4
Lahore (Pakistan)			2.9	3.5	12.6
Manila (Philippines)			5.5	10.8	29.9
Bangkok (Thailand)			4.7	9.9	68.6

significant investment in housing and services is unlikely, the fact that people are grouped together makes the delivery of some services relatively easier.

Lack of resources

The health budgets of many developing countries are small and often inadequate to meet the needs of the nation. Of the 86 developing countries for which data are available, in the case of 22 the average outlay on health is less than US $1 per head per year. Moreover, in the last few years economic necessity has resulted in a decline in health spending per person in more than three quarters of the nations of Africa and Latin America, and the decline is almost certainly more widespread than what available data suggest. Most countries of sub-Saharan Africa and Latin America enter the 1990s with a crippling burden of international debt. Debt servicing costs Latin America four times the value of exports. The total amount of debt for sub-Saharan Africa is 10 to 15 per cent of that for Latin America, but judging from the value of exports the debt burden works out to be twice as heavy.

The economic downturn has given rise to widespread poverty. During the 1980s average incomes have fallen by 10 per cent in most of Latin America and by over 20 per cent in sub-Saharan Africa. In many urban areas real minimum wages have declined by as much as 50 per cent. For the absolute poor, those who must spend 80 per cent or more of their income to purchase 80 per cent of the minimum calorie requirement, cuts in real income on such a scale can only mean malnourishment.

Politically strong urban sector

The cities of developing countries are very different from those of the Western democracies in the social and political sense. They house the legislature, civil service, the main government administration and the colleges and universities. In addition, the politicians, industrialists, leading businessmen and other power groups are all concentrated in the cities. Together, they control finance, all the mass media and most of the decision making processes. The modern urban sector demands, and is usually able to obtain, services as sophisticated as those of the West, even though this often means depriving the rural areas of even the most rudimentary service. On average, in many developing countries up to 80 per cent of the health budget may be spent on cura-

tive services based on hospitals which are invariably sited in urban areas. Also, it is not unusual to see that large teaching hospitals are consuming half the total health budget in recurrent costs.

The urban/rural maldistribution of resources

In most countries there is a concentration of health personnel in the urban areas, and a large proportion of vacancies in the rural health services remain unfilled (table 1.4).

The inequality in health care between urban and rural areas is reflected in the different mortality and morbidity rates, life expectancy rates and other health indices between the two areas. The pattern of expenditure in health manpower development is often such that it tends to perpetuate this inequality. For example, there is increased production of physicians as compared to medical auxiliaries who are the key persons in delivering health care in rural areas.

Health planning and policy based on an imported Western model

The present health systems of many of the developing countries have grown out of a nucleus of services established during the colonial era. Of necessity such beginnings were based on the experiences of the metropolitan country. Thus, the health systems have been capital intensive, based on large hospitals with emphasis on health care delivered by physicians and specialists. Growth of service after independence has invariably tended to perpetuate the Western model, as seen in table 1.5 which describes the growth of health services in Tanzania during the first ten years of independence.

Table 1.4 Distribution of doctors between the capital and the rest of the country – 1968

Country	Population: Doctor ratio		
	Nationwide average	Capital city	Rest of the country
Kenya	10 999	672	25 600
Thailand	7 000	800	25 000
Guatemala	4 860	875	22 600
Jamaica	2 280	840	5 510
Pakistan	7 400	3 700	24 200
Philippines	3 900	1 500	10 000

Table 1.5   Health budget of Tanzania and UK

	Tanzania (£)	UK (£)
Total health budget – 1961	2 million	981 million
Hospital Services	80%	56.8%
Local Health Authority Services	–	9.3%
Public Health	5%	–
Total health budget – 1971	7 million	1880 million
Hospital Services	79%	61.2%
Local Health Authority Services	–	10.4%
Public Health	8.5%	–

Table 1.5 shows that up to 80 per cent of the health budget of Tanzania was spent on hospital services, even though improvement of preventive services was the national goal. Increasing the health budget by three and a half times did not help because of the inherent nature of the model. Hospital services still continued to absorb 79 per cent of the enlarged budget and expenditure on public health could be enhanced by only 3.5 per cent. Fundamental policy decisions were necessary in order to create a health service more relevant to the needs of the country and to halt further development along the imported Western model.

Background to childhood illnesses in developing countries

Physical

A low standard of living in a harsh physical environment is common to all rural areas and many parts of the cities of developing countries. Housing is poor with inadequate ventilation and a large number of adults and children crowd into a small room, often with cattle or other domestic animals. Transmission of respiratory disease is common under such conditions and in young children upper respiratory infection is recurrent.

Environmental sanitation is virtually non-existent. Water is brought from a distant source, usually by women and children, and is not enough to maintain a good standard of personal cleanliness. Drinking water is invariably unsafe. It is not uncommon to see clothes being washed or morning ablutions performed on the banks of streams from which drinking water is obtained. Cattle are also brought to drink from the same source. Even in urban areas where sewage disposal systems and piped water supplies have been established, these do not reach out to the slums and shanty towns which have become the 'septic fringes' of the cities and where infective illnesses have become endemic.

Economic

Agriculture is of a primitive kind with poor yields per acre. Moreover, a large part of the harvest is destroyed by rodents and insects because of inefficient storage. It has been estimated that in most peasant societies fully 40 per cent of the calories consumed by man and cattle are utilised for the day to day toil on the land, leaving very little margin for anything else. Such subsistence nutrition is inadequate for growing children and pregnant and lactating women so that growth failure and undernutrition are prevalent in those groups. In addition, there is ignorance about nutrition and its importance in health so that even available foods are not utilised fully, giving rise to a high incidence of nutritional deficiency. The interaction of poor nutrition with infection usually develops into a cycle where one accentuates the other leading to illness.

Productivity of the average peasant household is small and constitutes one of the important causes of rural poverty. Thus in India, the average size of the holding is 3.04 ha but about 70 per cent of the holdings are below this average (Agricultural Labour Inquiry Report, 1954). In parts of tropical Africa where the plough has not yet been introduced and most cultivation is done by the hoe, the area per household is not more than 0.8 to 3.04 ha (Kenya Statistical Abstract, 1972). In many parts of Southeast Asia, in the Philippines, Ethiopia and parts of Latin America, the landless labourers, who form a quarter to a third of rural households, constitute some of the poorest sections of the rural populations. In a study of rural poverty in India it was shown that 40 per cent of the rural population had per capita consumer expenditure which was inadequate to provide enough calories.

Besides the subsistence sector representing almost all the rural population, there also exists the modern cash economy in the cities which attracts many from the rural areas in the hope of employment. In many instances urban unemployment and poverty represent an overflow from the rural areas.

It is not often appreciated that the situation in the cash sector is frequently precarious, because only a small number of products and services tend to predominate. Thus, cocoa in Ghana, copper in Zambia, coffee in Brazil and tea in Sri Lanka are the main sources of foreign exchange. Even in India tea, cotton and jute account for up to half the exports. The second characteristic of the cash sector is 'the big firm small country syndrome'. A great deal of the economic activity is in the hands of large multinationals with huge economic resources so that it is impossible for a small country to exert pressure on such companies to bring them in line with their domestic economic policies. For example, in 1966 the United Fruit Company controlled 100 per cent of export banana acreage in Guatemala, 70 per cent in Costa Rica and Panama and 56 per cent in Honduras. In such a situation it is the only large employer in the country.

Medical

Even though medical knowledge and technology have advanced considerably in recent years, the problem of making them available to rural communities has not been adequately solved. Effective systems of delivering health care to the rural masses and to the urban poor have been evolved by only a few countries. The rural communities are spread out over large areas in small villages or scattered homesteads. Roads and other means of communication are often poorly developed. The terrain may be difficult and, above all, the system of medical care is so entrenched in curative medicine within urban pockets that only minimal effort is made towards protecting and promoting the health of the majority of the population.

During the past two decades the health centre with a system of satellite centres around it and mobile teams operating from various outposts has come to be the core of a system for delivering health care to the people. Many developing countries have invested large sums of money on creating an infrastructure based on the health centre/sub-centre complex. The concept of the health centre as a unit for the total health care of the community and not just a curative centre looks attractive on paper but there are many obstacles to its full realisation. Evaluation of the work of the health centre in several countries has shown that often it turns into an extension of the out-patient department of the district hospital and produces no real impact on the health of the people it serves. In theory the health centre is expected to serve between 60 000 and 100 000 people, but in practice it serves the needs of only those in its immediate neighbourhood. In a survey of catchment areas of rural health centres in Tanzania it was found that over half of all out-patients came from within a distance of 8 km and 80 per cent of all attendances were from within 16 km. Analysis of service contacts in health centres in India revealed that 75 per cent of service contacts are for curative care. The preventive and promotive activities tended to be few and very little was done to improve environmental sanitation.

Until recently, the policies of most developing countries laid stress on the extension of the existing system of health care into the rural areas with a view to providing wider coverage of the population. The health centre and its satellite sub-centres were logical developments of such policies. But experience of the last two decades, as described above, has revealed the weakness of such a strategy. In Asia and Latin America where medical education has expanded a great deal, the rural areas have remained unaffected because of the preference of the professional for working in hospitals rather than in communities.

The failure of the above policy based on the 'trickle down' effect has led many nations to review their health strategies. It is obvious that spending more in the same way is not the answer. Secondly, national health plans in many countries have little relationship to what actually happens in the health sector. Whereas the health plans emphasise preventive and curative activities in rural areas, the major spending of the health budget continues to be on curative hospital-based activities in urban areas. This 'implementation gap' is due to a number of factors. There is the general difficulty of diverting resources from the politically powerful to the rural poor. Most national planning begins in the capital city which dominates the regions and the provinces which in turn dominate the district and local authorities. Finally, most health planning has to accommodate the prevailing medical opinions which are often moulded by forces within the society.

In spite of these difficulties, several countries have been able to expand their health coverage in a relatively short time through fundamental changes in the health care delivery systems. A study of the health policies of countries that have succeeded in extending health coverage to rural areas, such as Cuba, China, Tanzania and Venezuela, reveals that the following factors have contributed to their success

(1) Their health systems are directed towards the 'grass roots' and are fundamentally different from those which draw clients to a hierarchy of centralised services. Many of the basic illnesses of the peasant society do not need complex technology. These grass-root services have the objective of promoting good diet during pregnancy, simple antenatal and obstetric care, breast feeding and proper weaning of infants, clean environment, immunisation, prompt treatment and rapid referral in time of illnesses.
(2) Community involvement and total responsibility for their own health.
(3) Use of village health workers selected from within the community and who are resident in the villages they serve.
(4) The conventional health system acting to support the village health workers through training, supply of drugs and consultations.
(5) Closer links between village health workers and other aspects of community development. This takes account of the fact that the health of a community is influenced by several non-health factors like food, clean water, housing, clothing and basic education.

Whilst the different components of a national health service – village health workers, auxiliaries, the professionals and specialists working from a hierarchy of institutions, and community participation – are being assembled into a co-ordinated system, some important questions remain to be considered. How is the rural health service to be financed? If it is to be mainly financed from local resources, then the moral and political issues of making the rural poor pay for themselves whilst a major proportion of the national health budget is spent on the privileged urban population need to be fully debated. The possible solutions are: (1) re-allocate health resources equitably as was done in Cuba; (2) reserve a large proportion of the national health budget for the development and capital costs of rural health services as presently done in Tanzania; (3) re-design the government health service to make it more supportive of the rural health services as in Venezuela. The second issue is that of training so that the professional feels responsible not only for those who come seeking help to the hospital but also for the health of the community at large. This means a change of attitudes so that there is a sense of pride

in the achievements of the entire health team rather than in the individual's clinical skills.

Social

An important feature of rural life is physical and social isolation. Because of poor roads and communications the contacts between inhabitants of various villages are few and far between. The residents of one village may also be subdivided amongst themselves because of a caste system or a feudal system of ownership of land.

Many sociologists have emphasised the role of the joint family, matri- or patri-local as the basic social institution of the peasant society. The relationships between members of a family are a result of living closely together. They work on the family farm together, share the same household and undergo the same privations. Several families relate to each other through the social institutions of kinship and marriage. Many activities which in a complex society will be classed as 'economic', 'educational', 'political' etc. are carried out as part of the performance of kinship role. Kinship and belonging to a clan gives a man the right to land. It also determines the politics of intrigue against other clans. Even religion may be a matter of kinship because there are clan deities and ancestral cults. When the peasant society undergoes change, additional social structures like the village committee, the farmers' club, the women's organisation are grafted onto the previously existing social system in which kinship has a key role. Many sociologists believe that social change will be acceptable as long as there can be a 'fit' between the family and the social system. Acceptance and spread of innovations must be considered in the light of the existing system.

Each clan or extended family evolves a complicated system of rearing children. Foods allowed to the pregnant women, the taboos they should observe, the methods of delivery, breast feeding practices, methods of weaning, etc., are all governed by the traditional methods of child rearing. Similarly, each clan has specific attitudes towards health and disease, mainly bordering on the supernatural so that for protection of health or in illness recourse is taken to wearing amulets, propitiation of ancestral spirits, incantations of a priest or the help of a witch doctor. The 'germ theory' of causation of disease has not reached the majority of the rural people, and it will be some time before an increase in education and development of mass media can carry scientific concepts of health and disease to the villages.

Prevention of childhood mortality and morbidity

Sickness and death amongst children in the developing world are usually not due to rare tropical disorders. They are caused by preventable illnesses which, until recently, used to be widespread in all the countries of Western Europe and have now been controlled and contained. Thus, the three main causes of hospital admissions in children – the Big 3 – are protein-energy malnutrition, respiratory infections, and diarrhoea. They account for between 30 and 40 per cent of all paediatric admissions. The next six most common illnesses are anaemia, measles and other common infectious diseases of childhood, malaria and other parasitic diseases, tuberculosis, burns and accidents and poisoning. Together with the Big 3 these illnesses constitute the Dominant 9 of paediatric problems in the developing world.

It is very striking that only a handful of illnesses take such a heavy toll of young lives in developing countries. All of them are 'diseases of poverty' and indicate the low living standards and lack of adequate services in the villages and in urban slums. Wherever socio-economic improvement has occurred either as a result of political change or by means of a service programme, rapid improvement in mortality figures has followed. From the biomedical point of view two factors need to be mentioned

(1) Undernutrition and infection make a lethal combination. Health surveys of pre-school children in developing countries have shown that about half the children in a community may be undernourished. Resistance to infection is reduced in such children so that they are frequently ill. Each episode of illness causes further deterioration of the nutritional status and tends to take a severe form. In this way a vicious cycle is created culminating in dangerous illness.
(2) Paediatric pathology in developing countries tends to be multiple. Thus the child who is admitted to hospital for a respiratory infection may also have anaemia and malarial parasitaemia, and in addition suffer from undernutrition.

Health programmes for the prevention of childhood mortality

To promote health and reduce mortality an adequate system of delivering health care to the rural population must be organised. The basic requirements of such a system are

(1) A service to look after the very ill and the ambulatory sick.
(2) A service for the control of common communicable diseases like tuberculosis, malaria, leprosy and the common infectious diseases of childhood.

It is not generally recognised that a large proportion of the decline in mortality in industrial societies of the West has been achieved through control of communicable diseases. For example, in England and Wales mortality declined by 15 per cent between 1851 and 1900. Falling mortality in five diseases accounted almost entirely for this decline – tuberculosis for nearly half; typhoid, typhus and pyrexia for about a fifth; scarlet fever for a fifth and cholera, dysentery and diarrhoea for nearly a tenth. The continued decline after 1900 was also due mainly to a decrease in deaths from infectious diseases. Between 1901 and 1947 the standardised mortality rate from all causes fell by over a half. A third of this reduction was due to fall in mortality from infections such as measles, whooping cough, diphtheria, smallpox, scarlet fever, tuberculosis, typhoid, paratyphoid, dysentery, influenza and syphilis; a further third was from reduction in deaths due to respiratory infection and diarrhoeal diseases. Thus fully two-thirds of the reduction in mortality in the first half of this century in England and Wales was due to decline in deaths from infectious illnesses.

(3) A service for supervising the health of vulnerable groups, mainly children under the age of five and pregnant and lactating women.

Such a service will comprise antenatal clinics, delivery beds and under-fives' clinics. Once established, additions can be made in the form of home visiting, nutrition rehabilitation, school health programmes and family planning.

Recent experience of operating these services through minimally trained village health workers has demonstrated that such workers can be trained to select 'at risk' individuals and families and to organise medical or social services for their assistance.

(4) Regular medical audit by the district health
    team to assess the effectiveness or otherwise of
    the health activities.

Such a basic health programme can be expanded
and strengthened by the addition of other activities
as circumstances permit. For example, such
additional activities can be in the form of periodic
mass immunisation campaigns, improvement and
protection of the water supply, environmental sanitation and so on. It is, however, important to make
sure that all the different health activities in a district do not operate in isolation from each other
but are part of a well co-ordinated district health
programme.

Innovative and lively health programmes have
often become spearheads of change in traditional
society. Several instances are on record where a
successful health programme has led to community
awareness bringing in its wake improved agriculture and education, and a better standard of
living.

Further reading

Ebrahim G J. *Child Health in a Changing Environment*.
    London: Macmillan Press Ltd., 1982.
Webster A. *Introduction to the Sociology of Development*.
    London: Macmillan Press Ltd., 1984.
Mountjoy A, (ed). *The Third World: Problems and Perspec-
    tives*. London: Macmillan Press Ltd., 1980.
Harpham T, Lusty T, and Vaughan P, (eds). *In the Shadow
    of the City; community health and the urban poor*.
    Oxford: Oxford University Press, 1988.
Morley D, Lovel H. *My Name is Today*. London: Macmillan
    Press Ltd., 1986.
Richard P J, Thomson A M. *Basic Needs and the Urban
    Poor*. London: Croom Helm, 1984.

2 Nature of childhood illness in developing countries

All throughout childhood the important physiological processes of growth and development take place. Both are a result of interaction between the genetic endowment of the child and the environmental influences. The child's home, the neighbourhood and geography constitute the physical environment and the family, the kinsfolk, neighbours and community provide the socio-cultural environment (figure 2.1). The family encounters different environmental and infective hazards and protects the child from them. The family also applies cultural and nutritional ideas to the rearing of the child, ensuring that community expectations are upheld in their upbringing of the child. The family also makes use of available community facilities to their advantage. When the physical, social and intellectual adaptation of the family to the environment prove inadequate, illness and symptoms develop.

Effects of illness on growth

All illnesses in children interfere with the delicate balance between several physiological mechanisms which determines optimum growth. Nutritional intake, absorptive processes, cellular metabolism, endocrine function, circulation of blood and supply of oxygen and nutrients, removal of waste products and psychological mechanisms all interact in this highly complex process of growth in which new cells are being added to body tissues and acquire function. It is now widely known that during an illness there is breakdown of tissue cells and loss of nutrients from the body. At the same time food intake diminishes because of anorexia or nausea or because only fluid diets have been allowed during the illness. Thus, in all illnesses growth slows down. In normal

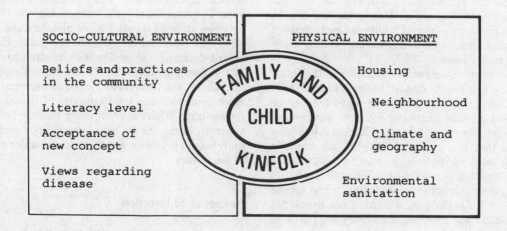

Figure 2.1 The child's environment

11

circumstances the lost ground is recovered by a period of rapid growth, the *catch-up growth*, during convalescence. During such a period of catch-up the velocity of growth may become several times normal. If the illness has been prolonged or chronic the catch-up growth will be minimal or even absent. Also, if the child's nutrition is inadequate, catch-up growth will suffer.

Nutrition

Nutrition is one of the most important environmental influences affecting the health and growth of children in developing countries. Closely related to nutrition and interacting with it is infection. The undernourished child has less resistance to infection so that even the most trivial illness tends to become severe. On the other hand, each episode of infection will cause a further deterioration of nutritional status resulting finally in clinical malnutrition. In recent years several longitudinal studies of children in different parts of the world have helped to clarify the interplay of environmental influences and especially the effects of common childhood illnesses. All the studies describe a common pattern of adequate growth in the first three to four months of life followed by severe faltering in the latter half of the first year and the early part of the second year with incomplete catch-up thereafter. For example, in Uganda it was noted that growth retardation in the first year of life accounted for 91 per cent of the deficit in body weight and 98 per cent of the deficit in body length at three years of age. Even though the average rate of weight gain in the second and third years of life was similar to that of English children, the ground lost in the first year was never recovered. In the Gambia also the main effects of environmental stresses on growth are seen to occur between the ages of six and eighteen months. In addition, there are seasonal influences with cycles of severe impairment in the rainy season and recovery during the dry season.

To a large extent growth retardation in the latter part of the first year is due to the low *energy density* of the diet. Traditional weaning foods tend to be bulky and provide comparatively few calories per unit weight. For example, in the Gambia it has been reported that the energy density of the common weaning foods varied from 33 to 42 kcals/100 g as compared to that of the breast milk at 68 kcals/100 g. In Uganda it has been noted that in the second year of life those children who were not breast fed consumed 30 per cent fewer calories compared to the ones who were receiving breast milk even though the former ate half as much more solids.

Frequency of illness

As placentally derived immunity begins to decline, the infant becomes susceptible to a variety of infective hazards in the environment. In the harsh tropical environment with poor standards of hygiene and bad living conditions, infection is more frequent. In a longitudinal study covering the first three years of life in 40 children in rural Uganda, it was found that the frequency of common illnesses far exceeded that suffered by the average child in the West (table 2.1).

Table 2.1   Illnesses in the second year of life: Total number of illnesses recorded in 1 year per 100 children at risk

	Uganda (1969–70)	Newcastle upon Tyne (1948)
Upper respiratory infections	74	13
Lower respiratory infections	258	124
Diarrhoea	107	20
Skin sepsis	160	8
Measles	36	18
Roundworms	33	–
Hook worm	48	–
Malaria	257	–

Source: Parkin J M. In *The Child in the African Environment* (1975)

In a similar study of 100 families in the urban setting in South India, it was found that the highest incidence rate of illness occurred in infants in their second six months of life at 21.9 illnesses per person-year. The total illness rate was also high for children between 12 to 24 months of life and declined gradually with increasing age. Of the total illnesses recorded amongst these families children under the age of five accounted for 47 per cent. Respiratory infections and diarrhoea together accounted for more than half the total episodes of illness in the community. Whereas respiratory disease tended to occur uniformly at all ages, over 80 per cent of all diarrhoeal episodes were in children under the age of four years.

Response to infection

In a child the response to infection may be different from that in adults, and is usually due to different levels of immunity. A good example is tuberculosis which takes the glandular, or the more disseminated form in the child compared to the fibro-caseous form in the adult. Several illnesses which cause so much morbidity and mortality in children are not major hazards in adult life. Again this can be explained on the basis of immunity derived from exposure to these diseases in childhood. Viral infections such as measles, chickenpox and mumps are diseases of young children. Malaria is common in the latter half of the first year and in early childhood. As immunity develops, clinical malaria becomes less common in school age, even though many children will show malaria parasites in the blood.

Response to infection is also determined by the nutritional status of the host. In measles, for example, not only is the disease more severe in malnourished children but they also tend to excrete the virus much longer than in the case of well-nourished children. Nursing care during illness, including nourishment offered to the sick, is important for securing early recovery. In communities where there is generalised ignorance about the causation of disease and many illnesses are thought to be due to supernatural influences, visitation of a deity or witchcraft, the care provided at home is inadequate or even harmful.

In many societies superstitions exist regarding foods which a sick person is allowed to eat. Some foods are believed to have 'cold' and some 'hot' effects on body organs, so that according to the nature of the disease certain foods are allowed and several others are prohibited. Eggs are not allowed in measles and milk is prohibited in diarrhoea. In some illnesses purges are administered to clear out the digestive system. The overall effects of such beliefs and practices is to deny the sick child a proper diet. It is not unusual to see many children recover from intercurrent illness in a precarious nutritional state. Diarrhoea and measles are thus common precipitants of malnutrition.

Adaptation to the environment

Childhood is a period during which the growing organism is learning to adapt to the physical and biological environment. The child's physiology is adapting to obtain nutrients for growth from the local staple and other foods. These may be plantains and root crops in Polynesia, maize and rice in tropical Africa, rice, millet and sorghum in Asia or maize, rice and wheat in South America. Depending upon the main staple and the way it has been processed prior to consumption, the child may or may not be susceptible to deficiency disorders or toxicants. At the same time, the body's biological processes are responding to the demands made for adaptation to the microbial, viral and parasitic agents in the environment.

Children and pregnant and lactating women are the main vulnerable groups in a community. The demands of growth, conception and lactation produce physiological stresses. In addition, immaturity of body systems in young children and lack of acquired immunity to microbial agents make them specially vulnerable to infection. In all developing societies, women also carry the additional responsibilities of running the home, processing the staple by grinding, winnowing and other means for cooking, and the fetching and carrying of water. Because of such physical and biological stresses women and children suffer the highest incidence of morbidity and mortality in the community. Specific health programmes like antenatal care and child welfare clinics with the objective of health supervision and personal protective measures for these vulnerable groups result in rapid improvements in their health. The dramatic fall in infant mortality in England and Wales during the first half of the present century has been largely due to the development and spread of the infant welfare movement. In the same way, the introduction of under-fives' clinics has produced similar benefits in several developing countries.

Further experience with health surveillance programmes like the under-fives' clinics has shown that disease does not occur by chance but tends to be associated with certain groups and families. For example, it has been said that in the community services in Britain, 50 per cent of the time of the clinic doctors and health visitors is taken up by 5 per cent of families who are 'at risk' of illness. Often it is social pathology which is at the root of medical problems. Inadequate parents, adverse social circumstances, disrupted families and lack of resources create situations in which optimal care within the family is not possible. Regular health surveillance of mothers and children through the antenatal and under-fives' clinics helps to identify such 'at risk' families for special care and supervision.

The changing pattern of disease

Disease patterns undergo change. The socio-economic development of a community, expansion of scientific thought and use of technology can bring about a change in the physical environment of the community and in the life style. This is reflected in the pattern of common illnesses. Thus, in 1913 the medical officer of health in Dar-es-Salaam considered malaria as the main public health problem followed by plague, ankylostomiasis, enteric fever, smallpox and tuberculosis. Today, only malaria and tuberculosis continue to be major health hazards and the rest have been controlled.

In a developing community infection is the main health hazard. Experience in several industrialised societies of the West has shown that the decline in mortality has largely been achieved through control of infectious diseases. In England and Wales between 1848 and 1872, one death in every three was due to infection and in children between the ages of one and four, more than half the deaths were from infectious disease. Since then there has been a dramatic decline in mortality and up to the year 1971, three-quarters of the reduction in mortality has been due to a fall in the number of deaths due to infectious illnesses. Much of the decline began before the present developments in health services or the discovery of antibiotics or the development of vaccines. Three factors appear to be mainly instrumental in bringing about this improvement in health. These are improved nutrition, thereby improving the resistance of the host to infection; reduced exposure to infective agents because of improved hygiene, thereby reducing the incidence of food and water-borne diseases; and the development of vaccines and chemotherapeutic agents in more recent times.

When the bulk of infectious illnesses in a community has been controlled there remains a hard core of genetic, developmental and social problems. This has been well demonstrated in the thousand family survey in Newcastle-upon-Tyne in England where during the period of study (1947 to 1962) rapid improvements in infant and child mortality occurred. In that city, amongst 5000 children entering school in 1952 the common disabilities expected were mental dullness, speech defects, behavioural disorders and growth failure. In 1962, of 760 children leaving school at the age of fifteen, the prevalence of disability was intellectual retardation (5 per cent), established respiratory disease (3 per cent), epilepsy and other neurological problems (2.5 per cent) and malformations (0.7 per cent). Surprisingly, 8.5 per cent had had a formal contact with the law by this age. Another striking feature was that only 47 per cent of the families could be described as whole and sound. In 45 per cent of the families there were various adverse factors and 8 per cent were described as seriously sick families.

Mechanism of disease

Health can be defined as a state in which the organism is in complete accord with the surroundings and there is a proper co-ordination of the different functions which characterise the living animal or plant. Disease is a change in that condition and as a result the organism usually suffers discomfort.

Disease is due to either the impact of the environment or because of biological processes intrinsic to the individual. In the preceding pages the important role of environmental hazards, chiefly microbial and parasitic infections, has been discussed. We have seen how control of the environment through public health measures, personal hygiene and immunisation has brought about a continuing decline in mortality in many of the industrialised societies in Western Europe. At the same time the individual's response to invasive agents has been improved by better nutrition and safe water. The common exogenous agents in the causation of childhood illness in the developing world are (1) deficiency diseases (2) infection – bacterial, viral and parasitic and (3) trauma.

The *response of the host* to any of the above environmental agents is determined by a variety of factors. The least studied are nutritional status, the maturity and previous experiences of the host, and the ability to adapt to the environment. The latter is determined by the genetic constitution of the individual and the endocrine system. For example, in a large part of tropical Africa, the sickle-cell gene is common. In the heterozygote it aids survival in an environment where malaria is holoendemic. Homozygotes not only suffer from anaemia and complications related to ineffective erythropoiesis, but they are also more susceptible to a variety of infections. Similarly, glucose–6-phosphate dehydrogenase deficiency is widespread. In Africa this genetically determined condition makes the population sensitive to drugs like primaquine. In Mediterranean countries it gives rise to haemolysis after ingestion of fava beans and in the Far East it is associated with neonatal jaundice. In the last instance, severe jaundice leading to kernicterus is often precipitated by practices like preserving the infant's clothes with mothballs.

There are often *multiple causes* for disease. For example, nutritional deficiency in pre-school children is widespread in the developing world. In some of them it is severe enough to cause the clinical syndromes of marasmus and kwashiorkor. It is not uncommon to find that these two strikingly different syndromes occur in children living not very far apart in the same villages and having very similar diets. It is postulated that in the child with marasmus there is metabolic and biological adaptation to deficient nutrition whereas in the case of kwashiorkor, such an adaptation fails to occur often because of intervening infection. Similarly, in a large proportion of children admitted to hospital with diarrhoea there is also co-existing malnutrition. They are as much in need of nutritional rehabilitation as of rehydration.

In a discussion on the mechanics of disease it is also necessary to draw attention to the possibility of *iatrogenic illness*. In most countries there is intensive promotion of drugs, vitamin supplements and infant foods. All kinds of claims about 'major scientific break-throughs' and about the superiority of the products are made by their manufacturers. It is useful to bear in mind that side-effects of drugs or idiosyncracy to new drugs can cause serious disease. Similarly, nutritional disorders can result from many of the so-called 'super' baby foods.

The phases of childhood

Childhood has several phases, each with its own priorities and problems. During *intrauterine life* the foetus is well protected from the external environment and is not easily available for clinical examination or treatment. All care must reach him through the mother. The state of health of the mother affects his health. The state of nutrition of the mother affects his nutrition, and the mother's body chemistry governs the foetal environment. Hence, adequate antenatal care of the mother is the best way of ensuring the care of the foetus.

The *perinatal period* is beset with hazards and in many developing countries perinatal events make a major contribution to infant mortality. Lack of antenatal care and unsupervised childbirth are two important etiological factors in the high perinatal mortality. Their effects are seen in the very high incidence of low birth weight and neonatal tetanus in developing countries. Besides her health during pregnancy, the mother's previous experience of disease and adequate nutritional state determine the health and vitality of the offspring. Hence the importance of health throughout childhood and adolescence.

In the cultural life of all rural societies, pregnancy and childbirth call for the performance of many rites which are not possible when the birth occurs in a health centre or a hospital. Thus in rural areas traditional midwifery flourishes and only 10 to 15 per cent of all births may occur in an institution. The resultant high mortality in the newborn period only serves to enhance the beliefs in the supernatural and the fear that giving up of traditional ways may bring down the wrath of ancestral spirits or of the deity on the community.

In *early infancy*, up to the age of four to six months most babies do well. Breast feeding is common in all rural societies and is an excellent source of nutrition as well as protection from infection. In areas where breast feeding has declined there is invariably an increase in infant mortality.

Towards the latter part of infancy, the immunity derived from the mother begins to decline and the infant becomes susceptible to a variety of infections. Growth faltering is also common because now the mother's milk cannot supply all the nutritional requirements. In many cases weaning commences at about the age of three to four months and weanling diarrhoea is now recurrent with its debilitating effect. Late infancy is the period to watch since many of the serious health problems of the child commence about this age period.

The *toddler* is passing through another crucial phase. Growth failure is often well established. In many cases the mother is pregnant again and he has been taken off the breast. His diet will now consist of mainly farinaceous foods grossly deficient in calories, protein and other essential nutrients. It is true to say that the very high second year mortality is an indicator of malnutrition in the pre-school period. In some communities the pre-school mortality may be 40 to 50 times that seen in Western countries. Intervention to change the predictable course of events is necessary at several points and over a long span even going back to the childhood of the mother.

The *school age child* has developed immunity against many of the common pathogens, including the common infectious diseases of childhood and malaria. The demands of growth are less; even though school children show a lag in their growth curve as compared to Western standards, it is rare to see clinical malnutrition at this age. Parasitic infestations like ascariasis and ankylostomiasis are common and in many areas of tropical Africa the entire school age population may suffer from schistosomiasis.

In the school age population, the actual schoolgoing children may be very few. These few may enjoy the benefits of school meals and a school health service; but the vast majority exist on the fringe of the health service provided by the local authority for the area. Their time is spent mainly on the family plot helping with various jobs and

they grow up essentially in the traditional pattern
of the family and the community. Adolescence
abruptly ushers the child into new responsibilities.
Marriage is early in most rural societies and in the
case of girls, it brings a continuous cycle of pregnancy and lactation, resulting in the various forms
of maternal depletion syndromes like anaemia,
osteomalacia, etc., so common in the adult females
in developing countries.

Further reading

Forfar J O, (ed). *Child Health in a Changing Society*.
  Oxford: Oxford University Press, 1988.
Learmonth A. *Disease Ecology*. Oxford: Basil Blackwell,
  1988.
Leisinger K M. *Health Policy for Least Developed Coun-
  tries*. Basel: Social Strategies Publishers Co-operative
  Society, 1984.
Mata L J. *The Children of Santa Maria Cauque. A Prospec-
  tive Field Study of Health and Growth*. London: MIT
  Press, 1978.
McKeown T. *The Origins of Human Disease*. Oxford: Basil
  Blackwell, 1988.
Miller F J W, Court S D M, Walton W S, Knox E G.
  Growing Up in Newcastle-upon-Tyne. Oxford: Oxford
  University Press, 1960.
Puffer R R, Serrano C V. *Patterns of Mortality in Child-
  hood*. Washington DC: Pan American Health Organis-
  ation, 1973.
Taylor, C E *et al*. (eds). *Child and Maternal Health Services
  in Rural India – The Narangwal Experiment*. Vols. 1
  and 2. Baltimore and London: Johns Hopkins University
  Press, 1988.
van Ginneken J K, Muller A S, (eds). *Maternal and Child
  Health in Rural Kenya*. London: Croom Helm, 1984.

3 *Social and cultural factors in health*

Part 1 Social background

The common illnesses in developing countries are often called the 'diseases of poverty'. Malnutrition, anaemia, tuberculosis, leprosy, worm infestations and many other infective and parasitic diseases are more common amongst the poorer classes. Lack of individual and community resources, poor development of services, high rates of illiteracy especially amongst women, low technology and inadequate community organisation act together as the determinants of the diseases of poverty. Their effects on the individual and the community are inter-related in such a way that the adverse influence of one factor is enhanced and perpetuated by that of another. Medical care in the narrow sense of diagnosis and treatment can only alleviate symptoms and cure illnesses when they arise. It will have little effect on the incidence of illness. In order to come to grips with the determinants of disease in a community it is important to study factors influencing the social environment, the availability and effectiveness of services and the inter-personal relationships within the community. In many ways an understanding of those factors is as helpful as that of organic pathology.

Definition of poverty

Different people have defined poverty in different ways. From the medical point of view a practical definition is 'the state in which an individual or family has to spend more than 80 per cent of income on food'. The basic biological needs are for food, clothing and shelter. When more than 80 per cent of the income is spent on food to satisfy hunger, then clearly very little is left for the other needs which will remain largely unmet.

Poverty rarely exists by itself. Low wages and lack of adequate land resources are usually associated with insecurity of employment, illiteracy, bad housing, large families, exploitation and a host of other factors. The insecurity caused by poverty gives rise to fatalism with a characteristic personality on the one hand and chronic undernutrition with recurrent ill health on the other. The overall effect is that there is a high incidence of illness with little energy or will to change the situation.

The extent of poverty

This definition of poverty applies to a disturbingly large segment of the population of an average developing country. For example, in one study of poverty in India, the authors concluded that in the year 1968–69 up to 40 per cent of the rural population and 50 per cent of the urban population – in all 224 million people out of a population of 530 million – lived below the minimum level of calorie consumption. Similar large numbers have been described in many countries of tropical Africa, especially those affected by the Sahelian drought, and in central South America.

An important cause of poverty in rural areas is lack of land resources. It is estimated that in many countries up to a quarter of all rural households are labour households, most of whom have no land of their own to cultivate and are dependent on the personal labour of their members. Even in those instances where a small piece of land may be available for cultivation, their main dependence is on wage employment as casual labour in agriculture. In urban areas, most of the poverty seen is due to the overflow of rural poverty into cities. When such families have lived long enough in urban areas they acquire characteristics of their own and create a culture of urban poverty.

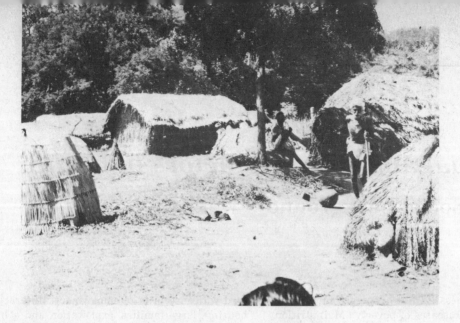

Figure 3.1   Rural poverty – landless agricultural labourers

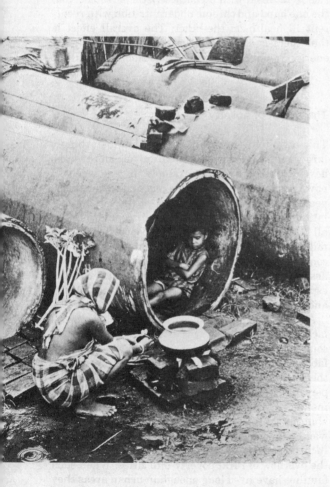

Figure 3.2   New arrivals in the city : a search for shelter

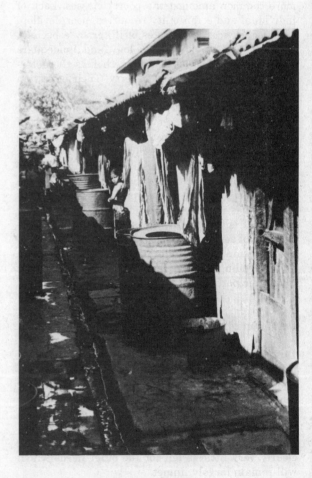

Figure 3.3   A typical urban slum

The culture of poverty

The family in the culture of urban poverty no longer cherishes childhood as a specially prolonged and protected stage in the life cycle. Initiation into sex occurs early. At the same time most marriages tend to be common law unions which are often short-lived. When such marriages break up the children often move with the mother. Thus, the family tends to be mother-centred and tied more closely to the extended family of the mother.

Characteristically in the culture of poverty there is an attitude of hopelessness and despair arising from the awareness of the impossibility of ever achieving success in the prevailing values. The individual growing up in this culture tends to develop a strong feeling of inferiority, dependence and fatalism. Most families have experienced too many illnesses amongst their members and gone through many tragedies and crises to ever hope for a better existence. In their move to the city many have left their social institutions and cultural traditions of rural life behind. In the shanty town and slum they now feel excluded and drift away from the major institutions and agencies of the larger society. Such a process of fragmentation from the larger society gives rise to lack of organisation, lack of leadership and under-utilisation of the capacity for self-help.

These observations are helpful in planning health services. Many of the successful programmes of health improvement have also created community organisation through establishment of local committees, provided leadership, generated dialogue with the community and identified targets. Such social developments provide the foundations on which integrated development of a community can take place.

Social factors and health in the industrial society

The industrial society provides opportunities for studying the influences of a whole range of social factors on health. In their progress towards industrialisation commencing from feudalism through to capitalism, many industrial countries passed through a phase in which there was widespread poverty and urban misery. These were reflected in their mortality and morbidity rates and some of these have been discussed in previous chapters. Education, class struggle and social awakening have resulted in several improvements so that relief of poverty and the care of vulnerable groups feature strongly in the national policies of most nations. In spite of such progress, social stratification as a vestige of the past continues and there are wide differences in the health experiences of different social groups.

Of all the many useful indices of health and welfare the best general index is the infant mortality rate. It is an expression of many factors – genetic, nutritional, life style, health habits, water supply, housing, environmental stress and the quality and availability of health services. Of all these the key factors are maternal and infant nutrition and here the real disposal of family income and how it is spent over two generations is what matters. The influence of health development in the past 30 years on social groups in Scotland is shown in table 3.1 and in England and Wales in figure 3.4.

In spite of a national health service which is available on demand and free, together with several social service benefits in the UK the improvements in health for different social groups have been very different. For example, in England and Wales in 1959–63 standardised mortality ratios for social class IV and V were higher than for I and II in the case of 49 causes of death out of 85 for men and 54 out of 87 for women. If the mortality experience of social class I in 1959–63 had applied to social class V only just over half the deaths in that social class would have occurred.

When infant mortality as a whole was declining in Britain, the percentage difference between mortality in class I and V should have remained at least about the same. A great deal of welfare legislation like family allowance, food subsidies, national insurance, maternal and child welfare services and local authority housing grants was undoubtedly more beneficial to the poorer sections of the population. These improvements were expected to reduce the social gradient in infant mortality. Moreover, there was a greater scope for reduction of mortality from infections in class V than in class I. On the contrary, the real decline has been greater for social class I. Death rates from diarrhoea and pneumonia have been five times greater in class V than in class I, showing the importance of social circumstance.

Table 3.1 Infant mortality rate of Scotland over 30 years analysed according to social class

Class	I	II	III	IV	V	Rate for all classes
1942	34	41	65	67	94	69
1952	18	25	35	39	46	35
1962	14	18	25	30	38	27
1972	10	13	18	20	28	19

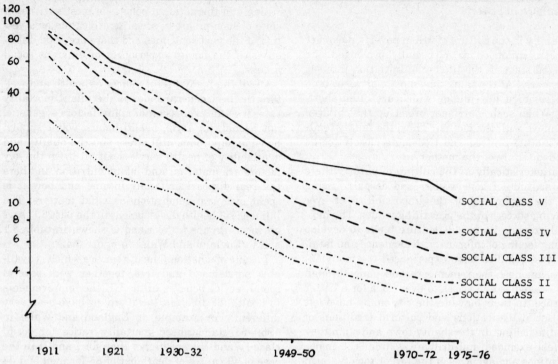

Figure 3.4 Influence of social class on infant and child mortality on IMR in England and Wales

Effects of social class

The effects of social class are felt in several ways besides better nutrition. It differentiates individuals in terms of material well-being. It determines the sort of job they will have, the income they derive from it, housing, opportunities for promotion, education of the parents and their children, and the opportunities their children will have. In many cases cycles of disadvantage occur from one generation to another in spite of social interventions of different types.

With regard to their relation to health, everyday experiences like the quality and type of occupation, housing conditions, and opportunities for self-improvement have important influences on physical and mental well-being. Family crises tend to be more frequent in circumstances of overcrowding, inadequate income and lack of education. In many communities it has been observed that illness, including infective illness, is more frequent after episodes of crises of one sort or another in the family. Add to that the effects of bad housing with insufficient space, squalor and lack of amenities in the neighbourhood and it is easy to understand the different health experiences of the poorer classes.

In one longitudinal study of 300 Mexican children, 22 were eventually found to develop malnutrition. The families did not differ in structure, economic status or socio-cultural characteristics. The biological characteristics of the parents were also similar. However, there was a significant difference in the characteristics of the home environment. The homes of the affected children were more disorganised. The emotional climate was different and there was less attention to the infant's needs from as early an age as six months. These differences persisted and even grew with the infant.

Different value systems

Individuals in a group have, in the course of time, come to establish particular attitudes about things and to people both within and outside their groups. They have also developed ways of responding to each other and to people outside the group. Often there is suspicion and hostility expressed towards individuals, including health workers, who may be recognised as outsiders. Members of a group share similar conceptions about appropriate attitudes and ways of behaving and dressing. These common ways of doing things distinguish the individuals in the group from others.

The norms and values in a social group are maintained by the process of 'social control'. An individual's membership of a social group requires submission to such control, and its influence is more powerful than generally realised. Different social classes have their norms and values maintained by the processes of social control operating within them. The norms and values of social classes at either end of the spectrum can be so radically different that often they are described as two nations within a nation. Since many health professionals usually belong to the highest social classes, it is not surprising that they find communication with their patients and establishing rapport with them difficult.

Role of health services

Modern clinical medicine is able to alleviate pain and reduce mortality without fundamentally alter-

ing the determinants of disease in the community. This is in contrast to the experiences of Western Europe where improvements in living conditions, both within the home and in the environment, had already occurred before the arrival of medical technology. Here clinical medicine helped to consolidate the ground already covered and to cause further improvements so that the effect was cumulative. Such changes are now occurring in the developing world and a review of strategy is necessary.

Figures 3.5 and 3.6 show the association between infant and child mortality in England and Wales and the advances in medical technology on the one hand and social improvements through legislation on the other. It is clear that improvement in mortality was already taking place before the advent of the vaccines and the development of antibiotics. Much of this improvement was due to social legislation providing for improved sanitation, alleviation of poverty through social benefits and the statutory provision of services for mothers and children by local health authorities at the beginning of this century.

An important concept of modern medical practice

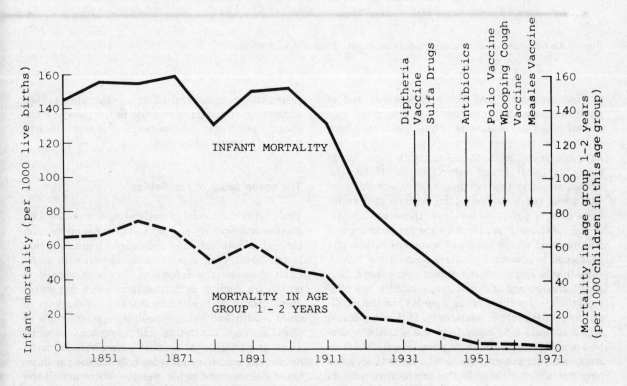

Figure 3.5 Influence of medical developments on IMR in England and Wales

INFANT MORTALITY IN ENGLAND AND WALES

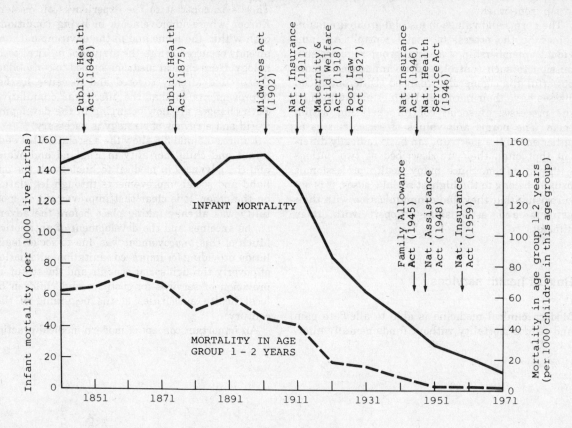

Figure 3.6 Social legislation and infant mortality England and Wales

in Western Europe and North America is that of public responsibility for health. It has given rise to two major developments. Firstly, services have evolved in the past 50 years or so to provide adequate coverage, with basic health care, for as many as possible and especially for those who cannot afford to pay for them. Even though inner city areas and some industrial regions still suffer from lack of adequate services, these are mainly of the specialist type. Health care for mothers and children and school health services are sufficiently developed to provide a uniform standard of health surveillance and screening almost everywhere. Secondly, the concept of public responsibility has widened the responsibility of the hospital and the paediatrician for the larger community. Hitherto medical action comprised no more than the services of doctors to sick patients. But now the paediatrician feels responsible for not only those who come to seek his help but also for those in the community who do not, and for the healthy children. This widening of

responsibility has resulted in a continuing review of the role of medicine and the health needs of the society, and has given rise to many changes in attitudes in medical education.

The seven faces of paediatrics

The traditional model of medical care was based on disease or deformity and worked towards prevention through identification of the cause by investigation or treatment. Such a model worked well with many adult illnesses and infections. But with regard to child care such a model neglects some important areas. Many of the fundamental requirements of child health include non-medical matters such as food, housing, sanitation and competent parents. Thus, the traditional form of paediatrics in many developing countries provides only for the paediatrics of sickness and is not enough. There is still the very large area of comprehensive child care to be covered through the paediatrics of prevention; paediatrics of community health; paediatrics of life-style and habit at home; paediatrics of education through school health services; the paediatrics of development through identification and care of the handicapped; and the paediatrics of mental health through the promotion of mental health of the family.

Teamwork in health – the new style of doctoring

It is difficult to define which of the above areas of paediatric care should receive priority. It will depend upon the social values and the state of development of the community. However, two things are certain, namely beginnings should be made in each of the seven areas and secondly, each area will require its own team of workers. A co-ordinator is needed to define the needs of each kind of paediatric care and to support each team with regard to continuity of training and the supply of equipment and materials. In most instances the paediatrician takes on the role of co-ordinating and counselling because he is nearest to most child health problems. The application of such a model of paediatric care at the district level means moving away from the traditional hospital-centred model with its focus on disease to a model based on the promotion of health.

Are paediatric priorities necessary?

In all countries hospitals exist as legacies of the past and are already consuming an undue share of the health budget. Moreover, medical technology has become increasingly complex and expensive. Medical science is international and innovations in technology travel rapidly all over the world, often aided by the vested interests of the promoters of such technology. Application of expensive technology in hospitals deprives other activities of resources and personnel. Given such a situation, it is inevitable that of the seven facets of paediatrics mentioned above, only a few can make progress and even then by only short steps. It is not surprising that the main development in child care in the Third World

has been away from the real problem. It is inevitable that determination of priorities is necessary so that development in child care can be channelled towards defined goals.

Who decides priorities?

In most countries it is the usual practice for the health ministries to put out guidelines on different aspects of health care. Such guidelines describe the policies and often suggest the strategies to be adopted, often with political goals. Medical schools and research institutions define specific problems, develop solutions and at times carry out evaluations. All these help in judging the direction to be taken. For the identification of specific goals in a district the only effective way is to establish a continuing dialogue with the community in order to identify those areas in which health and social improvements are necessary, taking full account of the national policy and medical scientific information.

In conclusion, health care is no longer thought of as a technical service available only to those who can afford it. In the medicine of poverty, social needs and health problems are so closely linked that health care is part of the social services in the same way as education. Protection of the weak from exploitation, removal of hunger, provision of safe water and sanitation can contribute more to health than the building of large hospitals. It is only through community-based services that social action can be mobilised to achieve these goals.

Further reading

Conyers D. *An Introduction to Social Planning in the Third World*. Chichester: John Wiley and Sons, 1982.

Chavez A, Martinez C. *Growing up in a Developing Community*. Guatemala: INCAP, 1988.

Doyal L. *The Political Economy of Health*. London: Pluto Press, 1979.

Townsend P, Davidson N, (eds). *Inequalities in Health*. Harmondsworth: Penguin Books, 1988.

Turshen M. *The Politics of Public Health*. London: Zed Books, 1989.

Part 2   Cultural background*

Culture, customs and child health

The bulk of child health work in developing countries presents cross-cultural problems to varying
extents, especially with health personnel trained
abroad who, as a result of their training, have
become cut off from traditional culture and values.
Nowhere is this more evident than in the field of
health education. Western trained workers who
work among traditional societies often complain
about the resistance or lack of response to their
attempts at health education. This is related to the
fact that attempts to alter people's ways of life,
beliefs and customary behaviour are never made *in
vacuo*, but usually in competition with, and against
the resistance of deep-rooted and time-hallowed traditional beliefs and customs. Health education that
aims to modify harmful practices is most likely to be
successful if it is based on knowledge of the people's
customs, beliefs, and practices; in other words the
local culture pattern.

Understanding culture
The nature of culture

It seems natural in the West to greet a long absent
friend with a hand shake. But this is not natural to
everybody. The Thais greet one another by raising
their hands, with palms pressed together, to their
foreheads; the Japanese bow to one another; the
Arabs embrace one another; the Andaman Islanders
weep; and the Malays hold both hands together
momentarily before they sweep their hands to their
chests.

A cheese sandwich might be an American idea of
a meal, but the Aborigines of Malaysia prefer the
bamboo rat, the Malays consider a meal incomplete
without rice, and the Chinese will not eat cheese or
dairy products.

In other words, there is no one right way of doing
things. Instead there are many different ways of
doing things. The manner in which we greet one

*By Paul C. Y. Chen, Department of Social & Preventative Medi-
cine, Faculty of Medicine, University of Malaya

another, eat, love, worship, dress, sit, work, rear our
children, is the product of having been raised in a
group in which these customs and ways are accepted
as the only correct ones. The differences in the way
people do things in different parts of the world are
a reflection of their distinctive cultures. There are
over three thousand different cultures in the world
today.

What people learn from their social group makes
up the culture of that group, and includes knowledge, beliefs, art, morals, ideas, customs and any
other capability and habit that has been acquired
by man as a result of shared experiences. Culture
may be divided into material and non-material culture. Material culture consists of man-made objects
such as tools, furniture, clothes, buildings, farms,
and in fact any physical substance that has been
changed and used by man. They are the concrete
result of ideas and practices. Non-material culture,
on the other hand, consists of words people use (language), thoughts, customs, the beliefs they hold, and
the habits they follow. Most of what we will deal
with, in relation to child health, can be classified as
non-material culture.

Man and only man has culture. He is unique
among all animals in his ability to create and maintain culture. Only man uses symbolic communication (language) and can exchange detailed direc-
tions, share discoveries, and organise elaborate
activities. Thus each chimpanzee stands (or rather
crouches) on his own two feet and must face the
world starting from scratch, whereas man stands on
the shoulders of his ancestors and brings to bear on
his problems a wealth of accumulated wisdom – his
culture. Culture is neither inherited nor instinctive
– it has to be learnt. Man is born without culture
but learns the accepted ways of doing things more
or less unconsciously. We pick up customs, habits
and words, spontaneously and unconsciously. In
other words, culture is transmitted socially and not
biologically.

Culture patterning

The smallest units of culture, the simplest functional units, are known as culture traits and are
the bricks or basic units of which all cultures are

composed. No society ever exhibits in the behaviour of its members, all the culture traits that exist. Each particular society selectively picks and combines some culture traits with others to form what appears to it to be the acceptable pattern or combination. For example, after childbirth, the Malay mother is traditionally required to avoid fruits, vegetables, several varieties of fresh fish, meats and eggs, with the result that her diet consists of rice, salted fish, spices and coffee. On the other hand, Chinese mothers in Malaysia, are enjoined to consume eggs, meat, chicken, ginger and rice wine.

Many people assume that what they do is a total expression of human nature. They do not realise that other human beings have found quite different patterns of dealing with the same problem. The range of variability in culture patterns is not infinite but is impressively broad. As each society develops its culture through the ages, it rejects or ignores many culture patterns particularly those that appear mutually contradictory and inherently incompatible. It selects those culture patterns that are in accord with a set of basic assumptions about the universe and are consistent with one another so that the culture is then a harmonious working whole – an integrated culture.

Each culture is thus made up of a multitude of selected culture traits integrated into a meaningful system in which all parts have a special relationship to the whole. No one of these culture traits exists in isolation but plays its role in contributing to a total way of life. A strange custom, which may appear incomprehensible at first, should be examined within the total cultural setting and in the context of the basic assumptions about the universe. When two cultures confront each other, one system of culture patterning seems to dissolve or fragment the second system.

Traditional view of ill-health
Supernaturalism

Although each culture conceives of the cause of ill-health somewhat differently, there seems to be the commonly recurring theme in most traditional societies that the causes of ill-health have both a supernatural component as well as a natural component. This is in contradistinction to western medicine in which the causation of ill-health is seen as belonging in the realm of the natural. To western medicine a child has pulmonary tuberculosis because the tuberculosis organism has established a focus in the lung of the child. To traditional medical

systems, however, in addition to natural causes, the causation of ill-health is often perceived to stem from the supernatural. Why did this particular child become ill? Has not some supernatural being been responsible? Was not the child particularly susceptible as a result of a loss of soul substance?

Supernaturalism finds its expression in the form of spirits some of which (including most gods) are thought to be benevolent whilst others are described as malevolent and evil. It is believed that some of these spirit beings can be reared as familiar spirits by sorcerers for use in witchcraft while others are inherently present in the environment. It is also believed that ill-health results when malevolent spirits will it to be so. Such supernatural theories of ill-health are widespread in traditional societies. The African Azande, the Philippine Ifugao, the Malaysian Kadazan, the Australian Aborigines, the American Navaho, and the Papuan, all subscribe to beliefs in witchcraft and evil spirits and attribute the cause of many illnesses to supernatural causes.

Supernaturalism also finds expression in the form of belief in a vital soul substance which exists independently of spirit beings and man. It is known under a variety of different names. To the Melanesians and Polynesians, it is *mana*; to the Crow Indians, it is *maxpe*; to the Malay and Iban of Malaysia, it is *semangat*; while to the Semai of the Malay Peninsula, it is *ruai*.

Supernatural and natural factors are usually linked to form a hierarchy of etiological factors as is the case in the Malay concept of disease causation (figure 3.7). It is believed that natural factors may act on their own as when the wrong food is taken resulting in abdominal colic. On the other hand ill-health due to natural agents can be precipitated by the next level of factors, namely, supernatural precipitating factors, as when a spirit makes a food harmful, or when a spirit interferes with the normal course of events so that a man is killed by falling from a tree – a fall which would not have happened otherwise. Of course a supernatural agent can act on its own to cause ill-health as when a spirit possesses a man's body. The third and highest level of factors, the supernatural predisposing factors are by themselves not thought to be disease producing. An individual who has suffered a loss of soul substance is not thought to be ill *per se* but is believed to be extremely susceptible to supernatural precipitating factors, such as evil spirits, as well as natural factors. Foods which would otherwise be considered harmless may become harmful to people who have lost soul substance. Another predisposing factor is socially disapproved behaviour. In many cultures health and illness are inextricably connected with

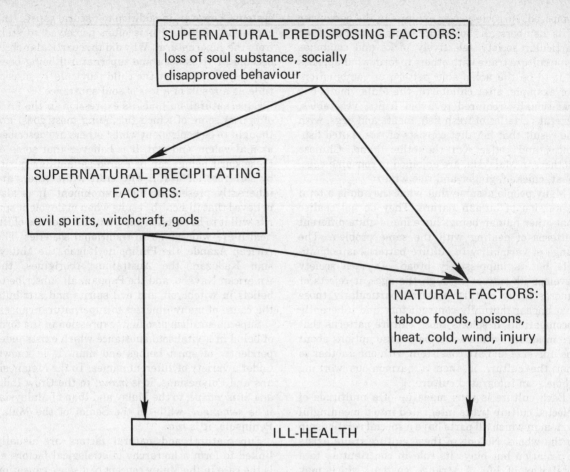

Figure 3.7   Traditional concepts of the causation of ill-health

socially approved behaviour and moral conduct. In some rural areas of the Middle East, illness may be attributed to failure to fulfil some religious ritual or ceremony.

Traditional medicine

The foregoing dualistic supernatural-natural concept of disease causation is often reflected by the recognition of two types of medicine-men. Among some peoples such as the Zulu, the herbalist is acknowledged to be the expert on natural remedies, while the diviner, who is invariably held in much higher esteem, is the acknowledged expert in diseases of supernatural origin. In other cultures the two are embodied in one category of medicine-man.

In treating any illness, the first step that the medicine-man takes is to find the cause. Determining the nature of the illness is not nearly as import-

ant as discovering the cause, as the cure is directed at counteracting the cause rather than of symptom relief. This is important as each cause warrants a different mode of treatment. Thus if the patient has broken a taboo, a purification ritual is called for. If soul substance has been lost or kidnapped, it has to be traced, recovered and returned to its owner. If the patient is a victim of witchcraft, counter magic must be used. If the patient is possessed by an evil spirit, exorcism must be resorted to. If a spirit or god has been angered, it must be appeased, often by the offering of sacrifices.

Despite the wide variety of culture patterns that characterise traditional societies, healing ceremonies concerning possession by evil spirits invariably take the form of exorcism. Exorcism is most simply attempted by way of magic spells. The offending spirit may also be exorcised in a variety of other ways. The Navaho Indians chant prayers for four days; the Malays tempt out evil spirits by offering a tray of foods, betel leaves and other delicacies and invite the evil spirit to take a new home; the Shona of Africa, the Iban of Sarawak, and the Gururumba of New Guinea, suck out the offending spirit or object; the Semai of Peninsular Malaysia conduct an elaborate 'sing' to coax the spirit out.

In treating loss of soul substance, the medicine-man may send his own soul substance in search of the missing soul substance and return it to its rightful owner. During this process he will enter into a trance when he may act out all the adventures that his soul substance encounters as it fights kidnappers and evil spirits in order to recapture the missing soul substance. To attract the wandering soul, certain articles such as saffron rice which are believed to attract soul substance, are thrown about and incense may be burnt.

Treatment often involves participation by kinsfolk as among the Tiv of Nigeria, the Navaho of the United States and the Malays of Malaysia.

It is often difficult for a health professional to understand why, when scientific medicine is available, traditional peoples often continue to patronise 'ignorant medicine-men'. The answer is that traditional medicine often brings good results. There is no doubt that the main benefits are psychological. Undoubtedly in many instances harm results, not so much for what is done as from what is neglected in terms of organic disease. But the medicine-man is rarely blamed. It is explained away in terms of negligence of the sick and his family in adhering to ritual taboos, incomplete and misleading information given by the sick and his family, and the extraordinary power of the offending spirit or sorcerer.

The alternatives

It is because of belief in supernaturalism that traditional peoples often view western medicine as a system that merely provides symptomatic or supportive therapy. To their minds the underlying supernatural cause remains untreated and ready to precipitate a relapse. Illnesses perceived to be due to natural agents are readily presented to practitioners of western medicine whereas illnesses thought to be due to supernatural causes are largely handled by traditional medicine-men. Illnesses that have no functional impairment are in the main seen by practitioners of western medicine whereas illnesses with severe functional impairment are largely managed by traditional medicine-men. Where functional impairment is severe the need to neutralise an underlying supernatural cause

becomes urgent and the tendency is thus to seek the aid of a practitioner who can deal with the supernatural.

Although several widely differing systems of medical care may be available to individuals in a society, many view these differing systems as complementary rather than opposing and are quite prepared to move from system to system in search of a cure. This is particularly so in chronic or severe illnesses. To the physician, this may seem strange and illogical. On the other hand, physicians trained in western scientific medicine often appear dogmatic to some traditional peoples. To a westerner, a thing is either true or false. If it is false it is completely rejected; if it is true it is accepted completely. To some traditional peoples, there is room for a gentle harmony that binds together what may seem incomprehensible or even contradictory.

Culture and child health

There are several aspects of culture that are of particular and direct relevance to child health, namely pregnancy, childbirth, child rearing, food and nutrition, and ill-health. Beliefs, customs and practices in relation to these aspects of the cycle of life will affect the way child health services must be organised and implemented.

Pregnancy and childbirth

In many traditional cultures, a mother's prestige is linked to her ability to have children, preferably in large numbers. Maternal depletion syndromes as a result of this continuous burden can be important causes of nutritional deficiency diseases and may lead to premature ageing and early death. Maternal survival is of paramount importance to that of the young child. The spacing of pregnancies not only permits nutritional repletion of the mother between births, but also ensures that the young child is not deprived of maternal attention and breast milk. In some cultures, such as the Ngoni of Malawi, sexual intercourse is not permitted during a prescribed period of time during lactation, and this has the effect of ensuring child spacing. The belief is that parents will do direct harm to their children by neglecting to observe this rule, and that if a child is born soon after an earlier one, it will 'destroy' the first child who must be weaned abruptly. As a result he often suffers *kwashiorkor*, the 'disease of the displaced child'.

Childbirth in many traditional cultures is conducted by traditional birth attendants who are popularly known as *curiosas* in Mozambique, *dayas* in Jordan and Egypt, *dais* in India, Pakistan and Bangladesh, *hilots* in the Philippines, *mohtamyaa* in Thailand, and *bidan kampung* in Malaysia.

These traditional birth attendants are highly respected for their skills and knowledge. Their influence begins long before birth. They often are the repository of traditional beliefs and practices influencing pregnancy, childbirth, the puerperium, and childhood. They advise on social behaviour, diet, customary rituals, and illnesses.

Where labour is normal and there is minimal interference in its course, as among the Shona of Zimbabwe, childbirth is in certain respects well-conducted. However if labour is slow or becomes obstructed, dangerous rituals may be carried out. Among the Mah Meri of Malaysia childbirth is hastened by a 'pusher' whose task is to expel the foetus by force. Among the Iban of Sarawak, bleeding, inversion of the uterus, prolapse of cervix and rupture of uterus have been caused by 'pushers'. Childbirth is often attended by a group of women who are there to assist or encourage the woman in labour. They may sit around and chant little songs of encouragement. Among the Igbo of Nigeria the birth attendant determines the right time to bear down and the group of women bear down in sympathy with the woman in labour.

Some of the practices advocated by traditional birth attendants, particularly dietary taboos such as among Malays, may be harmful. However not all practices are harmful. Some practices, such as the seclusion of the mother and baby in the place of birth for a stated period after childbirth varying from 10 to 44 days allows the mother to rest, permits her to learn how to handle and feed the baby, and helps the toddler to adjust to the arrival of a rival, the new baby. Other practices, such as the use of talismans as prophylactics by the Nyamwezi of Tanzania, are harmless.

In several countries, such as Pakistan, India and Malaysia, the traditional birth attendant is being trained to recruit family planning acceptors. In other countries, particularly in the Middle East, she is being trained in simple hygiene and asepsis, and new roles are being found to turn an unaccepted attendant into a useful ally.

Child rearing

In industrialised cultures a 'family' is usually limited to the circle of immediate relatives belonging to the nuclear family. Thus the terms father, mother, brother and sister have restricted meanings. In many traditional cultures, on the other hand, a wide circle of classificatory fathers, mothers, brothers and sisters constitute the kin group recognised as the 'family'. A child thus may have several 'mothers' upon each of whom he can depend for love and food during periods when he is deprived of his own mother by her employment in the fields, illnesses, or even death. Thus in one Malay village it was observed that out of 464 children under 15 years old, 117 were not living in the original family circle. About 11 per cent of the children were 'adopted', permanently or temporarily, by other people within the same village.

Mother-child relationships are warm and close. This is reinforced by breast feeding when the child is in close contact with the mother and can be easily comforted and fondled. In many cultures, the mother carries the young child wherever she goes. Among the Magars of Nepal, the mother carries the baby in a cloth sling across her back or in a basket on her back. Toilet training is usually gradual and done without fuss. Toddlers may ride about on a parent's hip or that of an older brother or sister. Young boys may spend considerable periods with their father while he is grazing the cattle, farming or hunting, while young girls learn the domestic arts by tagging along with their mother.

In some cultures, punishment in the form of 'shame' is the predominant way of social control of the young child. In others rewards for success and approved social behaviour is the predominant mode of control. Among the Melanesians and Papuans 'shame' can lead to severe behavioural disturbances, running away and a refusal to continue. The task of correcting school pupils in New Guinea is made very difficult when pupils 'turn off' because they have been shamed.

Food and child nutrition

In traditional cultures all over the developing world, breast milk, together with the foetal stores, are all that infants get and need for the first six months of life. In reality anything else that is given to infants during this period of life has to be considered a hazard liable to lead to diarrhoea. In fact, in most traditional cultures children continue to be breast fed for periods of one to four years. Breast feeding has economic advantages over artificial feeding, the cost of adequate quantities of processed cow's milk preparations being completely beyond the means of most parents. Unfortunately more and more mothers are turning away from breast feeding as a result of incessant commercial promotion.

Many of the problems of child nutrition are encountered during the period when the child is a toddler. Not only must there be a transition from infant foods to adult foods, but a number of food taboos can begin to limit the variety of foods available to him. Among the Samburu of Kenya cleanliness is highly esteemed and eggs are regarded as hen's excrement, while fish, donkey, dog, elephant, bush pig and monkey are all considered as unclean foods. Among the Malays fish is thought to cause ascariasis in toddlers. Among the Semai of Malaysia a young child is denied the meat of animals with 'strong spirits' such as the leaf monkey, bats, civets, ant eater, deer, turtle, tortoise, bear and the larger birds. However as they approach adulthood, these items are slowly added to their diet. In some cultures, protein deficiency may arise when customs do not provide for setting aside a portion of meat or fish for small children as is the case in Western Samoa.

In many cultures the withdrawal of various foods is considered an essential element in the treatment of childhood illnesses. Among the Guatemalans there is a strong tendency to deny foods of animal origin to children for fear of stimulating worms, and to withdraw protein-containing foods almost entirely when diarrhoea develops. This may be fatal if the child is already undernourished. Among the Malays children who are ill may be denied sour fruits, papaya, and other fruits rich in carotene and ascorbic acid, as well as protein foods such as eggs, most kinds of fish and meat.

Another problem is posed by the cultural practice of reliance on a staple food which leads people to believe that it is also the best food for children, who are fed diluted forms of the staple food. Among Malays, who consider rice as a 'super food', infants may be fed a dilute gruel of rice water in place of milk particularly if the mother has succumbed to replacing breast feeding with preparations of cow's milk and is unable to afford adequate quantities of cow's milk.

In many traditional cultures men, who are the productive members of the family, have the largest share of food and the best choice of scarce supplies of protein. Women and little children come last and must do with the left overs. In addition there is often a long interval between meals when mothers must go to the fields to work. Little children are unable to eat enough of the bulky staple cereal to carry them from one meal to the next, and hunger may be temporarily suppressed by the consumption of snacks such as biscuits and sweets, with the result that appetites are very often poor at meal-times.

An equally important problem in child nutrition is that posed by the food prejudices of urban cultures, who often discourage the consumption of protein sources that appear 'unclean' to them. For example, the Orang Asli (aborigines of Malaysia) are often discouraged from eating rats and other rodents, which form an important source of protein, when they come into contact with urban peoples, who do not realise that the 12 species of forest rat and 12 species of squirrel in the Malaysian jungle are as clean as many farm animals eaten by urban peoples. There should be an emphasis on the valuable elements in indigenous diets. The widespread use of baobab and other fruits containing appreciable amounts of ascorbic acid has been observed among the Gwembe Tonga, who have learnt to eat those fruits which are nutritionally best for them. Other examples of indigenous wisdom include the Somali habit of giving lightly cooked liver to pregnant women who are anaemic, and the Malay practice of giving liver to children who suffer from night blindness, an early sign of vitamin A deficiency.

Management of cultural variation

The variety of culture patterns that impinge on child health is great. Nevertheless it is essential that the health worker should be able to sort out the useful from the useless and to manage systematically any cross-cultural problems that confront him.

The first step is to learn as much as possible about the unfamiliar culture. Health workers can do this by reading the available socio-anthropological literature and by investigating those aspects of the culture that concern them most. Close contacts and friendly relationships with indigenous healers and birth attendants as well as religious leaders are often helpful in this matter. Having done this, they should then divide the various beliefs and practices into four categories.

The beneficial

Those that are psychologically and physiologically beneficial should be actively encouraged. Examples include breast feeding, sexual taboos that ensure the spacing of pregnancies, and the use of liver for early signs of vitamin A deficiency and anaemia.

The harmless

Cultural beliefs and practices that are harmless should not be interfered with. Thus, the various talismans used as prophylactics, the magic spells pronounced by medicine-men, and many of the ceremonial rituals designed to ward off evil spirits should not be interfered with, although they are unaesthetic to outsiders.

The uncertain

Where the psychological and physiological effects are doubtful, and difficulty is encountered in classifying a belief or practice, it should not be interfered with pending further observation. Examples include many of the herbs and drugs advocated by medicine-men.

The harmful

It is only when there are harmful psychological and physiological effects that cultural beliefs and practices should be actively changed. Examples include the dietary taboos advocated after childbirth among Malays, the use of dilute gruel of the staple cereal in place of breast milk as an infant food, and interference in the course of normal labour by 'pushers'.

The health worker will be chiefly concerned with harmful practices which will require modification by health education. This he can achieve by encouraging related beneficial practices while at the same time attempts are made to change the harmful practice. For example, Malay parents believe that papaya, which is a rich source of carotene, is 'cold' and should be avoided by children with night blindness. On the other hand, they believe that the liver of the dogfish is useful for night blindness. In such a case, the paediatrician can encourage the use of all forms of liver as a regular dietary item, and at the same time systematically encourage the Malay to eat increasing quantities of papaya.

Further reading

Harjula R. *Mirau and his Practice*. London: Tri-Med, 1980.

Howard M C. *Contemporary Cultural Anthropology*. Boston: Little Brown and Company, 1986.

Landy D. *Culture Disease and Healing*. London: Collier Macmillan, 1977.

MacCormack C P, (ed). *Ethnography of Fertility and Birth*. London: Academic Press, 1982.

McElroy A and Townsend P K. *Medical Anthropology*. Massachusetts: Duxbury Press, 1979.

Section II

Nature and Nurture

4 *The genetic constitution*

At any given time the individual is a product of the continuing interaction between his genetic endowment and the environment. Physical as well as psychosocial constitution is determined by this interaction. The differences which occur in individuals during health and disease are dependent upon the varying proportions contributed by the genetic inheritance on the one hand and environmental factors on the other. Thus, a genetic component can be identified in every disease, including those illnesses which are predominantly determined by the environment, such as measles. It has been shown that during an attack of measles those children who fail to mount a strong immunological response, as judged by a raised lymphocyte count, have a higher incidence of morbidity and death. Such a lack of lymphocyte response can be due to environmentally determined causes like nutritional deficiency but is also due to genetic predisposition.

Genetic component of disease

It is possible to postulate a spectrum of disease processes beginning with those that are mainly determined by the environment going on to those in which the environment provides the trigger for disease to occur in a genetically predisposed person and continuing to those conditions that are mainly determined by genetic factors. Control of the environment will have a different effect on the prevalence of disease in these three groups of conditions (figure 4.1). In a harsh environment infection is a major determinant of ill health. The genetic constitution may determine the individual's response but it is largely overshadowed by the infective process. The environment provides the trigger for a disease process in some conditions such as G-6-PD deficiency. The individual with such a deficiency

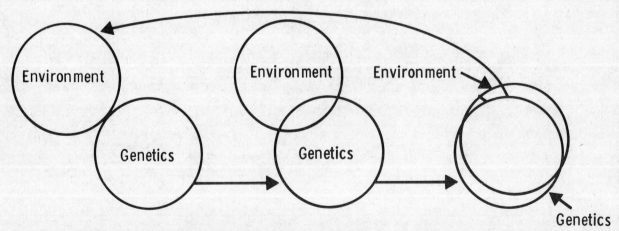

Genetics and environmental factors determine the etiology of a given trait

Figure 4.1 Interaction of genetic and environmental factors

may go through life without any illness unless he is exposed to a provoking stimulus such as fava beans, certain drugs or chemicals such as naphthalene. Finally there are pathological states chiefly determined by the genetic make-up of the individual for example chromosomal anomalies and haemoglobinopathies.

The genetic component of disease can be demonstrated even in some childhood malignancies. Certain tumours have long been known to run in families. Retinoblastoma can be inherited as an autosomal dominant trait or children may inherit conditions such as neurofibromatosis or xeroderma pigmentosa which carry a high risk of malignant transformation. It has been calculated that the risk for a sibling in childhood malignancy is twice that in the general population, which is 1 in 600, and the risk is higher for a twin of the same sex. This increased risk in siblings may be due to sharing of environmental factors both before and after birth, or due to shared genes or due to a combination of both.

More recently, HL-A antigens have been shown to be associated with several connective tissue diseases. It is known that HL-A genes are closely linked to those related to the immune response and thus serve as useful markers of the individual's response to antigens.

The gene-environment interaction occurs even prior to conception and can involve the genes located on the chromosomes of the gamete as in the case of individuals exposed to radiation or certain chemicals. Such a change determines whether the subsequently fertilised ovum will have a deleterious gene which was previously not expressed though carried by the parent, whether a new genetic mutation will occur or whether the chromosomes will be in normal or abnormal numbers. After conception, normal foetal genetic endowment may be adversely affected by abnormal intrauterine environment as in the case of: (1) infections such as rubella, venereal disease, malaria and so on, (2) inadequate nutrition of the mother or (3) drugs or X-rays administered to the mother or by altered blood chemistry as in diabetes.

The biological mechanisms of inheritance

Each individual develops from a single cell, namely the fertilised ovum. This single cell carries instructions for all the millions of cells that will develop from it to make the body. The sources of these instructions are the equal quantities of genetic information derived from the ovum and the sperm cell which fertilised it. These instructions as we know are stored in the thread-like chromosomes in the nuclei of the two cells.

Most of the time the chromosomes are so fine that they are invisible even with the higher power of the microscope. At the time of cell division, however, the chromosomes coil up into short, thick strands which can be identified because of their characteristic lengths and shapes. The chromosomes carry genes which determine inheritance. Each chromosome most probably consists of just one very long molecule of deoxyribonucleic acid (DNA). In its shape the molecule of DNA resembles a rope ladder twisted into a spiral form. The rungs of the ladder are of two types. One type is made up of a bonding of thymine and adenine each jutting out from opposite sides of the ladder. The second type is made up of guanine and cytosine. There are ten rungs in one complete spiral turn of the DNA molecule. The order of the paired units along the molecule varies according to the instructions that are being coded. A sequence of several hundred paired units is usually needed to code each instruction.

One gene corresponds to a length of DNA containing up to 1000 rungs. Since the rungs may be in any sequence, the number of possible arrangements for 1000 rungs is infinite. The precise order of the rung is a code determining genetic instruction. The DNA molecule codes instructions for the synthesis of proteins which make up a large proportion of the tissue structures. Proteins are also necessary for the different chemical processes which keep us alive. When a particular protein is required the DNA in the nucleus of the cell produces a duplicate molecule called ribonucleic acid (RNA) which leaves the nucleus and enters the cytoplasm where it activates the assembly of amino acids into polypeptides. This process is summarised in figure 4.2. There are only 20 amino acids but the sequence in which they are combined helps to form a vast array of proteins. Three base pairs, or rungs, on the DNA nucleus are required to specify one amino acid. Theoretically, one average chromosome can give rise to 100 000 different polypeptides, in chains consisting of 400 amino acids. But this is not necessarily so. It is now believed that structural genes comprise only a few per cent of the chromosomes. A large proportion of the remaining chromosome material performs a regulatory function.

Of the 46 chromosomes, two are sex chromosomes. The remaining 44 form 22 homologous pairs so that one of each pair is inherited from one parent. Each member of the pair has a high degree of similarity with the other which allows them to recognise each

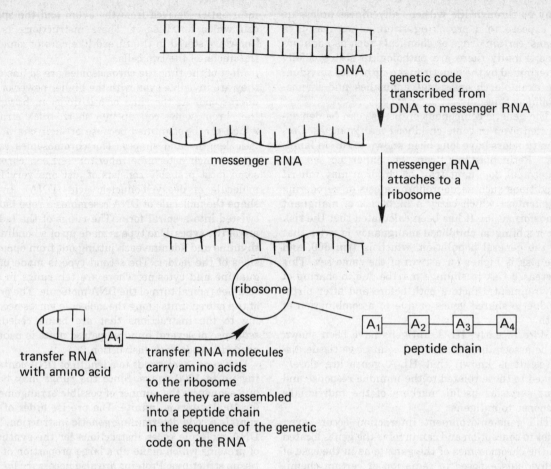

Figure 4.2   A simplified outline of protein synthesis

other and participate in the process of meiosis. The degree of similarity between the two members of the pair is not absolute. It is believed that 10 per cent of the structural genes of one member of a homologous pair will specify polypeptides that are slightly different from those specified by the companion genes of the other chromosome. The remaining 90 per cent of structural genes are present as pairs of identical genes, one of each pair to a chromosome. During meiosis, there is crossing over of chromatin material from one member of the pair to another. This allows for a different combination of maternal and paternal instructions. In this way every ovum and every sperm cell carries a unique combination of genetic instructions, and nature ensures that every individual inherits a different combination of genetic instructions.

During the process of meiosis modifications to chromosomes and genes can occur. This is known as mutation. Such a change involves chromosomal

rearrangements, breakages and junctions. A gross change of this kind will have considerable morphological effects but is usually not inherited. On the other hand, point mutations can also occur at a single gene locus and involve one or more of the bases in the way of deletion, addition, substitution or transposition. Any change in a single base unit will mean that subsequent bases will become out of phase and a new series of templates are formed specifying the production of a totally different polypeptide. The majority of such point mutations lead to single amino acid substitution in the polypeptide. The nature of proteins is such that even a single amino acid substitution can alter the physico-chemical properties of the whole protein molecule. A good example is the sickle-cell haemoglobin where a minor change in the amino acid sequence leads to a chain of events resulting in a variety of pathological processes.

Not all the genes are active at any one time. Some

are permanently inactive, for example, those concerned with the synthesis of haemoglobin which are switched off after birth in all cell types except in the erythroblast. Some genes are active only during certain phases of the life of the individual, for example, those concerned with the synthesis of foetal haemoglobin. Some genes produce their effects in one sex only, for example, the genes related to the male type of baldness.

Hormones are known to influence protein synthesis and could conceivably fit into a repressor or promoter mechanism. All messenger RNA does not necessarily pass into the cytoplasm, and at any given time more than half is to be found in the nucleus. This has led to the suggestion that mRNA molecules may be transported out of the nucleus after they have become bound to a protein moiety to form ribonucleoprotein complexes.

Genetic disease

Genetic disorders can be classified into three groups – the chromosomal disorders, the Mendelian single gene disorders and the polygenic disorders.

Chromosomal disorders

Chromosomal disorders occur when there is too much or too little chromosome material on account of defective meiosis. Most chromosomal aberrations are either due to an abnormal number of chromosomes or due to one or more chromosomes having abnormal configuration because of translocation, deletion or insertion of extra material. The abnormalities can involve both the sex and the non-sex chromosomes.

As a group, the chromosome disorders share several features. Complex physical abnormalities occur causing both internal (for example, congenital heart disease) and external (for example, of the face, neck and hands) malformations. Trisomy 21, 18 and 13 are examples of disorders involving the chromosomes. There is usually mental retardation with severe disability and shortened life span. If the aberration involves sex chromosomes, the individual will appear normal in the first decade of life and will go undiagnosed until there is delay in sexual maturation in the second decade of life. The majority of them will have a normal mental and physical state. They will commonly present as 10 per cent of infertile couples, approximately 30 per cent of those seen for abnormal sexual development and nearly 50 per cent of females with primary amenorrhoea.

Chromosomal aberrations are almost always sporadic, the affected individual usually being the only one in the family with the disorder. The frequency with which they arise in different ethnic groups is also similar since the frequencies of mutations and faulty meiosis are not different between races. Most are maternal and possibly paternal age dependent. The frequencies of various chromosomal abnormalities are shown in table 4.1.

Many pregnancies with chromosomal aberrations do not go to term. It has been estimated that approximately one in three spontaneous abortions in early pregnancy are chromosomal in origin and the frequency with which chromosome abnormalities produce still-births is unknown.

Single gene disorders

More than 2000 single gene disorders have been described. They are of three classes – (1) the autosomal dominant, (2) the autosomal recessive and (3) sex-linked.

Autosomal dominance

Autosomal dominance implies that the mutant gene is situated on an autosome (non-sex chromosome) and this mutant gene is capable of giving rise to an abnormal characteristic in a single dose in spite of the presence of a normal partner gene in the pair. Autosomal dominant conditions represent almost half of the 2000 to 3000 genetic diseases described and affect between 1 to 1½ per cent of the newborn population. Examples of autosomal dominant conditions are: achondroplasia, neurofibromatosis, tuberous sclerosis, Marfan's syndrome, Ehlers-Danlos syndrome, osteogenesis imperfecta, adult-type polycystic disease of the kidneys, acute intermittent porphyria, large bowel polyposis, etc. The most frequent in Western countries are the group of genetic hyperlipidaemias. Their incidence in developing countries has not been well documented.

In autosomal dominance there is a 50 per cent risk in each pregnancy for an affected offspring regardless of sex. For accuracy of diagnosis and counselling it is important to examine the parents and members of the family from prior generations bearing in mind that quite variable expressions of autosomal dominant genes can occur with mild to severe forms being manifested. If the autosomal dominant condition is found in the child but not the parents, that child represents a new mutation for the gene. The parents are not at risk of recurrence

Table 4.1 Frequency of chromosomal abnormalities

Chromosomal abnormality	Associated developmental abnormality	Frequency (per 1000 live births)
Trisomy 21	Mongolism	1.5
E	Edward's Syndrome	0.2
D	Patau's Syndrome	0.1
Deletion of short-arm B	Cri-du-chat	0.05
Miscellaneous autosomal abnormalities (unbalanced)	Physical and mental maldevelopment of varying degree	0.02
Sex chromosomal abnormality	About half will show abnormality of sex and/or mental development. The rest are clinically normal	2.5
Autosomal abnormality (balanced)	Clinically normal but may be infertile	5.0
Autosomal variant	Clinically normal	25.0
Variation of 'Y' chromosome	Clinically normal	15.0

for subsequent pregnancies but the affected child will obviously carry a 50 per cent recurrent risk for his offspring.

Many of the new mutations are parental age dependent. It is a good practice to examine closely all newborns one of whose parents is above the age of 40 years.

In most of the thousand or so known autosomal dominant disorders, no specific biochemical defects are known and it is believed that these genes are mainly concerned with the synthesis of structural proteins. Hence diagnosis relies heavily on accurate clinical examination.

Autosomal recessive disorders

In recessive conditions both genes of the pair are abnormal. The parents of the affected child are clinically normal but carry the mutant gene in a single dose. The risks in each pregnancy are one in four for an affected offspring and two in four for a carrier child similar to the parents and one in four for a genetically normal baby.

The most common autosomal recessive disorders in the developing world are the haemoglobinopathies, mainly sickle-cell anaemia and thalassaemia. Other examples of the over 900 autosomal recessive disorders include cystic fibrosis, oculocutaneous albinism, phenylketonuria and the adrenogenital

syndromes. Several of the inborn errors of metabolism fall into this group of disorders. In a large proportion of autosomal recessive disorders there is severe disability and early death or mental retardation unless treatment is available from birth.

The genes concerned in autosomal recessive disorders are those responsible for the production of enzyme proteins. The defect results in an alteration in one or more amino acids in the sequence of the specific enzymes or other proteins reflecting a change in the corresponding gene.

The carriers of the mutant gene are symptom-free and appear normal. The incidence of the disorder is governed by the marriage practices of the community. Since close relatives share their genes, a high level of consanguinity increases the risks of a homozygote. First cousin marriages are the practice in many societies. Similarly, by tradition village communities tend to practice endogamy or exogamy which is usually restricted to a group of villages. Such practices tend to maintain the incidence of an inheritable condition within the community.

In a majority of recessive disorders the birth of an infant with the disease is the first clue to the carrier state of the parents. Hence careful documentation of the family history and examination of the infant born in families with previous neonatal deaths and mental retardation is an important method of early detection.

The newborn responds to severe illness with a limited number of symptoms. Even though in most instances these symptoms may be due to more common conditions, screening tests to rule out inherited errors of metabolism may be necessary when the symptoms do not clear soon. Table 4.2 describes some of the common symptoms associated with genetic-metabolic disease in the newborn and the screening tests which can be performed in a side-room laboratory.

Sex-linked disorders

Of the 2000 to 3000 major genetic diseases, approximately six per cent are of the sex-linked type. The more frequently seen condition in the developing countries is glucose-6-phosphate dehydrogenase deficiency. It is an important example of pharmacogenetic abnormalities in which ordinarily non-toxic drugs and chemicals become harmful. Other examples of sex-linked genetic disorders are the

Table 4.2 Symptoms in severe genetic–metabolic disease in newborn infants

Symptom	Screening test	Disorder
Diarrhoea	Reducing substance in stool and in urine	Congenital lactase deficiency
	Reducing substance in stool; glycosuria	Glucose–galactose malabsorption
Vomiting	Ferric chloride test on urine	Phenylketonuria
	Non-glucose reducing substance in urine	Galactosaemia
		Hereditary fructose intolerance
Jaundice	Non-glucose reducing substance in urine	Galactosaemia
	Non-glucose reducing substance in urine	Hereditary fructose intolerance
	Ferric chloride and nitrosonaphthol tests on urine	Tyrosinaemia
	Reticulocyte count Red blood cell morphology	Spherocytosis
Hypoglycaemia	Ferric chloride test on urine	Maple syrup urine disease
	Dinitrophenyl-hydrazine test	
	Neutropenia	Methylmalonic
	Acidosis	Acidaemia
	Non-glucose reducing substance in urine	Galactosaemia
	Non-glucose reducing substance in urine	Hereditary fructose intolerance
Coma	Dinitrophenyl-hydrazine test	Maple syrup urine disease
	Acidosis	Propionic acidaemia
	Acidosis and neutropenia	Methylmalonic acidaemia
Unusual odour, musty	Ferric chloride test	Phenylketonuria
Sweaty feet	Acidosis Ketonuria	Isovaleric acidaemia
	Ferric chloride test Dinitrophenyl-hydrazine test	Maple syrup urine disease
	Ferric chloride test Nitrosonaphthol test	Tyrosinaemia
Abnormal hair	Ferric chloride test	Phenylketonuria
Sparse, kinky hair		Menke's syndrome

Duchenne type of muscular dystrophy, haemophilia A and B, partial colour blindness, nephrogenic diabetes insipidus and some forms of immuno deficiency.

The carriers of the disorders are females who are symptom-free and there is a 50 per cent risk of an affected male in each male pregnancy and 50 per cent risk for a non-affected carrier female in each female pregnancy.

Polygenic inheritance

Contrary to the popular belief that genetic disorders are determined by chromosomal aberrations or by mutations in a single gene, it is polygenic inheritance which is responsible for a large proportion of the genetic component of disease. Here several genes contribute to a predisposition which acts in concert with environmental factors to cause disease. Neural tube defects, congenital dislocation of the hip, congenital heart disease, pyloric stenosis, cleft lip and/or palate, allergies, psychosis, hypertension, peptic ulcer, coronary artery disease and most cases of gout fall under this category. These diseases are due to small contributions from a number of genes and so the inheritance patterns are more complex. As a rule there is a greater risk in family members depending upon the closeness of the relationship and the sharing of genes. To give an example, in the case of hare lip with or without cleft palate, when the general incidence in the community is in the order of 1 per 1000, the incidence in first degree relatives of an index case is 30 to 50 per 1000, in second degree relatives it is 7 per 1000 and in third degree relatives it falls to between 2 and 3 per 1000. In a family with one affected child the recurrence risks are 2 to 5 per cent for subsequent pregnancies. Hence careful documentation of all cases is necessary in order to anticipate difficulties in future and for counselling the family.

Many of the individual characteristics like height, weight, intelligence quotient, lean body mass, blood pressure, and age of menarche are dependent upon

Table 4.3   Recurrence risks of some common disorders

Pyloric stenosis	1 in 20 for brothers and sons and 1 in 40 for sisters or daughters of affected males
	1 in 5 for brothers and sons and 1 in 10 for sisters or daughters of affected females.
Cleft lip ± cleft palate	1 in 30 for sibs or sons and daughters of affected persons.
Congenital dislocation of hip (diagnosed in newborns)	1 in 40 for brothers and sons and 1 in 10 for sisters and daughters of affected females.
	In the case of affected males, there is a higher risk for relatives.
Talipes equinovarus	1 in 50 for sibs of affected persons
Down's syndrome	In regular trisomy 21 the risk for sibs of affected persons is 1 in 100. The risk is higher if a translocation is present.
Congenital malformations of the heart	For all types of heart malformations taken together the risk is about 1 in 30 for sibs of affected persons.
Diabetes (onset under 30)	1 in 20 risk of early onset diabetes for sibs of affected persons.

With several of the above conditions the risk of recurrence is raised when there is already more than one affected person in the family.

polygenic inheritance. In many instances an informed guess can be made by noting the family characteristics.

Genetics and the practising physician

The physician needs a working knowledge of the principles of genetic inheritance in order to be able to help the families under his care and the wider community. A knowledge of the frequency of the common genetic disorders is useful in order to anticipate the number of patients with such disorders each year in the district. It is estimated that about 0.5 per cent of all live-born infants have a chromosomal anomaly deleterious to health. It is also estimated that about one per cent of live-born children will be affected by conditions determined by mutant genes. Individual gene mutations are rare events and so the conditions they cause also tend to be rare.

It is necessary to have a wide coverage of the community with maternity services. When the majority of births in the community take place under supervision, genetic disorders are more likely to be diagnosed and documented. Success in genetic counselling depends on the detail and accuracy of such documentation. A knowledge of the pattern of inheritance in the community obtained from the family histories of many index cases is helpful in making prognosis and determining risks for future pregnancies.

For some of the more widespread conditions like the haemoglobinopathies and G–6-PD deficiency, it is advisable to establish facilities for screening of the population and for the counselling of parents with affected children.

In the case of the individual family with an affected child, genetic counselling is required for management and prognosis as well as with regard to risk of recurrence. Most difficulties in counselling arise from the variability of manifestations. Hence accuracy of diagnosis is most important. The risks according to Mendelian laws of inheritance for dominant and recessive conditions have been discussed above. The recurrence risks for some common conditions are shown in table 4.3.

After establishing the diagnosis, a history of the family, including examination of as many affected members as possible, is necessary to build up a pedigree tree. Figure 4.3 is an example of symbols commonly used for drawing up a pedigree, and figures 4.4a-c give typical examples of pedigrees obtained in autosomal and sex-linked disorders.

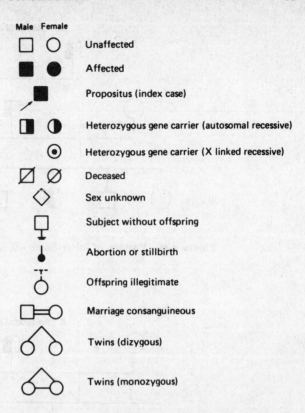

Figure 4.3 Symbols commonly used in a pedigree tree

Criteria for recognising single gene disorders

Autosomal dominant (figure 4.4a)

(1) The disorder affects persons of both sexes equally.
(2) Every affected individual has one affected parent.
(3) Every affected individual transmits the disease to one child out of two.

Variations in the pattern of transmission do arise from time to time. These are due to the following:

(1) *Mutation*
The normal gene in the gamete from one of the parents becomes transformed into a pathological one as a result of mutation. In such a case no individual in the previous generations will be found to carry the disorder. In the case of the affected person the usual criteria for dominant autosomal transmission will continue to apply to the offsprings. Mutation, however, is an extremely rare occurrence.

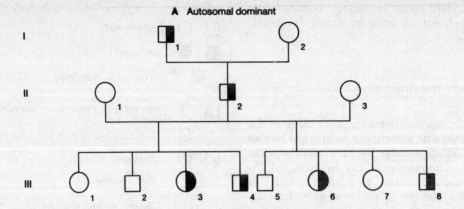

Figure 4.4a   Pattern of inheritance – 1. Autosomal dominant

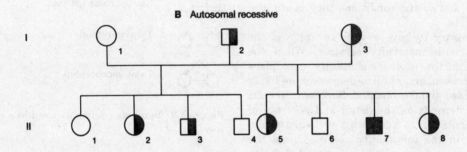

Figure 4.4b   Pattern of inheritance – 2. Autosomal recessive

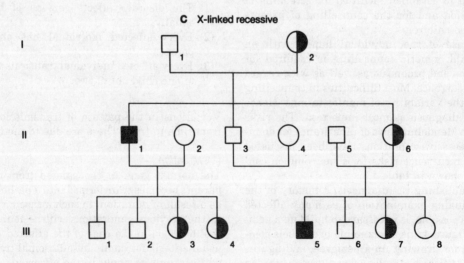

Figure 4.4c   Pattern of inheritance – 3. Sex-linked

(2) Difference in penetration and expressivity

A known dominant trait occasionally skips a generation. The individual may look phenotypically normal but nonetheless carries the 'dominant' gene which will be transmitted to the next generation. Gene penetrance is said to be incomplete in such cases. A number of autosomal dominant conditions are known to skip generations.

In certain conditions individuals with a dominant pathological gene do not show all the abnormalities. For example, a person with a gene for polydactyly may show the abnormality in one, two, three or all four limbs. Alternatively the age of onset of a dominant disorder may be in the newborn period or in later life. These are examples of differences in the expressivity of a dominant gene. Hence the need for accuracy of diagnosis, and meticulous care in recording details of family history when developing the family tree of inheritance of the condition.

Autosomal recessive trait (figure 4.4b)

In the majority of cases the affected individual is born to normal parents. The following criteria help to identify the individual with an autosomal recessive condition

(1) Affected individuals are born to normal parents.
(2) Both sexes are equally affected.
(3) In an affected sibship the proportion of those affected is one out of four.

Although the defective gene may be transmitted from generation to generation, the disorder generally appears within a single group of siblings. Many of the recognised inborn errors of metabolism follow this pattern of inheritance.

Sex-linked inheritance (figure 4.4c)

Three types of sex-linked disorders may be recognised: X-linked recessive; X-linked dominant and Y-linked disorders.

X-linked recessive inheritance is relatively easy to recognise. A recessive sex-linked gene always expresses the disorder in males since they carry only one X chromosome, while females must be homozygous for it to be expressed. Such a disorder affects only male children of the union of a carrier woman to a normal man. One out of two daughters of such a union will be a carrier and one out of two sons will have the disorder.

The above description of the pattern of inheritance is a guide to help the practising physician in counselling families with genetic disorders about risks to future children. The steps involved in estimating risks correctly may be summarised as follows.

Accurate diagnosis   + Meticulous family history
↓
Mode of inheritance
↓
Estimation of risks improved by: Risks
Knowledge of the natural history
of the disorder
+
Results of laboratory tests

The laboratory tests relate to biochemical tests for abnormal substances (for example raised creatine kinase activity in muscular dystrophy), or for defective gene products (for example sickle cell haemoglobin). More recently new developments in the science of genetics have led to newer tests like DNA probes for gene analysis. Such tests help to confirm carrier states as well as enable prenatal diagnosis to be made in a number of conditions, for example thalassaemia.

New genetics

The remarkable progress in molecular biology and genetics made in the past decades is often referred to as the New Genetics, to distinguish it from classical genetics based on the Mendelian Laws of Inheritance. New laboratory techniques and therapeutic developments have come about as a result of these advances.

DNA analysis

The two strands of DNA can be dissociated by heating. They come together again on cooling. The reassociation of separated strands is a highly specific process and will occur only between DNA (or RNA) strands which have complementary or almost complementary base sequences. Thus, if a gene carried on a strand of DNA is to be investigated, a length of DNA with a known complementary sequence of bases may be used to identify it instead of having to search along the entire length of the DNA. This is the principle on which laboratory techniques for gene probing are based.

DNA can be obtained by using the standard

techniques from any tissue containing nucleated cells including blood and chorionic villi. Once extracted the DNA is stable and can be stored indefinitely. A number of restriction enzymes have been identified in bacteria. These enzymes recognise specific DNA sequences and cleave double-stranded DNA at these sites. Using a battery of restriction enzymes the DNA can be cut into manageable fragments for analysis. The DNA fragments produced with the help of a battery of restriction enzymes can be arranged in order of size by electrophoresis.

Another important development has been the discovery of the enzyme reverse transcriptase. The enzyme is used to synthesize DNA (called copy DNA) from any messenger RNA. If radioactive bases are added to the reaction the copy DNA becomes radioactively labelled. Such labelled pieces of DNA can be used as probes to look for complementary sequences on DNA fragments.

In the laboratory DNA analysis has not only improved the accuracy of diagnosis as well as the calculation of risk for future pregnancies, but also early diagnosis, for example by chorionic villus biopsy at a gestational age of 10 weeks. The pregnancy may then be terminated if need be. Thus in a number of Mediterranean countries programmes were set up to combat B-thalassaemia using prenatal diagnosis. Within three years a 60 to 90 per cent fall in births of infants affected with thalassaemia major has been recorded. In Sardinia a fall of 70 per cent has occurred.

Recombinant DNA technology

This development is based on the observation that several bacteria carry closed circular DNA molecules called plasmids within their cytoplasm. The plasmid contains sites where a number of restriction enzymes can open up the circular DNA and convert it into a linear molecule. A foreign DNA with a known sequence can be fragmented by the same restriction enzymes. The plasmid and the DNA fragments are then mixed in solution and some join each other. The joint is made firm by means of another enzyme called DNA ligase. The recombinant plasmid is then mixed with bacteria and a proportion enter the bacteria. Bacteria containing the recombinant plasmid are selected out and cultured in colonies.

The expression of recombinant DNA in a cell was first achieved with *Escherichia coli*. Since then expression systems have been devised for many types of cells, including yeast. Using the recombinant technique a number of therapeutic agents have been produced. Human insulin, growth hormone and hepatitis B vaccine are well known examples.

Further reading

Cherfas J. *Man made Life*. Oxford: Blackwell Scientific Publication, 1982.

Emery A E H. *An Introduction to Recombinant DNA*. Chichester: Wiley, 1984.

Kingston H M. *ABC of Clinical Genetics*. London: British Medical Journal, 1989.

Roberts J A F, Pembrey M E. *An Introduction to Medical Genetics*. Oxford: Oxford University Press, 1985.

Weatherall D J. *The New Genetics and Clinical Practice*. Oxford: Oxford University Press, 1985.

5 Nutrition and its disorders

A major part of paediatric practice in the developing world is concerned with adequate and proper feeding of children. The paediatrician should not only be able to diagnose and treat nutritional disorders in children brought to the hospital, but should also be actively involved in setting up community programmes for the promotion of good nutrition. The number of children seen in the hospital with malnutrition is a rough measure of the prevalence of malnutrition in the community. It also provides a measure of the efficacy of the services and programmes in the community. The role of the paediatrician and the health team is to raise community awareness about the prevalence of malnutrition and to disseminate knowledge about the proper feeding of children. The paediatrician should also be involved in studying the etiologic factors leading to poor nutrition. In a continuing dialogue with the community and its leaders these factors should be discussed fully and strategies evolved for dealing with them. Such strategies will involve not only health education and services for the surveillance of vulnerable groups, but also methods of identifying those who are 'at risk' of malnutrition. People will eat better if they produce more, and improvements in agricultural technology, methods of storage and the choice of crops for cultivation are also important in combating malnutrition. Community participation is better in an atmosphere of mutual trust and harmony. Social activities which increase cohesiveness in the community, like women's organisations, young farmers' clubs, parents' clubs, are helpful in this respect. The interest and involvement of the health team often helps to hold together these various activities of community development.

Feeding of infants and young children
Breast milk

Breast milk is *the* most important source of nutrition for the newborn and the young infant,

as well as the toddler. Successful establishment of lactation after the birth of the baby is so important that any baby whose mother does not secrete breast milk will have a poor chance of survival. Most babies do well on breast milk alone during the first four to six months of life. Their weight gain is comparable to that of their counterparts in Western countries.

During pregnancy, the body metabolism of the mother alters so that energy stores are laid down (in the form of fat) in preparation for lactation. If the mother is on a marginal diet, poor or no body stores will be laid down and it is likely that she will have to draw upon her own tissues for the demands of pregnancy and lactation. Thus, with regard to maternal nutrition, pregnancy and lactation are part of one integral physiologic process, and the preparation for lactation must begin in pregnancy.

Lactation is a greater strain on the mother's nutrition than pregnancy. As pregnancy advances the mother's activity slows down; on the other hand, after the birth of the baby she may rapidly have to resume all her household duties, in addition to having to look after the baby and secrete enough milk to keep up with his increasing demands. A healthy mother produces an average of 850 ml of milk daily, which is equivalent to 600 calories daily. The protein content of milk is about 1.2 g per 100 ml so that the average baby receives approximately 10 g protein per day. The efficiency of protein conversion in the human mammary gland is not known, but if by analogy with the veterinary world it was 50 per cent, then the mother should receive at least 20 g of protein per day in addition to her normal intake.

Dietary energy is converted into milk with an efficiency of about 90 per cent. Based on these assumptions, and also on the fact that the body lays down stores during pregnancy, it is recommended that an additional 500 calories a day is an adequate supplement for a nursing mother. The nutritional needs of lactation are chiefly for calories and not so much for protein. These requirements can be quite easily supplied from a predominantly cereal-based diet so long as it provides adequate calories.

The high efficiency rate of conversion of food energy into breast milk in the mother, and the relatively low requirements of protein added to the ability to store energy during pregnancy enables mothers to breast feed their infants for prolonged periods even when subsisting on marginal nutrition. The concentration of various major constituents of breast milk like protein, carbohydrates, fat, calcium and iron remains unchanged within a wide range of intake and over a prolonged period of lactation. For example, in New Guinea it was found that the composition of milk was much the same after 18 to 24 months of lactation as it was at 6 to 12 months. However, if the mother's diet is inadequate, the total output of milk is reduced. Even then many studies have shown that mothers of low socio-economic class are able to secrete 400 to 800 ml of milk per day in the first year of lactation, the output falling to between 200 and 450 ml per day in the second year.

Physiology of lactation

At the time of puberty, the mammary gland grows and develops under the influence of the sex hormones. The fully mature mammary gland consists of a system of lacteals and ducts radiating from the nipple and the areola and leading to the acinar epithelium, with a supporting network of reticular and adipose tissue together with involuntary muscle fibres (figure 5.1).

During pregnancy, the high levels of oestrogen and progesterone in the blood stimulate further growth and development of the acinar epithelium in the mammary gland. Soon after parturition, the levels of oestrogen and progesterone fall. At the same time the pituitary gland secretes another hormone called prolactin, which stimulates the formation of milk in the epithelial cells of the mammary gland. How parturition brings about the secretion of prolactin from the pituitary is not exactly known;

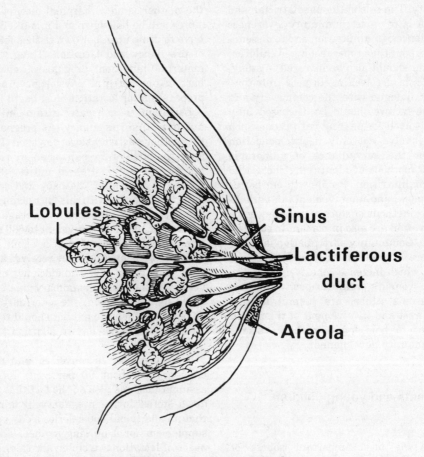

Figure 5.1   Milk secreting structures of the human mammary gland

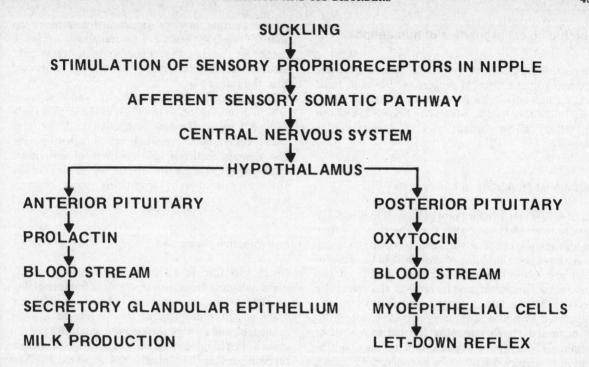

SUCKLING

STIMULATION OF SENSORY PROPRIORECEPTORS IN NIPPLE

AFFERENT SENSORY SOMATIC PATHWAY

CENTRAL NERVOUS SYSTEM

HYPOTHALAMUS

ANTERIOR PITUITARY

PROLACTIN

BLOOD STREAM

SECRETORY GLANDULAR EPITHELIUM

MILK PRODUCTION

POSTERIOR PITUITARY

OXYTOCIN

BLOOD STREAM

MYOEPITHELIAL CELLS

LET-DOWN REFLEX

Figure 5.2 Neurohormonal pathways of lactation

it is most likely due to a removal of inhibition rather than stimulation of secretion.

Tactile stimulation of the skin of the nipple and the areola by the baby during the act of suckling causes reflex stimulation of the pituitary along the sensory branches of the vagus nerve. Oxytocin is released from the pituitary as a result of the stimulation, and causes contraction of the involuntary muscle fibres of the mammary gland, thereby causing the emptying of the gland. Under the effect of oxytocin the other breast may also show an escape of milk, which has led to the common term 'let-down reflex' (figure 5.2).

Once established, milk secretion in the breast is maintained by the complete and regular emptying of the breast by the baby. In a healthy mother, within physiologic limits, the quantity of milk secreted by the breast depends upon how much it has been emptied by the baby. If the baby fails to empty the breast completely during a feed, the amount of milk secreted and available for the next feed will be a little less and so on until a proper balance is established. Similarly, if a baby is fed on one side only, the milk in the other breast will decrease progressively and may dry up completely.

Just as nervous and hormonal mechanisms in the mother initiate and maintain her supply of milk, various reflex mechanisms are present in the baby which enable him to take his nutrition from the breast. Some of the more important reflexes are

(1) *The rooting reflex.* When the side of the baby's mouth is touched by the nipple, he turns his head towards the nipple and takes it in his mouth.

(2) *The suckling reflex.* The baby does not suck at the nipple as one does on a straw, but actually 'milks' it between the tongue and the hard palate, by rhythmically compressing it with the tongue against the palate.

(3) *The swallowing reflex.* This requires the closure of the nasopharynx and the co-ordinated action of the muscles of deglutition.

Recent research has demonstrated the presence of other reflex mechanisms which help and act in conjunction with the reflexes mentioned above. Thus, babies one week old are able to recognise the smell of their mothers' milk and will selectively turn their heads towards the source of the smell. There is also evidence that chemoreceptors at the back of the throat are able to influence respiration in accordance with the electrolyte content and osmolarity of the feed.

The biological properties of human milk

Since the early 1970s there has been a growing interest in the biological properties of human milk and its protective role for the nursing infant. This has, in turn, helped to widen our knowledge of the physiology of the infant and of developmental biology.

Nutritional properties of human milk

Exclusively breastfed infants grow well and usually double their birthweight by the time they are four to six months old. For such rapid growth to occur there has to be a doubling of the traffic in the absorption and assimilation of nutrients, growth of the gastrointestinal tract, and increase in the metabolic activity for the laying down of tissues. All this is supported by a food containing not more than 1.2g/dl of protein. Such reasoning has led to a shift of emphasis away from protein, and to the identification of 'energy density' as a key factor. At 6 cal/g solid matter breast milk is an excellent source of energy. This knowledge has led to a number of innovative approaches for the improvement of the energy density of weaning foods for the prevention of malnutrition (see page 56).

What is more significant is the realisation that the newborn infant does not handle large amounts of 'foreign' protein well. In studies where pre-term infants were fed formulae prepared from unmodified cow's milk the blood levels of phenylalanine and tyrosine as well as of other amino acids were found to rise. In some instances the levels became as high as those seen in phenylketonuria and tyrosinaemia, and remained elevated for several weeks. In such cases there is a potential risk of damage to the growing brain. Thus each period in the life-cycle of an individual has its typical metabolic needs. The amino acid composition of a given protein is also important. For example studies in small infants with birthweights <1500g indicate that breast milk fortified with human milk protein is tolerated well at intake levels of between 3.0 and 3.5g/kg per day.

In the newborn, especially if pre-term, the levels of pancreatic lipase and bile salts are low. Efficient fat absorption depends upon alternate mechanisms for the digestion of dietary fat, for example gastric lipolysis due to lingual and gastric lipase compensating for low levels of pancreatic lipase. An additional compensatory enzyme is the bile-salt stimulated lipase in human milk. Thus in the case of human milk the digestion of milk fat begins long before the milk reaches the small intestine of the infant. Free fatty acids are an important source of energy for the infant, and the lipase of breast milk ensures that free fatty acids are readily generated from the infant's food.

Trace elements like iron, copper, and zinc occur in higher concentration in colostrum than in mature milk. All trace elements in human milk occur as complexes bound to specific proteins called ligands. The ligands facilitate the transfer of individual trace elements across the mucosal epithelium of the neonatal gut thereby improving their bioavailability.

Anti-infective properties

Up to one-third of all protein in human milk is immunological protein in the form of immunoglobulin, lactoferrin, complement, lysozyme and so on. They act in synergism to form a shield against pathogens and foreign antigens. A great deal of the protection provided is specific against environmental pathogens as they colonise the maternal gut. The identification of the gut-mammary axis explains the presence of antibodies specific for the maternal gut flora in the IgA of breast milk. This observation has helped to define the mammary gland as a significant arm of the mucosal immune system.

Human milk is live. It contains cells varying in number from 5×10^5 to 1×10^7 per ml. Macrophages constitute 30 to 50 per cent of cells in early milk. Neutrophils and small phagocytic cells make up another 20 per cent or so of cells in the first few days of lactation, the remainder being lymphocytes. The latter include T cells, B cells and various T cell subsets. All these cells are active. They can ingest and kill micro-organisms; secrete immunoglobulins, interferon, lysozyme, complement components and lactoferrin. In animal experiments the lymphocytes in breast milk have been shown to gain entry into the gut associated lymphoid tissue of the suckling. In the case of the human infant, secretory IgA levels in the saliva and urine are higher in breast fed as compared to formula fed infants. The antibody response to BCG and triple antigen vaccination is greater in breast fed infants compared to those fed on formula. These studies provide evidence that the cells and other factors in breast milk have immunoregulatory influence on the developing immune system of the infant.

The *metabolic* response of breast fed infants to a feed is different from those on formulae. The pattern of secretion of insulin and of a number of gut hormones in response to feeding is different in breast fed infants. This difference in the metabolic response is still demonstrable at age nine months between exclusively breast fed infants and those who were weaned before they were three months old. Hormones like enteroglucagon, gastrin and cholecystokinin have trophic effects on the gut. However, the most potent trophic agent is the Epidermal Growth Factor (EGF) present in breast milk. EGF stimulates DNA synthesis along the entire length of the gastrointestinal tract as well as promoting maturation of cell function.

Suckling the infant more than six times a day maintains high basal levels of prolactin in addition to surges of the hormone at every feed. High levels of prolactin suppress ovulation so that exclusive and 'on demand' breast feeding has come to be recognised as the most practical and effective means of contraception at present in the developing world.

After reviewing data from 13 prospective studies carried out in Australia, Canada, Britain, the Philippines, Mexico, Egypt, Thailand and Chile, the Bellagio Consensus stated that the maximum effect on suppression of ovulation is achieved in the first six months postpartum when a mother is breast feeding exclusively and remains amenorrhoeic. The degree of protection from another pregnancy is as high as 98 per cent. However, if regular menstruation has commenced the degree of protection falls to 75 per cent, but is still much higher compared to non-breast feeding controls.

The role of breast feeding in encouraging mother-infant *bonding* is now well recognised. The eye-to-eye contact, body warmth and closeness as well as the mutual sense of pleasure and satiety make breast feeding an especially intimate experience for the mother and the infant.

Promotion of breast feeding

A number of old-fashioned hospital routines and practices are known to interfere with the successful establishment of breast feeding. Many such practices have no scientific basis. Thus the practice of nursery care of the newborn instead of rooming-in, pre-lacteal feeds, night feeds and top feeds are all empirical. Their replacement by routines which are more conducive to breast feeding is needed. A 10-point programme for adoption throughout the health service has been proposed as follows

(1) Have a written policy on breast feeding that is routinely communicated to all health workers.
(2) Train all health care staff in the skills necessary for implementing the policy.

(3) In antenatal and other clinics all attending parents should be informed about the benefits of breast feeding.
(4) Mothers should be encouraged and helped to initiate breast feeding within half an hour of delivery.
(5) When mothers are separated from their infants for any reason, they should be shown how to maintain lactation.
(6) Newborns should be offered no food or drink other than breast milk unless medically indicated.
(7) Practise rooming-in 24 hours a day.
(8) Encourage breast feeding on demand.
(9) Give no artificial pacifiers or dummies to infants.
(10) Foster the establishment of breast feeding support groups and refer mothers to them on discharge from the hospital or clinic.

Problems in breast feeding

Causes of a feeding difficulty may be in the baby or the mother.

Causes in the baby

These are mainly related to factors which interfere with the smooth working of the above reflexes.

(1) *Absence of reflex mechanisms*
In the case of immaturity of the central nervous system, as in prematures, in cases of cerebral birth trauma, developmental defects of the central nervous system, or with loss of consciousness, the reflex mechanisms are non-functioning. The newborn is not able to feed and it may become necessary to maintain his nutrition by a nasogastric tube until such time as these reflex mechanisms appear.

(2) *Physical inability to suckle*
In certain physical abnormalities of the oral cavity the baby is not able to carry out the 'milking' manoeuvre, for example, in cleft palate and micrognathia; the mouth may be sore, as in candida infection, or there may be muscle spasm as in tetanus neonatorum. (Difficulty in suckling is often noticed a day or two before the generalised spasms in neonatal tetanus and could lead to an early diagnosis.) In severe infections, the baby may become too weak to make the effort of feeding; similarly, in severe respiratory distress or congenital heart disease with failure, the baby may not be capable of suckling for prolonged periods and is not able to take enough.

Causes in the mother

These can be either local or general.

(1) *Painful cracked nipples* – this is usually a common cause due to a hungry baby sucking too vigorously on the breast. Infection may easily occur and if it spreads to deeper tissues may cause acute mastitis.

(2) *Retracted nipples or engorged breasts* – during feeding, the breast tissue presses against the baby's nose and interferes with his breathing, so that he cannot suckle well. Examination of the breasts in the antenatal clinic and ensuring that proper breast feeding has been established before discharge from the maternity ward is essential, so that such problems can be dealt with before the baby goes home.

(3) *Failure of lactation* – women from the rural societies of the developing countries do not suffer much from this problem, which is common in the educated elite and amongst the higher socio-economic groups. In most cases the causes are psychological, namely, anxiety and undue worry in the mother about her capabilities to produce breast milk. The mother's own upbringing and social and family background can also influence lactation.

The various social and emotional factors that can influence the secretion of milk in a mother are indicated in figure 5.3.

In recent years another major force leading to a rapid decline of breast feeding in many developing countries has been added to the above biological, social and cultural variables. This is the high pressure and at times unethical promotion of artificial feeding by manufacturers of baby foods. Many of these promotional practices are aimed at creating doubts in the mind of the mother about her ability to secrete enough milk. Some promotional literature holds out the promise that the canned formula is superior to human milk. In an indirect way mothers are also tempted by the thought of being free and able to take up gainful employment. Sometimes promotion comes under the guise of 'aid'. Free samples of powdered milk are given for distribution to mothers who attend the clinic. At the same time on the radio and television and other mass media there is continuous and seductive promotion. But the worst form of promotion is where mothers are offered 'gift packs' containing a feeding bottle and a sample of the product. The mother is told to try it and if she does not like it she could discard it. However, such a period of trial interferes considerably with the let-down reflex and the mother's milk dries up. After two or three days of trial the mother has no milk and she is 'hooked' on the formula. The health profession is another target of the promotional effort and is being wooed as well as fed a continuing flow of pseudo-scientific literature describing the scientific superiority of the manufactured product. The role of the paediatrician is therefore to safeguard the community from the effects of such promotional practices and to ensure that breast milk will be looked upon by the community as a highly desirable nutritional resource.

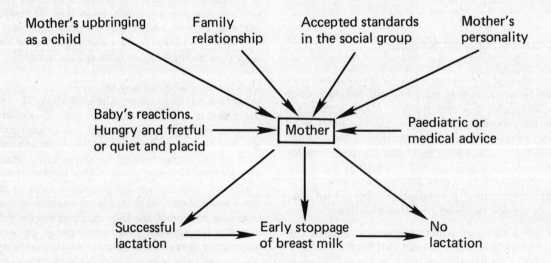

Figure 5.3 Factors influencing lactation

Practical problems in the management of breast feeding

As in all normal biological functions, various problems can arise with breast feeding. In the management of all these problems it is important to bear in mind that the 'let-down' reflex is crucial to the secretion and flow of milk. Any factor interfering with this reflex will have adverse effects on lactation.

Normal schedule

The normal healthy newborn baby needs 150 ml of milk per kilogramme body weight. At each feed he takes about 120–150ml of milk and usually settles on a three- or four-hourly schedule. Some babies are fretful and hungry and make more demands than others.

In a healthy mother with well-established lactation and a good let-down reflex, the baby with good hard suckling will empty one breast in approximately 15 to 20 minutes. One breast is offered first for 20 minutes, and the other for the rest of the feed. At the next feed the second breast is offered first, and so on. Thus, the baby is able to empty completely at least one of the breasts at each feed.

Most rural mothers feed their babies 'on demand' during the day as well as the night. This repeated suckling is good for the proper establishment of lactation. In addition, the repeated surge of prolactin in the mother's blood stream helps to suppress ovulation. Breast feeding is thus an important biological mechanism for the spacing of children.

Multiple pregnancies

In the case of twins or triplets, feeding should begin with the smallest baby, one breast being offered first, followed by the other. The same process is repeated with the other baby, beginning with the second breast, and so on. The demands of growth in these babies will soon outstrip the mother's capacity to secrete more milk. In such cases the breast milk will need to be supplemented by fresh cow's milk. In each case, cleanliness and hygiene are important and all feeds should be given with a cup and spoon and not a bottle.

Acutely ill mother

Whenever the mother has to be admitted to hospital on account of an acute illness, the baby should be taken in as well and nursed in a side room as a 'lodger'. The mother may continue to feed the baby as usual, or, if she is too ill, the milk may be expressed and given to the baby by a cup and spoon.

Tuberculosis in the mother

In all cases breast feeding should be continued. The likelihood of death from diarrhoea due to unhygienic bottle-feeding and malnutrition is much greater than that of contracting tuberculosis from the mother.

If several examinations of the mother's sputum do not reveal acid-fast bacilli, the baby should be given BCG and breast feeding continued as in any normal case. If the mother is coughing up tubercle bacilli in the sputum, the baby should be given INH syrup, 4–6 mg/kg body weight in 24 hours, and breast feeding continued. The mother will need simple health instruction like turning her head away from the baby whilst coughing and not spitting indiscriminately in the house. When the mother finally becomes sputum-negative, the INH syryp can be stopped and BCG can then be given to the baby.

The transmission of viruses through breast milk

Ever since the AIDS epidemic there has been a great deal of interest in the transmission of viruses in breast milk and some rather alarmist statements have been made by public bodies. In this section the scientific evidence about the presence of viruses in breast milk is being reviewed and practical approaches in the light of the evidence are suggested.

Human Immunodeficiency Virus (HIV)

There have been several case reports of mothers becoming infected after delivery through postpartum blood transfusion and then transmitting HIV infection to their newborns. Even though the number of adequately documented cases is small the studies have established that a potential risk of transmission of infection exists. Infants who are exposed to newly infected mothers are at greater risk because they get exposed to the virus in the absence of maternal antibody against HIV. Moreover, newly infected persons and those with advanced disease have higher titres of circulating virus or a higher proportion of lymphocytes infected, and are more infective.

After the first case report the Centers for Disease Control in the USA recommended in 1985 that HIV-infected women should be advised against breast feeding. This was the period of alarmism when a number of policy statements were being issued by national institutions in several developed countries. Within the USA this recommendation has had very little impact for the simple reason that only a small proportion of women known to be infected with HIV breast fed even before the statement. Moreover, the current medical practice in the USA is not oriented towards routinely detecting HIV infected women in pregnancy or in the postpartum period.

In 1987 the World Health Organisation recommended that "breast feeding should continue to be promoted, supported and protected in both developing and developed countries. In individual situations where the mother is considered to be HIV infected the known and potential benefits of breast feeding should be compared to the theoretical but apparently small risk to the infant of becoming infected through breast feeding. Consideration should be given to the socio-economic and ecological environment of the mother-child pair and the extent to which alternatives can safely and effectively be used." It is obvious that on the basis of available information breast feeding should remain the feeding method of choice for the mother infected with HIV.

Human T cell Leukaemia Virus (HTLV-I)

This virus is endemic in parts of Japan and the West Indies. It can be transmitted by blood and sexual contact, but transmission from mother to child accounts for many of the infections. An estimated 25 per cent of the children of seropositive mothers are infected. In some studies up to 10 per cent of the T cells in breast milk of carrier mothers had HTLV-I antigen. Since over 10 per cent of the cells in breast milk are T cells this would amount to about 1000 infected cells/ml of milk.

A number of prospective studies suggest breast feeding as a major mode of transmission. With the available data it would be reasonable to follow the same guidelines as for HIV, namely recommending breast feeding in developing countries where the advantages outweigh the risks, and discouraging the known HTLV-I infected mother from breast feeding in developed countries. HTLV-I appears to be more readily transmitted through breast milk than HIV but its effects on the infant are less pronounced. Only 5 per cent of carriers become affected after a latent period of several decades.

Cytomegalovirus (CMV)

In common with other members of the herpes virus family and the retroviruses CMV persists in host cells indefinitely. In different studies CMV has been isolated from breast milk in 14 to 44 per cent of seropositive mothers. The presence of a specific antibody in the milk does not prevent transmission. What is more important is the fact that neither symptomatic infection nor late sequelae have been documented in the infants.

Rubella

Both the wild and the vaccine strains have been isolated from breast milk. In women immunised soon after delivery 69 per cent pass the virus in milk. Either the virus or virus antigen is detectable in more than half of their infants and about a quarter may show a transient antibody to the rubella virus. No symptoms or adverse effects are recorded in infants.

Hepatitis B virus

Most vertical transmission of hepatitis B occurs at birth as a result of exposure to maternal blood and secretions during labour. In endemic areas like Taiwan most studies do not show any difference in infection rates between breast fed and bottle fed infants. With the advent of an effective and safe vaccine the theoretical risk of transmission of hepatitis B is of not much concern.

Failure of lactation

In many rural societies, social anthropologists have reported that if a mother were to die in childbirth, the baby would be taken over by the grandmother or a female relative and put to the breast. In many instances they were able to record successful establishment of lactation. Even though the use of galactagogues and local applications of herbs have been mentioned, the most likely factor in the stimulation of lactation is regular suckling by the infant.

On the basis of these observations, health workers have attempted to stimulate lactation in mothers where the milk has 'dried up', or in foster-mothers, with varying degrees of success. It is obviously easier to re-establish lactation in the mother when it has 'dried up' than in another female who is not lactating. Similarly, the time interval since the last period of lactation is also important. The following routine has been found useful

(1) Admission of the mother and baby to hospital for regular supervision.

(2) Reassurance of the mother and building up her confidence in her own ability to secrete breast milk.

(3) Attention to the mother's nutrition by providing a diet containing a high level of protein and calories.

(4) Putting the baby to the breast regularly for 5–10 minutes on each side, every three to four hours, followed by a 'top feed' of 120–150 ml milk with a cup and spoon. The quantity of milk given as 'top feed' is progressively reduced by 10–15 ml every week.

(5) Oral metoclopramide to the mother in a dosage of 10 mg twice daily, or chlorpromazine 25 mg b.d. to induce prolactin secretion by relaxing hypothalmic inhibition.

Weaning

As the baby grows older, the demands for nutrients increase and breast milk by itself is not sufficient to meet them. The growth rate which was comparable to that of infants in Western countries until the age of four months now begins to lag behind.

Usually about this age many mothers begin the introduction of other foods. Commonly, it is in the form of a 'porridge' made from the staple whilst breast feeding is progressively reduced.

The process of getting a baby used to the 'porridge' and other semi-solids is known as weaning and in any society it is an integral part of the child-rearing practices. Faulty weaning is an important cause of childhood malnutrition, and in many instances faulty weaning is conditioned by the agricultural practices, the traditional dietary patterns, and the folklore, prevalent customs and beliefs of the people. Any attempt at improving the weaning practices with health and nutrition education should take these factors into account.

The thin, watery 'porridge' has very little nutritive value. Moreover, since it is made from water which is usually contaminated, it is likely to give rise to episodes of diarrhoea. Several studies on bacterial counts in such gruels have shown that whereas the counts are tolerable when the gruel has just come off the stove, on keeping the bacteria multiply, and high counts are found in most samples. Hence it is necessary to emphasise that the gruel should be freshly prepared each time and its nutritive value needs to be improved by enrichment with fresh cow's milk, pounded groundnuts, egg yolk, edible oil and so on. During this time of weaning it is most important to see that the baby's nutrition is well maintained with breast milk and also for as long as possible afterwards. Studies in rural Uganda have shown that in the second year of life those children who had been taken off the breast received 60 per cent fewer calories compared to those who were still being breast fed. This deficit

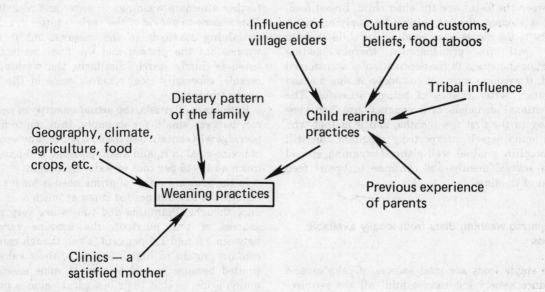

Figure 5.4 Factors influencing weaning practices

Table 5.1 Nutritive value of main staples

Foods	Water %	Calories per 100 g	Protein %	Fat %	Carbohydrate %
Rice, milled white	13	360	6.7	0.7	78.9
Wheat, low extraction	12	370	10.9	1.1	75.5
Maize, 90–96% extraction	12	360	9.3	4.0	73.5
Cassava flour	14	338	1.5	0.6	81.5

Table 5.2 Percentage loss through washing

	Thiamine	Riboflavine	Nicotinic acid
Husked rice	21%	8%	13%
Milled rice	40%	26%	23%
Parboiled rice	15%	15%	13%
Home pounded rice	7%	12%	10%

Table 5.3 Effect of boiling potato and rice

	Percent water		Protein/100 g of cooked product	
	Raw	Boiled	Raw	Boiled
Potato	76	81	2.1	1.4
Rice	12	70.88	6.8	1.0–2.3

was in spite of consumption of twice the quantity of solids in the case of the former. Thus, breast milk is an important source of energy in the second year of life. Commencement of weaning or the successful accomplishment is no criterion for stopping breast feeding. This should ideally continue until the age of eighteen months to two years.

With many rural mothers, weaning is usually abrupt and is generally precipitated by a new pregnancy. The mother fears that the 'heat' from the uterus may affect her milk and cause disease in the child on the breast, or that 'jealousies' may occur between the foetus and the older child. Breast feeding is stopped abruptly either by applying bitter herbs to the nipple or by sending the child away to live with the grandparents, thereby adding emotional distress to the deprivation of accustomed food. If weaning were not so sudden it would stand a much better chance of being successful. The nutritional demands of pregnancy are not very heavy in the first few months, and a mother who has found herself unexpectedly pregnant can still accomplish gradual well-planned weaning spread over several months and continue to breast feed most of the time.

Preparing weaning diets from locally available foods

The staple foods are good sources of calories and produce satiety but cannot fulfil all the requirements for proteins and other nutrients, especially in the growing child (table 5.1). This is especially

so in the case of cassava and plantains. Hence, as soon as the child has got used to the staple, a protein food and a source of energy in the form of edible oil should be added to provide adequate nutrition. Groundnuts and soyabeans are useful in this respect being good sources of both protein and energy.

During the preparation and cooking of food, the nutritive value may be altered by loss of nutrient or by absorption of water, so that the percentage of nutrient per portion eaten may be less than that in the raw food. For example, cassava is processed for eating by soaking in water, pounding, and several further alternate washings in water and pounding. This is done to get rid of the various bitter cyanide-containing alkaloids in the cassava, but it also washes out the protein and the final product as eaten is chiefly starch. Similarly, the washing of cereals, especially rice, removes some of the vitamins (table 5.2).

In the case of gruels, the actual quantity of cereal can be very small, for example, thin maize-meal porridge will contain less than 20 per cent by weight of maize-meal in it, and a stiff porridge will have as much as 40–45 per cent of water by weight.

In the growing infant a prime need is for *protein* though the amount needed is not as much as it was once thought. Plantains and tubers are very poor sources of this nutrient, the amount varying between 1.0 and 1.5 per cent. Even though cereals contain protein in higher amounts, their value is limited because of a deficiency of some essential amino acids, so that their biological value is much less than that of protein from animal sources. To offset this deficiency the missing amino acids may be provided from an animal source, for example, cow's or breast milk or egg, or by using another vegetable food in which the amino acids lacking in cereals are present in large quantities (table 5.4). In other words, by using food mixtures, the diet of the weanling can be made more balanced. Thus, adding boiled and mashed legumes or groundnuts to the child's porridge increases its food value.

For mixing purposes, foods can be divided into four main groups: (1) *staple*, which may vary from one geographical area to another; (2) *animal protein*, usually expensive and in rural areas of the tropics very scarce – also subject to taboos and religious prohibitions of various kinds; (3) *vegetable protein*, cultivated and stored easily but likely to need prolonged cooking, and (4) *dark green vegetables* (DGV). Foodstuffs from any of these main groups can be taken to provide a mixed diet, the biological value of which will depend upon its components and how varied the mixture is (table 5.5).

Table 5.4 Protein value of commonly available tropical foods

		Protein (g)	Fat (g)	Carbohydrate (g)	Calories
Group I	Staple				
	Cassava, fresh	0.7	trace	32.0	131
	Maize, whole	10.0	4.5	67.0	349
	Plantains	1.0	0.3	24.0	103
	Rice, white	7.0	1.0	78.0	349
	Sorghum	10.4	3.4	70.9	356
	Wheat, whole	11.5	2.4	62.0	316
	Potato, sweet	2.0	1.0	26.0	121
Group II	Animal protein				
	Fresh cow's milk	3.1	3.5	4.6	62
	Breast milk	1.0	4.5	7.1	75
	Fish, fresh	17.0	3.0	trace	95
	Egg, whole	13.0	11.0	0.9	153
Group III	Vegetable protein				
	Bambara nut	18.0	6.0	55.0	346
	Chick pea	22.0	5.0	55.0	353
	Cow pea	24.0	1.0	44.0	281
	Groundnut	23.0	47.0	10.0	555
	Lentil	24.0	1.0	50.0	305
	Peas	22.0	1.0	53.0	309
	Soyabean	35.0	18.0	20.0	382
	Sunflower seed	27.0	45.0	14.0	569

Amount in 100 grammes

Table 5.5 Food mixtures

	Biological value	Expense
Quadri-mix		
Staple – animal protein – vegetable protein – DGV	++++	++++
Triple mix		
Staple – animal protein – vegetable protein	+++	+++
Staple – animal protein – DGV	+++	+++
Staple – vegetable protein – DGV	+++	++
Double mix		
Staple – animal protein	+++	+++
Staple – vegetable protein	+++	++
Staple – DGV	++	+

Table 5.6   The nutrient content of common tropical foods

Food	Protein g/100 g	Calories /100 g	Limiting SAA* mg/g protein	Amino acids lysine, mg/g protein
Egg	13	158	54	59
Chicken	19	139	35	86
Fish (fresh, lean)	17	73	39	86
Fish, (dried, white)	29	125	39	86
Dried skimmed milk	36	357	37	80
Dried whole milk	25.5	500	37	80
Soyabeans	35	382	30	64
Average legume (e.g. cowpea)	22	340	20	72
Groundnuts (dry)	27	579	20	35
Wheat flour (70% extraction)	10	350	31	21
Rice (polished)	7	352	32	25
Maize (96% extraction)	9.5	362	25	19
Millet (*Pennisetum*)	9	365	28	21
Sorghum (Guinea corn)	10	353	27	19
Oats	12	388	32	27
Potatoes (Irish)	2	75	26	48
Sweet potatoes	1.5	114	26	48
Taroes	2	113	26	48
Yams (fresh)	2	104	26	48
Plantains	1	128	16	48
Bananas	1	116	16	48
Cassava flour	1.5	342	16	48
Reference protein	–	–	35	55

* Total sulphur-containing amino acids (cystine + methionine)

Table 5.7   The score of common vegetable proteins*

Food	Score	Limiting amino acid	
		Amino acid	Quantity mg/g
FAO provisional protein	100		
Groundnut	55	S-containing	150
Pigeon pea	38	Tryptophan	30
Chick pea	57	Tryptophan	50
Soyabean	72	S-containing	200
Mung bean	66	S-containing	140
Kidney bean	46	S-containing	120
Peas	58	S-containing	160
Broad bean	26	S-containing	70
Cow pea	66	S-containing	230

* 1 g of Reference protein has 35 mg SAA and 55 mg lysine

In any mix, the protein value will depend upon its content of essential amino acids. If one of the essential amino acids is completely lacking, the protein value of the diet will be zero. Thus, the value of the dietary protein is determined by that amino acid which is present in the least amount and is called 'the limiting amino acid'. In general, the limiting amino acid for cereal foods is lysine and those for legume proteins are the sulphur-containing amino acids methionine and cystine. When the amount of the limiting amino acid in 1 gm of a food is compared with the quantity of the same amino acid in 1 gm of an 'ideal' protein and expressed as a percentage, the *protein score* is obtained.

Table 5.6 gives the nutrient content of the commonly used tropical foods, and in table 5.7 the protein scores of some of the common vegetable sources of protein have been calculated.

In addition to the amino acid pattern and the protein score of the diet, the calorie content is also important. When calories are deficient, proteins are burnt as a source of energy instead of being used for body-building and growth. These two principles, namely, the protein score of the food and its calorie content, are brought together in one formula to give the *Net dietary protein calorie per cent* (NdpCal per cent) which then provides the protein value of a food mixture. In the calculation of NdpCal per cent, the calories derived from the protein in the food expressed as per cent of total calories are plotted against the protein score on a nomogram to obtain the value of NdpCal per cent (figure 5.6).

Breast milk has a NdpCal per cent of 8.3. It is estimated that a diet which supplies less than 8.0 per cent calories in utilisable protein is incapable of meeting the needs of a young child. As children become older, this figure can be lowered to 7 per cent, and in adulthood to 5 per cent, but for pregnant and lactating women a NdpCal per cent of 7 is needed.

For example, to calculate the NdpCal per cent in a double mix containing 100 g rice and 10 g legume:

	Protein	Calories	Sulphur-containing amino acids	Lysine
100 g rice =	7 g	352	224 mg	175 mg
10 g legume =	2.2 g	34	44 mg	158 mg
Total	9 g	386	268 mg	333 mg

Protein score* $= \dfrac{268}{9 \times 35} \times 100 = 85$

Calories derived from protein $= 9 \times 4 = 36 = 9\%$

From the normogram NdpCal per cent $= 7$

Based on 1 g of Reference protein = 35 mg SAA

The principle of calculating NdpCal per cent of food mixtures is useful in advising parents on weaning diets for children. It emphasises that mere mixing of foods is not enough. They should be mixed in the right proportion of utilisable protein and energy.

Practical problems with multi-mixes

A number of problems arise in preparing weaning diets based on multi-mixes. Food composition tables give the nutrient values of raw foods only. During processing and cooking changes occur in consistency and volume. Hence it is important to derive the raw weight equivalent of cooked foods in order to calculate the nutrient content. Secondly, cereals and legumes when cooked in water absorb it and increase in volume. Different cereals absorb different amounts of water. Rice and wheat increase between two and three times in volume and maize flour about six times. Legumes increase to three times the volume when cooked. This increase in bulk must be taken into account when feeding the small child whose stomach capacity is 200–300 mls. If the child is eating only two or three small meals a day the food must provide sufficient energy and nutrient density, especially during illness. The addition of 10g of edible fat or fat containing foods (for example mashed groundnuts, coconut, soya beans etc.) helps to overcome the problem of bulkiness. Fats and oils also improve the palatability and consistency of the food.

The concept of the Food Square (figure 5.5) has been proposed as a basis for teaching parents and health workers about weaning foods. Breast milk is an excellent source of energy and high quality protein. In many traditional societies breast feeding continues well into the second year of life. Hence breast feeding is the cornerstone of a sound strategy for weaning, and occupies the central position in the Food Square. As a rule of thumb, the staple cereal, a legume and oil in the proportion of 10:1:1 with a handful (30–40g) of green vegetables or seasonal fruit whilst continuing breast feeding will make a well-balanced weaning food for the second year of life.

Table 5.8 Double mix from common staples

			The value of each mix is 7–8 NdpCal% To 100 g of staple food, add weight of the supplementary food				
Supplements (g)	Wheat	Rice	Sorghum	Millet	Maize	Plantain	Cassava flour
Egg	25	25	25	25	30	20	55
Dried skimmed milk powder	5	15	10	10	15	15	30
Dried whole milk powder	10	25	15	20	30	25	55
Fresh fish	10	20	15	20	25	20	45
Chicken or lean meat	10	25	15	20	25	20	50
Soyabean	10	20	15	20	25	20	45
Legumes in general	10	25	25	25	25	25	Not possible

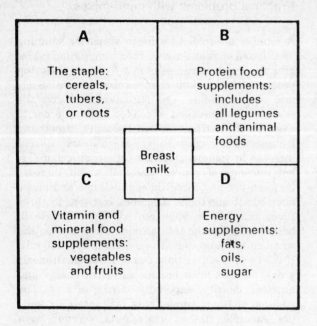

Figure 5.5 The food square

The problem of bulk is more serious at the younger age of four to six months, when a cereal gruel is first introduced. The development of the structures of the mouth at this age is such that the infant is incapable of chewing. Hence all foods offered must be of liquid consistency to avoid choking. On the other hand the natural property of starch, which is the main nutrient in all cereals, is such that on cooking in water the granules absorb water, swell and coalesce to form a viscous product. Thus all gruels of liquid consistency can have no more than 5 per cent of the cereal before they are too viscous for the infant to handle. The energy density of such a gruel is 1 cal/g as compared to 6 cal/g solid matter of breast milk. Any attempt to increase the energy content by adding more flour will make it too viscous. The addition of fats and fat containing foods is one way of increasing the energy content but is expensive. An innovative solution has been to alter the starch by malting the grain prior to milling. The process of malting consists of soaking the grain in water overnight (12 hours), allowing the grain to germinate (48 hours) drying the germinated grain (6–8 hours) and subsequently milling. Gruels cooked from flours of malted grain are less viscous and remain liquid at concentrations of up to 15 per cent. This is because amylase is released during malting and it digests the starch to dextrin and dextrimaltose. Further work with malting has shown that flour milled from malted grain retains the amylase activity, and can be used to sprinkle on gruels and slurries made from ordinary flour to make them less viscous. Stocks of amylase rich flour can be prepared at intervals and used on thick gruels for thinning, thereby increasing their energy and nutrient density for feeding young infants.

Fermentation

In many communities the traditional way of cooking requires the dough to be made and 'rested' for some time before cooking. During the period of resting fermentation takes place. It is believed that the products of fermentation have antibiotic properties. In communities where such fermentation is a common practice the incidence of diarrhoea is reportedly less.

Nutritional deficiency syndromes

Nutritional disorders are common in infants and young children in developing countries and constitute a major problem of world-wide public health importance. Whenever gross dietary imbalance exists, several deficiencies are likely to be present simultaneously. In a child with a clinically manifest deficiency syndrome of one kind a search should always be made for deficiencies of other nutrients as well. For example, it is not unusual to encounter anaemia and vitamin deficiencies in children suffering from protein – energy malnutrition.

Protein – energy malnutrition (PEM)

This term was originally introduced to stress that in all cases of nutritional growth failure there is a deficiency of both calories and proteins. It is now commonly agreed that proteins can be utilised in the body to provide energy and calories have a protein-sparing effect. Thus, adequate intake of both calories and proteins is necessary to protect against nutritional growth failure. It is also implied that what the child needs is food, even though the clinical signs indicate the predominant deficiency of one nutrient.

In its gross form protein – calorie deficiency presents either as kwashiorkor or marasmus or a mixture of the two, namely, marasmic kwashiorkor.

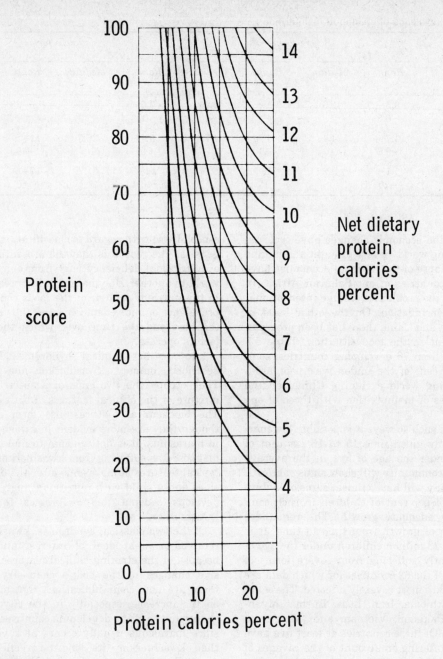

Protein score

Net dietary protein calories percent

Protein calories percent

Figure 5.6 Nomogram

Together these syndromes constitute the most serious health problem of children in the world. At any given time approximately 100 million children suffer from the moderate or severe form of PEM. In any one country the number of children suffering from the disorder will be influenced by the season, the availability of food, political and economic stability, the prevalence of infectious illnesses and so on. The peak of incidence is immediately after epidemics of diarrhoea and infectious illnesses such as measles and whooping cough, or in the so-called hungry months.

Community surveys during the 1970s in 17 different countries and involving 175 000 children revealed an aggregate prevalence rate of 20 per cent for protein-energy malnutrition. Since then marked

Table 5.9 The prevalence of childhood malnutrition

Area	Severe forms				Moderate forms			
	1970s		1980s		1970s		1980s	
	Range (%)	Median	Range (%)	Median	Range (%)	Median	Range (%)	Median
Latin America	0.5––6.3	1.6	1––8	2.25	3.5––32	18.9	6–33	12.8
Africa	1.7––9.8	4.4	1––11	4.7	5.4––45	26.5	11––48	22
Asia	1.1––20	3.2	1––12	6.2	16––46.4	31.2	17––60	42

socio-political and economic changes have occurred in the developing world. Severe drought and famine followed by collapse of the national economies have affected most countries of sub-Saharan Africa. In South America the problem is of huge international debts and hyper inflation. On the other hand in South-east Asia and China there has been progressive improvement in the food situation. Table 5.9 compares data from 76 developing countries, comprising 83 per cent of the under-fives' population of the developing world excluding China, on the prevalence rates of malnutrition with those of one decade ago.

As a result of such surveys it is possible to generalise that at any given time 15 to 16 per cent of the children under the age of five in the average disadvantaged community will show signs of growth failure, and many will have clinical signs of malnutrition. Only 24 per cent of children in such communities show adequate growth. The remainder suffer faltering of growth from time to time. It is estimated that 23 million children under the age of five are currently suffering from severe forms of malnutrition. Of the 62 countries for which data are available nine are most severely affected. These are Bangladesh, Ethiopia, Iran, Laos, Burma (Myanmar), Nepal, Pakistan, Vietnam and the Yemen Arab Republic. Of these countries at least five have seen marked suffering on account of the ravages of war. As the child population increases in the coming decade it is estimated that at the current level of prevalence there will be 178 million severely malnourished children in the world by the end of the century.

Classification and definition

A great deal of controversy surrounds almost every aspect of protein – energy malnutrition. This is especially so with regard to classification and pathogenesis. The reason is that the presenting features of nutritional deficiency vary from one part of the world to another, due mainly to the great variation in the nutrient content of the foods consumed, the prevalence of antecedent illnesses, the variability of the host and the time over which the causative factors operate.

Two distinct clinical syndromes have been described, namely, kwashiorkor and marasmus. They occupy the two ends of a spectrum, with a mixture of the clinical features of both in between. The biochemical features also form a spectrum though they are more evident in kwashiorkor than in marasmus. It is not unusual to find that a child diagnosed as suffering from kwashiorkor shows the typical features of marasmus after the oedema subsides and a child with nutritional marasmus often develops oedema and progresses to marasmic kwashiorkor.

Of the two classical syndromes, kwashiorkor has received a great deal of interest and attention because of the striking clinical features and extensive changes in the body's chemistry. However, there are now clear indications that marasmus is on the increase, especially in the city slums and shanty towns of the developing countries. Moreover, since marasmus usually occurs at a younger age than kwashiorkor, its long term effects on the developing body organs, especially the brain, are more severe.

The clinical picture

The clinical picture seen in practice is usually a mixture of kwasiorkor and marasmus.

In *marasmus*, the appearance is one of gross wasting. Thee is a loss of subcutaneous fat with thin, emaciated extremities. The skin hangs loosely over

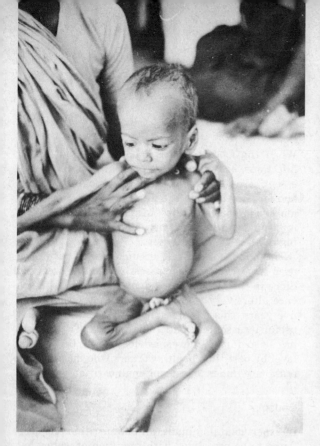

Figure 5.7 Marasmus

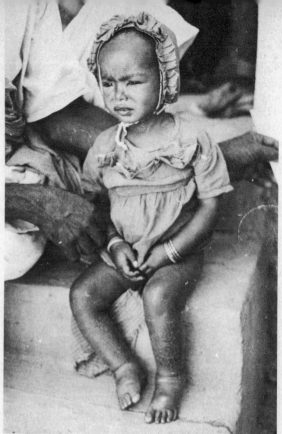

Figure 5.8 Kwashiorkor

the body, especially in the gluteal region. The child has an alert, staring look, the prominent eyes following the movements of the examiner. The appearance has often been described as the 'wizened old man' look. Even though obviously hungry and often seen sucking at his fingers, the marasmic child does not tolerate large feeds which can cause vomiting or episodes of diarrhoea.

Studies of body composition in marasmus show a marked increase in total body water; up to 89 per cent body weight compared to the normal range of 75 per cent at birth and 60 per cent at age four months. The high percentage of total body water indicates large deficits of body fat. The proportion of extra cellular fluid is also high due to losses of visceral and muscle protein. Total body sodium is also increased although less so than total body water producing hyponatraemia. By comparison the deficit of potassium other than that associated with decrease in cell mass is not excessive.

Endocrine-metabolic adaptation is the main physiologic response in marasmus. The BMR and oxygen consumption fall due in part to a decrease in the active forms of thyroid hormone at the cellular level. Rates of cellular division and protein synthesis also decrease. The levels of growth hormone are elevated. Insulin responses are blunted. These changes together with those of gluco-corticoids and catecholamines create a milieu in which glucose utilisation by tissue is minimised while levels of alternative sources of energy like ketones and fatty acids are increased. During rehabilitation these adaptive changes revert to normal only after a sustained period of nutrition intake. This explains why recovery from marasmus is a slow and prolonged process.

Kwashiorkor has been classically equated with protein deficiency, which is overly simplistic. The antecedent diet of the child with kwashiorkor is no different from that of the child with marasmus. Infection is often the critical variable, especially measles. The total body water as a percentage of body weight may be normal or increased. Sodium retention is common, and there are excessive losses of potassium.

In kwashiorkor, misery and apathy are notable features. The child is unhappy, not interested in his surroundings and continually crying. He has no appetite, does not engage in play or show interest in toys. These mental symptoms do not clear until the child is well on his way to recovery. In fact interest in the surroundings and the first smile are important milestones in his recovery.

Oedema is another important feature of kwashiorkor. It may be mainly localised to the lower extremities, or generalised. In spite of the retention of water, the weight of the child may be well below the standard for his age. The coppery discolouration of the skin stretched over the oedematous subcutaneous tissue, the characteristic dermatoses and the sparse hair with its greyish-red tint give the child a characteristic appearance, so that in many local dialects he has been described as the 'red' child. The muscles and subcutaneous fat are not wasted to the same extent as in marasmus. In addition, oedema may make the extremities look rounded and the face full – hence the term 'sugar baby'.

Infection is an added hazard, especially to the respiratory tract, the gastro-intestinal system and the skin. The vitality of the tissues is greatly reduced and any sepsis tends to spread rapidly. Many children with kwashiorkor show deep ulcers on the skin or in the mucosa of the mouth, the latter sometimes leading to cancrum oris.

The child may show signs of deficiency of other nutrients in the form of anaemia, xerophthalmia or angular stomatitis.

The major clinical signs of protein – energy malnutrition are described below and summarised in table 5.10.

Table 5.10 Major clinical signs of malnutrition

Marasmus		*Kwashiorkor*
+++	Growth failure	++
+++	Muscle wasting	+
±	Oedema	+++
±	Hair changes	+++
±	Skin changes	+++
±	Mental and psychological upset	+++
++	Anaemia	+++
+	Hepatomegaly	+++
++	Loose stools	+++

Growth failure

This is the most important and characteristic sign of defective nutrition, both the height and weight being well below the lower limits of normal. Weight and height charts are invaluable diagnostic aids for this purpose. If previous growth data are available, in most instances it will be possible to show that growth has slowed down for a considerable time before admission to hospital, and in most instances

it will be possible to relate the clinical onset of malnutrition to events or illnesses in the immediate past.

Muscle wasting

When the food supply is inadequate, and during infections, body tissues are broken down to provide essential nutrients for vital physiologic functions and for homeostasis. The wasting of muscle is more marked where the diet has been quantitatively inadequate, as in marasmus, but also occurs in varying degrees in kwashiorkor.

The mid-arm and calf circumferences have been used as parameters for assessing muscle wasting. Since in the healthy individual mid-arm circumference alters very little between the ages of one and five years, this measurement has been found most useful in assessing nutritional status. The concept has been further developed for use at the village level by part-time health workers who may be illiterate (see under Measuring malnutrition page 68).

Oedema

In experimental animals, all malnutrition has been found to be associated with retention of water, but clinical oedema as such is usually found only in protein-deficiency syndromes.

Oedema implies retention of sodium and though various explanations have been put forth, the etiology is still obscure. The various factors contributing to oedema in malnutrition are low serum albumin, anaemia and poor cardiac function. The role of other factors, such as anti-diuretic hormone, altered renal function, etc., is still not adequately defined.

Skin and hair changes

Skin lesions, though not invariably present, are characteristic when they occur and often diagnostic in the borderline case, so that they have often been useful in conducting nutritional surveys. The dermatoses usually begin as large areas of erythema and have led to the use of such terms as the 'red baby syndrome'. The red areas then become progressively dry, hyperkeratotic and hyperpigmented. Some desquamation also occurs and the picture has been variously described as 'crazy paving' or 'enamel paint'. Petechiae and areas of small echymoses may also occur and are usually a bad prognostic sign. Unlike the dermatoses of pellagra, which are limited to areas of the body usually exposed to sunlight, the skin lesions of malnutrition usually begin at pressure points and then spread. The skin may also become hypopigmented and light in colour, usually on the face, thus providing the typical appearance of a red baby on a background of fairer skin.

The epithelium peels off easily, leaving behind raw areas which readily become infected, causing indolent ulcers. Infection can spread rapidly through tissues wet with oedema fluid and devitalised because of chronic undernutrition. This is especially seen in the oral cavity where necrotic ulcers affecting the palate or the cheek are common, giving rise to cancrum oris.

The appendages of the skin, chiefly the hair on the scalp, also participate in the pathological process of undernutrition. The hair becomes dry and lustreless and is easily pluckable; curly hair may become straight and the colour may change from black to brown or red and even white.

Anaemia

Anaemia is a common accompaniment of clinical malnutrition. The generalised nutritional deprivation that affects the several physiologic systems of the body also affects haemopoiesis and the anaemia is due to a malfunctioning marrow rather than deficiency of a specific nutrient.

Malaria, hookworm and other helminthic infestations, as well as bacterial infections, also contribute to the anaemia and may require attention. Iron deficiency is widespread in pre-school children. Protein – calorie deficiency occurring in such children may make the anaemia worse by interfering further with marrow function. In some geographical areas, the anaemia of kwashiorkor has been found to be due to folic acid deficiency; the megaloblastic bone marrow responds well to treatment with folic acid and a well-balanced diet. In all cases, haematinics alone are of little use until such time as the underlying protein and calorie deficiency has been corrected.

Hepatomegaly

A fatty enlarged liver is common in most cases of kwashiorkor. Rarely, ascites may also occur; whether it is due to a derangement of liver function or part of the generalised oedema is not known. The liver enlargement may increase with increase in ascites initially on commencing treatment.

Serial liver biopsy studies have shown swollen liver cells containing fat, often resulting in rupture of the cell wall between adjoining cells. During treatment, the liver cells lose their fat content and assume a normal appearance. Increased amounts of fibrosis may be seen but there is no evidence to

show that kwashiorkor in early childhood leads to cirrhosis of the liver in later years.

Diarrhoea

Diarrhoea is one of the most troublesome complications of malnutrition. In many instances it acts as one of the immediate precipitating factors in the aetiology of clinical malnutrition. On the other hand, children with malnutrition are more susceptible to diarrhoea. Thus, often a vicious circle is established in which diarrhoea and malnutrition potentiate and aggravate each other.

The various causative factors of diarrhoea have been studied in detail in cases of kwashiorkor admitted to hospital. The earlier studies were on the secretion of digestive enzymes by duodenal intubation. It was found that in kwashiorkor the production of pancreatic and intestinal enzymes is markedly diminished. The enzymatic activity in duodenal fluids was one-tenth in the case of amylase, one-fourth in the case of lipase, and one-twelfth in the case of trypsin, as compared to the activity obtained in the same children on recovery. These studies clearly indicate that digestion of food may be inadequate in malnutrition. Later studies on jejunal biopsy in kwashiorkor have shown a mucosal pattern consisting of flat denuded villi – a picture not unlike the one seen in coeliac disease and other malabsorption syndromes. Serial biopsies in children responding to treatment have shown that the jejunal mucosa recovers and becomes normal as clinical improvement occurs. Thus, malabsorption may be superadded to poor digestion.

During treatment with milk-based diets, some children develop profuse diarrhoea. Studies on these children have shown a deficiency of lactase and other sugar-splitting enzymes. The sugars in the gut lumen are not digested but undergo fermentation by the gut bacteria and cause a profuse diarrhoea.

Associated deficiencies and problems

In most rural areas parents have to make a long trek on foot or by slow local transport to reach a source of medical care. There may be further delays because of waiting in long queues at the hospital or clinic. A considerable time may elapse before the child is seen by a doctor. Because of poor body reserves, the child with malnutrition cannot go without food for long periods and becomes hypoglycaemic. It is important to consider all children with an advanced degree of malnutrition as medical emergencies requiring immediate dietary therapy.

Infections like bronchopneumonia and tuberculosis are commonly associated with malnutrition. Skin sepsis, oral thrush and other similar forms of localised infection are also common. Diagnosis is made difficult by the absence of normal physiologic response to infection. There may be no fever or leucocytosis. Heaf and Mantoux tests are negative even in the presence of active tuberculosis. Often the only signs of septicaemia are hypothermia and low blood sugar. A careful clinical examination including a chest X-ray and careful observation are necessary to detect infection. In endemic areas the presence of malaria parasites and intestinal worms must also be routinely looked for and treated.

In an overcrowded children's ward, cross-infection can easily occur, especially with measles and other droplet infections as well as infection of the gastrointestinal tract. It is a common experience to see a child make a slow and difficult recovery from malnutrition only to succumb to measles or diarrhoea.

It is a general rule that nutritional deficiency is very rarely confined to just one or two nutrients. In most instances, the deficiency is generalised so that protein – energy malnutrition is usually associated with signs of vitamin and other deficiencies. Many of the illnesses which precipitate malnutrition also provoke loss of nutrients from the body. Hence deficiencies of iron, folic acid, vitamins A and D, and of the members of the B-complex group, are usually associated and need treatment. Moreover, with dietary therapy the metabolic activity of the body accelerates and a borderline deficiency may become overt. Provision of adequate amounts of vitamins is essential in the management of all cases.

Treatment

The objectives of treatment are

(1) To restore tissue regeneration and to supply nutrients in an easily digestible form.
(2) To replace additional body constituents lost in the course of the illness, for example, fluids, electrolytes, vitamins and minerals.
(3) To diagnose and treat infections so frequently associated with malnutrition.
(4) To treat other associated conditions such as parasitic infections, anaemia and others which affect the general health of the patient.

Restoration of tissue regeneration

This is best considered in two stages

(1) Recovery from the acute phase and initiation of cure.
(2) Catch-up growth with nutrition rehabilitation.

Recovery from the acute phase

The severely malnourished child is very ill. All the metabolic processes have slowed down, and additionally there is catabolism because of infection. The principles to follow are

(1) Provide maintenance intakes of protein and energy to achieve homeostasis taking care not to overload the physiological capacity of the patient. The aim is to regenerate the metabolic machinery which can then utilise the nutrients offered for tissue growth.
(2) Halt the catabolic processes by control of infection and small bowel overgrowth.
(3) Replenish specific nutrients.

Maintenance intake of protein and energy

In the early delicate stage nutrients must be offered relatively slowly and in a balanced way so that the disordered metabolism can be corrected. It does not help to present excessive loads to a fatty liver to metabolise, nor to a myocardium with degenerative changes for circulation, and so on for all body systems. Since the severity may vary from one individual to another careful clinical monitoring is necessary. Two hourly feeds of fresh cow's milk to provide 100 kcal and 1 g protein/kg body weight per day is a good starting point.

Control of infection

Because of lowered body resistance infection is common even though the usual clinical signs of pyrexia, leucocytosis etc. may be absent. Sudden changes in consciousness or hypothermia are indications of underlying sepsis. A broad spectrum antibiotic or a combination of penicillin and gentamicin are effective in most cases.

A search should be made to exclude tuberculosis, malaria and intestinal helminths in all cases. Mebendazole (100 mg as a single dose) is effective for helminths and metronidazole (7.5 mg/kg thrice daily) for amoebiasis and giardiasis.

Chronic diarrhoea with offensive watery stools is more likely due to bacterial overgrowth of the small bowel than lactose intolerance as previously thought. Metronidazole is effective and should be continued until the child has recovered from the acute stage.

Replenishment of specific nutrients

Some tissue constituents are more depleted than others. As tissue synthesis commences with feeding and control of infection the deficiency of micronutrients becomes a limiting factor for rapid recovery. Potassium and magnesium are almost always deficient which accounts for a wide range of metabolic disturbances. Potassium chloride 2–4 mmol/kg per day and magnesium chloride 0.5–1 mmol/kg per day should be given orally once urine flow is established. Usually potassium deficiency is only fully corrected after magnesium has been replenished. Zinc deficiency should be suspected if there is chronic diarrhoea. Full recovery is delayed until zinc deficiency has been made good. Moreover, zinc has a role to play in all cell mediated immune responses. Zinc acetate (2mg/kg per day) should be given in the acute state to all children with diarrhoea. Copper deficiency is common in all diets based on cow's milk, and copper (0.2mg/kg per day) may be given as acetate or chloride.

Even though iron deficiency is common it is advisable to give iron only after recovery from the acute state. Intramuscular iron should be avoided, and if the anaemia is severe it should be treated with a small (10ml/kg) transfusion of fresh blood. There is often a dramatic improvement after a transfusion.

Vitamin deficiency is very common, especially of the B group and of vitamin A in endemic areas. A multi-vitamin mixture should be given to all the children with malnutrition.

On the above regimen most children show improvement within a week with return of appetite, loss of oedema and return of alertness. These changes mark the initiation of cure and a gradual transition can now be made to high energy feeding.

Any of the 'milk' formulae shown in table 5.11 may be used to initiate cure.

Stage of catch-up

The change to high energy feeding should be made only after metabolic recovery, and even then gradually. If high energy intake is introduced abruptly there is a likelihood of profuse diarrhoea or congestive cardiac failure. An increase in pulse and respiration rates should be taken as warning of impending danger.

In the catch-up phase the aim is to achieve maximum recovery and weight gain, so that the child can recover the lost ground and growth can resume. The energy density of the feeds is increased by adding oil, and the volume of the feed is increased progressively to provide 250–300 kcal/kg per day (1000–1300 kjoules/kg per day). Supplements of minerals and vitamins must continue to provide all the constituents for the building of tissue. Easily digestible solid food is offered in between energy rich milk feeds. Minerals and other micronutrients are best obtained through resumption of a good

Table 5.11 Milk based formulae to initiate cure

	Calories	Protein (g)
Fresh cow's milk		
Milk (100ml)	64	3.3
Water (100ml)		
Oil 15g	135	–
200ml	100	1.6
Powdered whole milk		
Milk powder (60g)	255	15
Sugar (30g)	120	–
Oil (75g)	675	–
Water 1000ml	1050	15
Skimmed milk		
Skimmed milk powder (50g)	175	18
Sugar (30g)	120	
Oil (80g)	720	–
Water 1000ml	1015	18

Dosage for all 100ml/kg per day.

To the above add daily:
   Abidec 0.3ml (5drops) daily;
   Becosym 1 tablet daily;
   Folic acid 5 mg daily.
Once urine flow is adequately established add mineral mixture (30ml for every 1 litre of the milk diet) made up as follows:
   Potassium chloride 60g
   Magnesium chloride 60g
   Zinc acetate 600mg
   Copper acetate 60mg
      in 1 litre of water.

varied diet. In small units where it may not be possible to monitor the requirements of micronutrients this is usually the best approach. On this regimen most children respond with weight gain and marked improvement in appetite.

Nutrition rehabilitation

Once the acute phase is over and there is return of appetite it is time to plan for rehabilitation. There is no sense in investing a great deal of time and effort in the recovery of the child only to discharge him to the same home environment where malnutrition first occurred. Hence a careful history of the family background and social circumstances is needed onto which a strategy of nutrition education may be planned. Each family has a specific need. Bland health talks or nutrition demonstrations cannot be expected to be effective.

A busy paediatric ward with the demands for

intensive care of acutely ill children can hardly be conducive to teaching. Many centres prefer to discharge the patient to a convalescent unit during the stage of catch-up once recovery has commenced. Whilst the children are recovering a daily programme of health education, nutrition demonstrations and group work is arranged for their mothers and other family members. The emphasis is on the practical aspects of home economics, effective use of locally available foods and healthy child rearing. Time is also allowed for the mothers to engage in play activities with their children, and to learn about the importance of stimulation for consolidating the process of recovery in mental growth.

Complications

Several complications may arise during the management of the child with malnutrition. Their early recognition is essential so that appropriate steps can be taken before they endanger life.

Hypothermia

This occurs in the early days of admission and is mainly caused by the removal of the child from the warmth of the mother's body. In the hospital, the child sleeps in a separate bed, whereas previously he was in close physical contact with his mother whose body warmth prevented him from developing hypothermia, especially in the cooler hours of the night.

Unexplained and prolonged hypothermia may occur in a severe infection such as septicaemia. The body's responses to infective processes are altered in malnutrition, so that there can occur sudden collapse with hypothermia.

Hypoglycaemia

The child with severe malnutrition is not able to withstand prolonged periods of starvation, and hypoglycaemia has to be looked for in the early days of admission, until such time as regular food intake has been established.

During the first few days blood sugar levels tend to be unstable, and even though symptoms do not appear until blood sugar levels fall below 20mg/100 ml, blood glucose estimations should be done in any child who shows undue apathy, drowsiness or irritability.

Diarrhoea

Bacterial overgrowth in the small intestine or superadded parasitic infection like giardiasis or amoebiasis is the common cause of diarrhoea. It responds well to metronidazole which should be continued until the acute stage is over.

Intolerance to lactose and sucrose as a cause of diarrhoea is not as common as once thought. If present it is self-limiting and may improve spontaneously. In some cases, a change over to the low-lactose formula is necessary, in which case careful attention should be paid to the daily intake of vitamins, minerals and electrolytes. When the diarrhoea subsides, small milk feeds can be offered. If these are tolerated, the quantity is increased in small amounts to replace the low lactose formula.

Electrolyte imbalance

Animal studies have shown that water retention and change in the electrolyte composition of the fluid compartments of the body occur during malnutrition. Diarrhoea and vomiting may cause further complications. With recovery, the electrolytes return to normal, but in severe cases, especially when electrolyte loss has been an added factor, oral rehydration is usually effective.

Congestive cardiac failure

Autopsy studies have shown that the myocardium in kwashiorkor undergoes degenerative changes. During blood transfusion or intravenous fluid therapy, signs of congestive cardiac failure like engorged neck veins, increased respiration or pulse rate, should be looked for carefully. A heavy electrolyte load in the therapeutic diet is known to lead to salt retention, expansion of the extracellular fluid compartment and congestive cardiac failure.

Prognosis

The mortality rates in the various series reported from different parts of the world vary from 18 to 25 per cent. This high mortality is usually due to associated infections, other concomitant nutritional deficiencies and delay in seeking treatment. The presence of several clinical features together is known to indicate a bad prognosis. These are xerophthalmia, a haemorrhagic rash amongst the dermatoses of kwashiorkor, lactose intolerance, associated infections, or electrolyte imbalance causing low serum Na content.

Immediate outcome

The severely malnourished child is acutely ill. A better understanding of his fragile physiology and the sequence of metabolic events leading to it has helped to rationalise the treatment. The immediate outcome is now much improved with mortality figures of 5 to 10 per cent reported in several units compared to previous high figures of 20 to 25 per cent.

With adequate therapy, and if no complications arise, it is possible to get over the acute phase in about one or two weeks, at the end of which time appetite will have returned, the child will be eating solids, oedema will have been lost and the processes of recovery will have begun. As recovery proceeds, there is a period of catch-up growth, but it is likely that the child may not be able to regain totally all the lost ground, so that the eventual stature may be smaller than that of normal children in the community. The eventual reduced adult height in the case of females may give rise to obstetric difficulties in the future, especially in village communities where early marriages are common.

One of the most important after-effects of malnutrition is said to be on the central nervous system. The misery and the apathy of the acute phase of kwashiorkor is a reflection of the involvement of the central nervous system in the generalised nutritional deficiency. Psychomotor tests in children recovering from kwashiorkor have shown defects in sensory integration which could eventually interfere with learning processes. EEG changes seen in kwashiorkor are known to persist for several months after recovery. Further work is needed to establish whether ultimate recovery from the mental and intellectual after-effects of malnutrition is possible, especially because most of the children suffering from malnutrition come from poor homes with little parental stimulation.

In several ways, the after-effects of marasmus are more serious. The onset of the deficiency state takes place in early infancy when brain growth is incomplete. Studies on the DNA, lipid and other constituents of the nervous tissue in experimental animals have shown that malnutrition of early onset interferes with the development of the optimum number of cells in the brain tissue.

The *long term outcome* depends on the quality of the home environment. This is especially true for intellectual growth. Curative services have very little to offer for improving the home environment, but Mother and Child Health (MCH) services can achieve a great deal through home visiting, counselling and regular growth monitoring. On discharge from the nutrition rehabilitation centre the children need to be followed up by the MCH services on a regular basis.

The routine ward diet

When the oedema is lost and the child is well on his way to recovery, the routine ward diet can be introduced in stages, whilst still continuing with the high-protein milk formula.

Malnutrition is widespread in the developing world. Moreover, many of the children admitted to the paediatric wards for other illnesses usually show the presence of mild – moderate malnutrition. Hence it is important to pay special attention to the routine ward diet to ensure that adequate nutrients are provided. If the ward diet is inadequate, recovery will be slow and hospital stay is extended.

A specimen diet for the average paediatric ward is as follows

6.00 a.m. 1 slice (30 g) of bread spread with 2–4 g margarine or peanut butter. 1 large cup (200 ml) of tea containing approximately 60 per cent milk with sugar.

10.00 a.m. 1 slice (50 g) of paw-paw cut into small pieces and gruel (150–200 g) containing 45 per cent milk, 8 per cent maize flour, 12 per cent eggs and sugar.

12.00 noon 150 g rice or stiff porridge made from maize flour, 100 g mince meat containing 2 per cent cooking oil, 80 g soup containing 7 per cent carrot, 7 per cent turnip, 15 per cent spinach and bone broth.

3.00 p.m. 1 slice (30 g) bread and 2–4 g margarine, 1 large cup (200 ml) tea as in the morning. Half an orange.

6.00 p.m. 100 g rice, 100 g mince as at lunch or beans or groundnut stew and 50 g soup.

The above diet will provide just adequate nutrients for most one to three year olds. For older children the helpings served need to be proportionately bigger according to age and appetite.

Prevention of malnutrition

Nutritional deficiencies arise when the environment does not provide the essential nutrients in a balanced form for the requirements of the organism.

Normally there is a wide margin of safety and the body stores of nutrients help to tide over short-term dietary deficiencies. However, when the diet is defective over a prolonged period or if demands suddenly increase as during illness, nutritional deficiency syndromes occur. In laboratory animals clinical and biochemical features of kwashiorkor or marasmus can be created by offering them diets which are deficient in either proteins or calories. In the case of the human, however, even though the intake of nutrients plays the major role in the etiology, other factors such as infection, physical and psychological stresses and cultural and social environment are also important. In a majority of cases infection acts as a precipitating agent, either in the form of an acute illness or as recurrent minor episodes.

The interplay of several etiological factors which determines the intake and utilisation of food by the child is illustrated in figure 5.9.

The ecology of malnutrition

In most peasant societies, people eat what they grow. Agriculture consists mainly of subsistence farming and modern methods of farming are employed only in small pockets for the production of cash crops such as tea, cotton, coffee, rubber, etc. A large proportion of the working population of a country is likely to be engaged in subsistence agriculture, using simple technology for the production, processing and storage of food. The yield per acre is low, and even in a good year many families suffer 'hungry months'.

For example, in the Gambia a faltering in the growth of children has been noted during the rainy season. This is because the stock of food from the previous harvest is running low. Moreover, during the rainy season every member of the family must work on the land to plant crops for the next harvest and the care of the young child suffers as a result. In addition, there is an increase in the prevalence of malaria and diarrhoeal disease during the wet season.

There are several stages between the preparation of the land for planting and the consumption of food in the home. Each of these stages can be improved by using better technology or improving the agricultural institutions in the community. However, tradition, customs and culture determine these aspects of agricultural life, as in everything else, and there is resistance to change.

Certain groups in the agricultural population are at greater risk of food shortage. These are the landless agricultural labourers, or migrant workers who often suffer from a system of share-cropping or become grossly underpaid wage-earners.

Unchecked population growth in many developing countries has led to mass migration to the cities

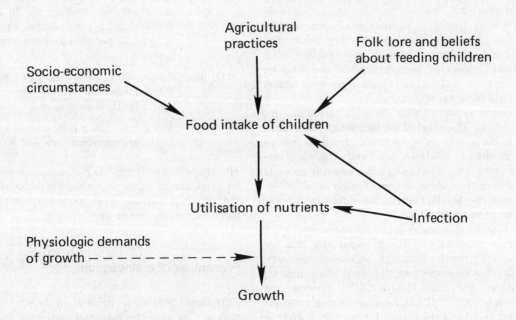

Figure 5.9 Factors influencing food intake and growth in children

causing rapid increases in urban population. Under the new conditions and stresses of city life, the old traditions of family life are rapidly breaking down, resulting in social and cultural isolation. A sudden departure from subsistence economy demands new skills in budgeting. Overcrowding and lack of sanitation in the 'septic fringes' of the large cities further complicate the problems of malnutrition in young children.

Working on the land to grow food for oneself and the family is such a major preoccupation in a peasant society that it is not surprising to see the importance given to food in all cultures. In ancient India different diets and foods were recommended for the different social classes. In some communities foods are considered to possess physiologic properties and are classified as 'hot' or 'cold', whereas in others certain foods are given pre-eminence and considered to be 'superior', for example, the plantain amongst the Baganda of Uganda. There may be taboos and superstitions regarding certain foods, especially for feeding young children and pregnant women. Thus, egg is not considered suitable for young children because it is 'hot' (India) or can cause worms (Malaysia) or may be a bad influence on the child (East Africa).

Attitudes and beliefs regarding food are woven into the matrix of the social life in rural societies and influence the kind of foods offered to a child at various stages of life. The first offering of a solid food or cereal is an occasion for a religious ceremony, as in Bengal; if for any reason the parents cannot afford the expense of the ceremony, weaning is postponed until such time as enough money can be raised, and during this period the child continues on milk feeds alone. Similar beliefs are also practised in times of illness or convalescence. In several systems of traditional medicine, dietary restrictions are an important aspect of management. It is customary to offer only clear fluids to a sick child, or to administer purgatives.

The interaction of these factors may determine the incidence of malnutrition in a community, as shown in figure 5.10.

The role of infection

During infective illnesses complex metabolic changes occur in the body. There is an increased flux of amino acids from skeletal muscle as a result of increased catabolism. The synthesis of visceral proteins in the heart and the brain is not known to be affected. Similarly the synthesis of protein in the liver is not altered, but there is increased gluconeogenesis. In addition, the liver utilises amino acids at an increased rate to produce acute phase plasma globulins and other factors involved in the immune mechanism.

The adverse effects of infection on child growth

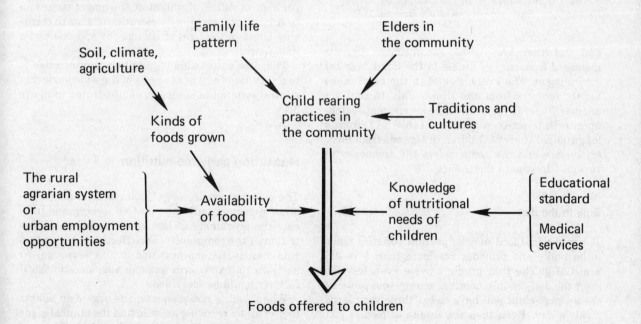

Figure 5.10 Factors influencing the feeding of children

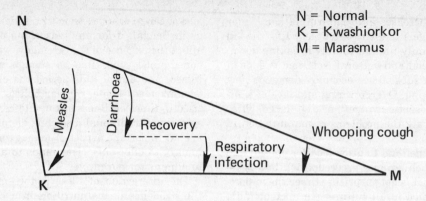

Figure 5.11 Infection and clinical nutritional deficiency syndromes

Table 5.12 Frequency of childhood illness in Uganda

	Total number of illnesses per 100 children	
	Kampala	Newcastle
Upper respiratory infection	74	13
Lower respiratory infection	258	124
Diarrhoea	107	20
Skin sepsis	160	8
Measles	36	18
Round worms	33	–
Hook worms	48	–
Malaria	257	–

Source: Rutishauser I H. In *The Child in the African Environment*, East African Literature Bureau, 1975.

and nutrition are further accentuated by the increased frequency of illness in the harsh tropical environment. The average child in the rural areas hardly recovers from one illness only to contract another. There is very little time for adequate catch-up growth to occur in between. Table 5.12, from a longitudinal study of children in Uganda from birth to the age of three, emphasises the frequency of various illnesses in the tropics.

Bulk in the diet

The traditional food in most peasant societies tends to be bulky and provides not more than 100–125 kcal/100 g. The thin gruels provide even less. To meet the daily requirements of energy and proteins the average child will have to eat three very large meals a day. Even then the intake of food is just adequate for normal weight gain and for mainten-ance of serum albumin levels, but not for catch-up

growth after an illness. The anorexia which accompanies most illnesses reduces food intake even further. If the energy density of the traditional foods were to be raised by 25 kcal/100 g through the use of fats and edible oils, it would provide an adequate margin of safety.

To summarise, the traditional weaning foods with low energy density, together with episodes of anor-exia during illness and the negative nitrogen bal-ance during episodes of infection result in cumulat-ive nutritional deficit. This is especially so between the ages of six and eighteen months. It has been demonstrated in several longitudinal studies of children that 91 per cent deficit of height and 98 per cent of deficit of weight at the age of three can be accounted for by the deceleration of growth occur-ring between the ages of six months and one and a half years.

The close association of nutrition and infection is to a very large extent the basis of the wide variety of clinical syndromes observed, as illustrated in figure 5.11.

Measuring early malnutrition

The classical syndromes of marasmus and kwashi-orkor represent only the tip of an iceberg and indi-cate the prevalence of less severe forms of malnu-trition in the community. For effective intervention it is obvious that malnutrition should be recognised early in its early form and the various etiological factors should be identified.

When food is not adequate, the organism adapts first of all by reducing growth, and the clinical signs on which diagnosis of early malnutrition is based are those of such an adaptation. Thus, weight gain slows down and so weight for age has been commonly used to assess the degree of malnutrition. The Gomez classification was first suggested in the late fifties as a method of diagnosing mild – moderate forms of malnutrition in the community and for the early detection of marasmus. The standard used is the weight of healthy American children under the age of five years, and the fiftieth percentile is taken as the standard. Malnutrition is graded into three degrees of increasing severity according to the percentage reduction in weight from the standard.

Gomez classification

First degree malnutrition   <80% of the standard
Second degree malnutrition <70% of the standard
Third degree malnutrition   <60% of the standard

The Gomez classification does not take height into consideration. Moreover, in some communities more than half the children will be classified as suffering from second or third degree malnutrition. Further experience in the community has shown that the best way of dealing with the problem of malnutrition is through service programmes that promote and monitor the growth of children. The concept of Gomez classification was modified to develop local weight charts. In more recent years the World Health Organisation has produced a weight chart for international use (figure 5.12). This chart is a mix of several concepts. It consists of a home chart, first proposed by Morley and used extensively in many countries. There is also a service chart to be retained in the clinic. This latter chart has several channels, each representing a proportion of weight deficit as follows

Channel A   Greater than 97th percentile
        B   Between 97th and 50th percentile
        C   Between 50th and 3rd percentile
        D   Between 3rd percentile and −3 standard
            deviation
        E   Between −3 standard deviation and −4
            standard deviation
            Less than −4 standard deviation

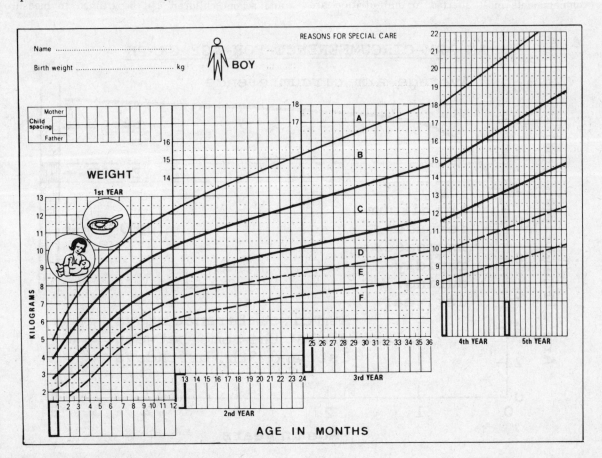

Figure 5.12   Weight-chart for international use (World Health Organisation)

With further experience it is now realised that the place on the growth chart where a child's weight falls is less important than the *shape* of the growth curve compared to the standard. Any flattening of the growth curve represents a decline in the velocity of growth. It indicates the need for early intervention to avoid a slide into the lower channels.

In countries with a long tradition of utilising auxiliary health personnel it has been found that such health workers can become proficient in the use and interpretation of growth records provided they receive adequate training. But auxiliaries are not available in all areas, and the new trend is to train part-time village health workers who are not always literate. There is thus a need for a much simpler way of assessing the nutritional status. Various anthropometric measurements have been simplified so that they can be applied at the village level. Of these, the mid-arm circumference as an indicator of nutritional status has been the most promising.

Besides growth in weight and height, the body compartments most affected in malnutrition are those of energy reserve such as subcutaneous fat and the protein store of skeletal muscle. Measuring these two body compartments can provide an indication of the nutritional status of the individual. In a large proportion of malnourished children there is wasting of muscle not only because of lack of protein in the diet but also because muscle is metabolised to provide energy. On the other hand, adequate muscle with lack of fat suggests lack of energy reserves.

Circumference of the mid-arm as an indicator of lean body mass has been used as one of the parameters for measuring nutritional status. It is known that in the normal child between the ages of one and five years the arm circumference changes very little. Here then is a parameter which is age independent (figure 5.13). In a study of undernourished children in Baghdad it was shown that children whose arm circumference was less than 75 per cent of the standard had a body weight less than 60 per cent of the Harvard Standard (Gomez third degree) in nine cases out of ten. The practical value of this study is that illiterate village health workers and school children can be trained to measure

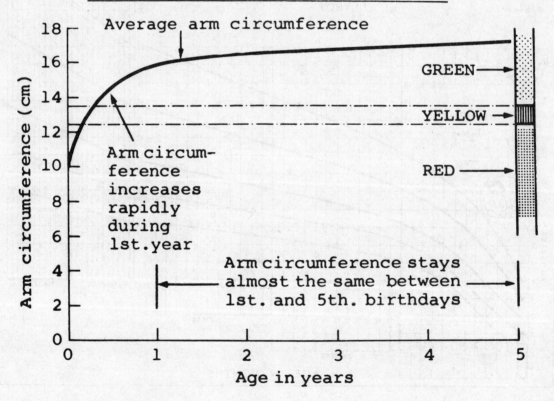

Figure 5.13   Arm circumference and age

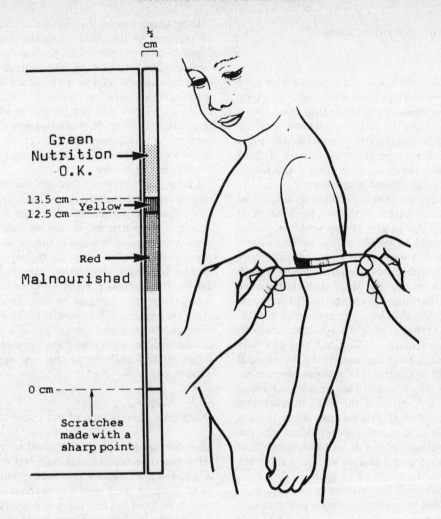

Figure 5.14 Measuring arm circumference

malnutrition in the community using a string or a strip of plastic with a mark and colours in green (over 14.0 cm), yellow (12.5 to 14.0 cm) and red (less than 12.5 cm) (figure 5.14). The concept is further modified to use a bangle or a bracelet in India.

Even though weight-for-age is the most commonly used parameter for assessing nutritional status it has been suggested that height-for-age and weight-for-height must also be taken into account for complete assessment. Low height-for-age indicates a chronic and prolonged period of nutritional inadequacy. Low weight-for-age indicates acute malnutrition, and low weight-for-height is an indicator of current nutritional status. Based on these parameters it is now usual to classify malnourished children as 'wasted', 'stunted' or 'wasted and stunted' (figure 5.15).

A recent collection of global anthropometric data

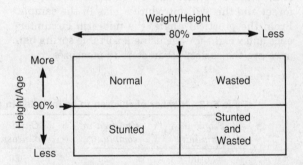

Figure 5.15 Classification of malnourished children

which included weight-for-height, height-for-age, and weight-for-age measurements showed that stunting is the dominant form of malnutrition, not wasting.

Making a community diagnosis of malnutrition

A community is a defined group of people who have things in common. They have a common life style, usually have common ways of earning their livelihoods and share the same belief systems. For the medical officer in the district hospital or the rural health centre the community is usually defined administratively, for example, a district and a sub-district, or by geographical boundaries.

When malnutrition is being commonly diagnosed in the paediatric wards or the out-patients, it is important that the extent of the problem in the community should be measured. As we have seen, for every case of kwashiorkor or marasmus there are many more with mild – moderate forms of malnutrition in the community. Many such children are not brought to the attention of the health workers.

Depending upon the resources available, weight-for-age, height-for-age, weight-for-height, arm circumference, or arm circumference-for-height may be used as parameters for measuring nutritional status of children. Clearly it is not possible to measure all the children in a village or town. One can measure only a fraction of the total number and these must be selected without bias so as to be a truly representative sample. Depending upon the size of the village or the town, the number of children included in the sample will vary from one in two to one in ten as shown in table 5.13.

It is best not to ask for children to be brought to a local clinic but to visit the houses and measure all children in the house under the age of five. If people are instructed to bring their children to a clinic on an appointed day it is likely that some will forget and this will introduce a bias in the sample. From the practical angle, the mid-arm circumference and weight-for-age using a portable spring balance are the easiest parameters to measure.

If by using any of the above methods more than 15 per cent of the children in the community are found to be undernourished, then serious food problems are likely to exist in that community. Further observations and studies with regard to methods of growing food crops, or choice of foods if they are being purchased, and the prevalent weaning practices are necessary. In most instances useful information can be obtained by talking to the community leaders and individually questioning some 10 to 15 parents in the village.

Information obtained through surveys and questionnaires described above provides an insight into the causes of malnutrition within a given community. Malnutrition is almost always a community-based problem and is the consequence of the prevailing state of cultural, social and technical development. Its eradication requires community action. Hence close rapport and exchange of information with the community and its leaders at all stages is important. The results of the data gathered through surveys and questionnaires must be discussed with the community leaders and all plans for intervention should be formulated in consultation with them.

Nutritional surveillance of the community

Most countries employ nutritional surveillance systems but these are largely national or regional in scope, and are intended for making policy decisions. Food scarcity and nutritional distress, however, tend to be localised and there is a need for operating community level surveillance methods. One simple method is based on the assumption that household food availability is the most important determinant of the nutritional status of the people. Food availability at the household level is influenced by local food production, and food prices. Food production is extremely difficult to measure, but rainfall is a

Table 5.13   Number of children to be included in a survey

People in community	Children in community	Children to measure	Number of houses	Houses to visit
100	20	20	5 to 7	All houses
500	100	100	25 to 30	All houses
1 000	200	200	50 to 70	All houses
2 000	400	200	50 to 70	Every 2nd house
5 000	1 000	200	50 to 70	Every 5th house
8 000	1 600	200	50 to 70	Every 8th house
10 000	2 000	200	50 to 70	Every 10th house
20 000	4 000	400	100 to 200	Every 10th house

useful indirect influence on agricultural productivity. Food prices are influenced by local food production, fluctuations in commodity prices in the country, and the international economy. A monthly walk through the local market noting the prices of the local staple foods, imported food items and luxury beverages will give an idea of the cost of food. To these indices are added the monthly percentage of babies born with low birth weight (<2500 g) in the district and the proportion of pre-school children with low weight-for-age (<60 per cent of the standard). These data together provide a useful practical guide and an early warning system of the changing nutritional influences in the community.

Intervention programmes

General

In the prevention of malnutrition in a community, the most crucial factor is the knowledge of simple principles of child feeding and nutrition in that community and in the various individuals and teams who provide services or leadership in that community. Thus, the health team, the community development worker, the agricultural extension worker, the teacher, and so on, should all be conversant with the problems of nutrition in its various aspects and should be able to provide practical guidance to the individual family in the community. Applied nutrition should form an important aspect of the training of these several cadres of workers. It is also important that the various teams working in the field should come together regularly for exchange of views so that they can all preach a common theme. Because the health team meets the problem constantly, it may be best suited to take the initiative in these matters and provide the base for practical guidelines to be evolved and implemented, in co-operation with local leaders of the community. Such a combined effort to define problems, to set out objectives, implement programmes and carry out evaluations with the help and interest of the community is more likely to succeed than any directives from above.

A community which can feed its children adequately is in a healthy state of social development compared to one which cannot. One must therefore attempt to search for solutions within the community and help to develop local resources. A first step is to raise the level of awareness in the community. A regular dialogue together with the feed-back of information about the prevalence of malnutrition and its causes helps to achieve this objective to some extent. In most cases it will be found necessary to have an agent of change resident in the community. The part-time village health workers have been found to be most effective in this respect. They are able to maintain the dialogue within the community and also bring with them useful information on the level of community concern and awareness to the health team.

The village health worker will of course be supported and given status by the health team. At the same time it is also necessary to strengthen the community's social organisation for the administration and support of local programmes. Creation of women's groups, young farmers' clubs or youth groups, and associating them with the activities of the village health workers provides a supporting framework for local programmes. Such social organisation creates a climate for community-based activities in improving agriculture, conserving water resources, preparing weaning diets from local foods in the form of multi-mixes, establishing child feeding programmes, identifying the beneficiaries of such programmes and so on. These community activities generate interest in the service programmes mentioned below. In return, the service programmes act like a network holding the community activities together and giving them a common purpose.

Service programmes

Most rural areas suffer from lack of services. The various issues related to inadequate development of rural health services have been discussed in section 1. In this respect it is important to bear in mind that basic health care, like education, is more of a social service than a technical one. The state of development of both services is a measure of the level of social development in a community. It should surprise no one that in the absence of health services there is widespread malnutrition and infective illness.

One way of combating malnutrition in a community is through the creation of services for primary care, however elementary they may be. The objective of such care is to help with the diagnosis and treatment of common ailments, and the supervision of vulnerable groups like pregnant women and young children. The two most important services are antenatal care and the under-fives' clinic. Both these services aim to provide health surveillance of the maximum number, the target being at least 80 per cent of the pregnant women and children in the area being cared for on a regular basis. They provide health education, immunisation and primary curative care for minor illnesses. They also help to identify individuals and families who are at risk of disease, and mobilise community resources for their special care.

There will never be enough resources to establish a conventional clinic at every village. Use of auxiliaries and village health workers will help to make these services more widely available, the aim being a service programme for every village.

Once the core service programme has been established and well associated with community-based activities in agriculture and water conservation, the development of other health related activities can be explored. These are nutrition rehabilitation centres, literacy classes, school health programmes, child spacing and so on.

A growing child health activity in many areas is the nutrition rehabilitation centre, which is being increasingly used as a tool against malnutrition in the community. The nutrition rehabilitation centre has the following objectives: (1) It provides convalescence for the child recovering from the acute phase of protein-calorie malnutrition, using locally available foods. (2) It is a place for the mother to receive simple instruction in nutrition and the feeding of her child by being actively involved in the preparation of the food and offering it to him. As the mother observes the gradual improvement in the child's condition, she realises that it is brought about by food, and not by medicines or doctoring. The mothers also participate in regular group discussions with the health educator; such discussions help to bring about a change in attitudes. (3) The mother who has received instruction in practical child feeding may become a source of information in her immediate neighbourhood when she goes home, and in this way the activity of the centre can indirectly benefit the community. Similarly, it is a readily-available demonstration area for visiting dignitaries, community leaders or teams from various government agencies in the area.

Evaluation of all services is necessary. However, it is important that in all evaluations the community should be involved as closely as possible, and the results of the evaluation should be freely discussed with the community and its leaders.

Vitamin deficiencies

The common clinical syndromes seen in children due to a deficiency of vitamins are visual loss due to deficiency of vitamin A, rickets and osteomalacia due to deficiency of vitamin D, pellagra and, in certain geographical areas, beri-beri. Most of these deficiencies are due to a monotonous diet consisting entirely of the staple, and cooking methods which may lead to loss or destruction of nutrients in the food.

Vitamin A deficiency

Vitamin A is believed to be necessary for maintaining the stability of cell membranes, but its most important association is with vision – the formation of visual purple in the retina and the integrity of the epithelium of the conjunctiva and the cornea. It has not been generally appreciated that vitamin A deficiency is a major cause of blindness in children in some countries. In a global survey sponsored by the World Health Organisation it was found that vitamin A deficiency was a cause of blindness, in varying degrees, in all of the 30 countries in Southeast Asia, Africa and Latin America visited by the team. In India it has been observed in several nutrition surveys that 15–20 per cent of all preschool children in the rural areas show signs of vitamin A deficiency.

Vitamin A deficiency often occurs in association with protein – calorie malnutrition and affects the same age groups. In India, clinical signs of vitamin A deficiency have been seen in 32 to 36 per cent of children admitted to hospital for protein – calorie malnutrition. In Indonesia, keratomalacia has been found in 29 out of every 44 children with kwashiorkor.

The defective weaning practices and poor supplementary feeding responsible for protein – calorie deficiency also operate in cases of vitamin A deficiency and illnesses such as diarrhoea, measles and respiratory infections act as precipitating factors for both.

Sources of vitamin A

Vitamin A is obtained in two forms, as vitamin A itself (present only in foods of animal origin such as milk fat, egg yolk and liver) and as carotenoids from plants which are converted into vitamin A in the epithelium of the small intestine and stored in the liver. The most important carotenoid is the ß-carotenoid which is widely distributed in nature, being present in green leaves, most green and yellow fruit and in some roots such as carrots. Table 5.14 below gives the amount of precursor of vitamin A available from cereals and vegetables.

Table 5.14 Nutritive value per 100 g edible portion

	IU
Cereals	
Maize	150
Rice	0
Wheat, whole	180
Wheat flour	49
Pulses	
Bengal gram	218
Lentil	450
Red gram	220
Leafy vegetables	
Amaranth	9 200
Cabbage	2 000
Coriander	11 530
Curry leaves	12 600
Spinach	9 300
Carrot	3 150
Other vegetables	
Brinjal	124
French beans	221
Cauliflower	51
Drumstick	184
Ladies fingers	88
Fruits	
Mango	4 800
Pawpaw	1 110
Tomato	585

Etiologic factors

In most cases the primary condition for the occurrence of low body stores of vitamin A is a dietary deficiency. Even though green vegetables with high ß-carotene content may be available, they are not offered to children because of a mistaken belief that they may cause diarrhoea. Some of the children with a chronic dietary deficiency may show clinical signs of xerophthalmia or Bitot's spots, either alone or in combination with a general picture of protein – calorie malnutrition. In others, there may be no overt signs, but intercurrent illnesses may lead to further sudden losses of vitamin A from the body and an acute deficiency is precipitated. Epidemics of measles, whooping cough and dysentery leave in their wake a number of children who have developed acute vitamin A deficiency.

Signs and symptoms of vitamin A deficiency

An early manifestation of vitamin A deficiency is night blindness, an association recognised since the earliest times, since its treatment by feeding liver is

mentioned by Hippocrates and an Egyptian medical papyrus. In the conjunctiva, there are changes in the epithelium causing a lack of lustre and drying – hence the term xerophthalmia. Similar changes may occur in the cornea, leading to the formation of scar tissue which impairs vision, or a 'liquefaction' of the cornea or keratomalacia leading to total loss of sight. The process may often be rapid, so that it is not unusual to find that a child seen in the outpatient clinic with xerosis and some corneal involvement has rapidly progressed to keratomalacia and total destruction of the cornea.

The effects of vitamin A deficiency on other tissues like the skin, mucous membranes and bone have been described, but the eye lesions are the most important from the clinical aspect.

Treatment

An adequate diet containing animal proteins and well balanced in other nutrients should be provided. For xerophthalmia vitamin A 5000 IU/kg per day is given orally in the oil-miscible form until recovery occurs. It is doubtful whether absorption of vitamin A occurs from oily preparations given by intramuscular injection. They are painful and may cause abscess formation and are better avoided, reliance being placed on oral medication. Water-miscible preparations can be given parenterally for rapid absorption, but in high doses may cause toxic symptoms.

Programmes of prevention

In a situation where clinical cases of xerophthalmia and keratomalacia are regularly seen in the hospital, it is reasonable to assume deficiency of the vitamin in the diets of the local community. Nutrition and dietary surveys in sample populations may help to confirm the suspicion. In such cases, preventive programmes within the framework of the existing MCH services are indicated. Nutritional rehabilitation of children admitted with established eye lesions is always necessary. The objectives and principles are no different from those in the case of children admitted with protein – calorie malnutrition, namely, to promote recovery in the child and provide health education for parents and communities.

Health education, either by itself or through clinics and nutrition rehabilitation centres, is a slow process and takes a long time to bear fruit. In the interim period, urgent measures are required to prevent the ravages of xerophthalmia in early life. Early studies of administering massive oral doses of vitamin A (200 000 IU) to the pre-school child in an oil-miscible form once or twice a year have shown that many of the eye complications can be prevented. Such a programme is easy to integrate in the under-fives' clinics or similar services for the pre-school child, with little extra cost.

Experience with large scale programmes of vitamin A supplementation has shown that not only is the prevalence of the clinical signs of deficiency reduced but also there occurs a concomitant reduction in mortality. It has been postulated that vitamin A protects against infection, especially of the respiratory tract. Invading bacteria must establish themselves on the respiratory epithelium before they can multiply and spread into the tissues. It has been suggested that adherence to epithelium is easier when there is a deficiency of vitamin A, and that healthy epithelium is able to resist adhesion.

Vitamin A has a number of functions. It is necessary for the synthesis of visual pigment in the retina. It helps to regulate the multiplication and differentiation of epithelial cells, and helps to maintain the different types of epithelium in a healthy state. It is active in a number of enzyme processes which metabolise foreign substances, including the elimination of toxins. It also plays a role in immune mechanisms.

Vitamin D deficiency (rickets)

Vitamin D, a fat-soluble vitamin, occurs in most animal fats, for example, milk, butter, egg yolk and liver. Liver fat is a rich source, so that cod liver oil has been the traditional means of treatment and prevention. However, in children of the poor socio-economic groups diet may contribute very little, so that they are mainly dependent upon exposure to sunlight for their vitamin D requirements. The ultra-violet rays of the sun acting on the skin convert the 7-dehydrocholesterol present in the skin to cholecalciferol (vitamin D_3). On absorption from the skin it accumulates rapidly in the liver where it is converted to $25\text{-OH-}D_3$. Further hydroxylation occurs in the kidney giving rise to $1\text{--}25\text{-(OH)-}D_3$ which is the active form of vitamin D and behaves like a calcium and phosphate mobilising hormone in the body.

Socio-cultural or climatic reasons may lead to inadequate exposure of children to sunlight, for example, children may be kept indoors all day to protect them from heat, as in Northern India, or they may not be able to play outdoors as in some city slums, or they may be kept swaddled and covered to prevent excessive tanning, as in some higher socio-economic groups in Ethiopia. It may appear strange that rickets can occur in countries where sunshine is plentiful. Its uneven distribution in Africa and Asia illustrates the socio-cultural factors in the etiology. In tropical Africa rickets is rarely seen, for example, in several nutrition surveys on children in Uganda and Tanzania rickets has rarely been noted. Analysis of hospital and dispensary records in countries of East and West Africa shows that rickets is not a major problem. However, in Ethiopia, Sudan and countries of North Africa, rickets is seen as a major deficiency disorder. In Ethiopia, 52 per cent of all infants examined in the Ethio-Swedish Clinic in Addis Ababa showed evidence of the disease, sometimes in severe form. In Morocco and Algiers 10 per cent and 11 per cent respectively of children attending hospital showed evidence of serious rickets. Comparable figures are obtained in Asia, the incidence being higher in urban children and often in combination with protein-calorie malnutrition.

Throughout the eighteenth and early part of the nineteenth centuries rickets was common in the towns and cities of Europe. With the industrial revolution the incidence in urban areas increased; in the slums of Glasgow and London rickets was almost universal. In the hospitals of Paris and New York rickets was a common diagnosis in hospitalised children. With the free supply of cod liver oil and common use of fortified milk preparations, rickets was virtually eliminated from the industrial cities of the West, only to appear again in more recent years in immigrant children in the UK. Several recent studies in Glasgow have shown that there was no significant difference between the diets of immigrant children who were healthy and those who were suffering from rickets. Similarly, a control group of native Scottish children were eating an average diet differing little in nutritional content, including vitamin D, from those of immigrant children, showing that non-dietary sources of vitamin D are important.

Vitamin D deficiency leads to rickets and osteomalacia. The basic lesion is retardation of bone formation, so that collagen is formed without concomitant impregnation with bone crystal. As a result, an excess of osteoid accumulates. In non-growing bone it leads to softening and deformity (osteomalacia), and in the growing child there are characteristic skeletal changes of rickets. There is a delay in the closure of the anterior fontanelle and a characteristic bossing of the frontal and parietal eminences. The epiphyses of the limb bones are enlarged because of accumulation of osteoid; this is best seen at the wrists and ankles. Similar increase of osteoid tissue also occurs at the costo-chondral junction, giving rise to 'beading' of ribs. Bowing of the legs may occur and in severe cases changes may also occur in the pelvic bones which, persisting into adult life, may cause obstetric difficulties in females.

The diagnosis is confirmed by X-ray appearances of the bones which, in advanced cases, may show characteristic cupping and fraying of the epiphyses. The serum alkaline phosphatase is raised and phosphorus is usually reduced, but serum calcium often remains normal. The bossing of the skull and X-ray appearances of the bones may need differentiation from other conditions, such as sickle-cell anaemia or congenital syphilis.

Treatment of rickets is with administration of vitamin D 2000 IU daily for two to four weeks, reducing to 1000 IU for several months.

Nutritional anaemias

Anaemia constitutes a major problem in child health in the tropics. It is one of the principal causes for hospital admissions and deaths; in addition it is often present with other illnesses such as pneumonia and protein-calorie malnutrition, and makes them more severe. Thus, in an analysis of 853 children attending Muhimbili Hospital, Dar-es-Salaam, as out-patients, the average haemoglobin was 6.78 g/100 ml. In surveys carried out in Africa, 6 to 17 per cent of men and 15–50 per cent of women have been found to have haemoglobin levels below 10 g/100 ml and in children the incidence of anaemia varied from 30 to 60 per cent.

From the public health point of view the most common type of anaemia is due to iron deficiency, though deficiency of folic acid or vitamin B_{12} also occurs, especially in pregnant women and young infants. In developing countries megaloblastic anaemia has been reported in 20 per cent of pregnant women and significant megaloblastic change in the bone marrow has been reported in 50 per cent of them, as compared to 2.5 to 5.0 per cent and 25 per cent in Western countries. B_{12} deficiency in association with folate deficiency is a frequent complication of pregnancy in India and South-east Asia and may lead to similar deficiency in the young breastfed infants of such mothers.

Iron deficiency in pregnancy may lead to poor stores of iron in the foetus. Milk, which may be the only source of food in early infancy, is a poor source of iron (0.075 mg iron/100 g), so that the infant relies heavily on his body stores for growth in the first year of life. The average 3.5 kg infant at birth has 190 mg of iron in haemoglobin and an additional

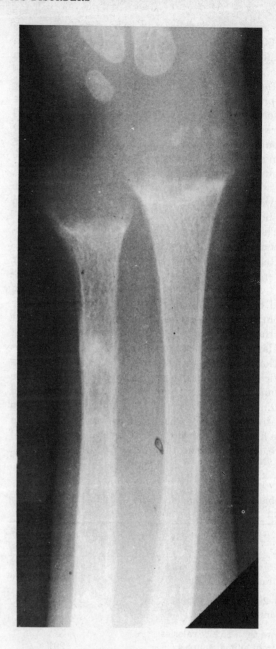

Figure 5.16 Rickets. Note cupping and fraying at the epiphyses

60 mg in tissue. During the first year of life he will need an additional 115 mg of iron for haemoglobin synthesis and also 50 mg for synthesis of myoglobin and iron-containing enzymes. Thus 165 mg or approximately 0.45 mg iron per day will be required. If these requirements are not met from body stores or from dietary iron, anaemia will result.

In developing countries the staple food largely

determines the intake of iron, because it accounts for 60–80 per cent of daily calorie intake. In Western countries, although the staple is generally low in iron, the inclusion of large amounts of other foods in the diet leads to adequate intake. The presence of proteins in the diet is essential for adequate absorption of iron. It has been observed by several workers that though the diet may be providing enough iron through vegetable and other sources, iron deficiency still exists. Recent studies have now shown that unless the diet contains enough proteins, this iron may not be absorbed. The relationship between proteins in the diet and absorption of iron is shown in table 5.15.

The intake of iron shown in table 5.16 is recommended according to proteins in the diet.

Repeated infections in the toddler may further interfere with utilisation of iron and lead to anaemia. Thus, the baby born with poor stores of iron and on a poor dietary intake of iron in the early months of life becomes progressively iron-deficient as the demands of growth are not met. Episodes of malaria and infections may add further complications and make anaemia worse, so that iron deficiency anaemia is common in the pre-school age group. As demands of growth slow down and immunity develops the haemoglobin tends to rise so that average haemoglobin levels in school children are higher compared with children under the age of five, though lower than the Western standards.

Many children will grow up to be iron-deficient adults, and in women with repeated child-bearing on an inadequate diet, the cycle is repeated again.

The MCH programme in the community in conjunction with the hospital services can play an important role in the prevention of morbidity and mortality due to anaemia. An integrated approach through the antenatal clinic, the under-fives' clinic and the out-patient services, utilising the principles of prevention, early diagnosis and treatment, rehabilitation and health promotion is required to make an impact on the prevalence of anaemia. A suggested plan is indicated in figure 5.17.

Iodine deficiency disorders

Iodine deficiency is a major risk factor for physical growth and mental development affecting at least 1000 million people who live in iodine deficient environments around the world: an estimated 300 million in China, 200 million in India, 100 million in Indonesia, 100 million in Africa and 60 million in Latin America.

Iodine poor soil and food are common in mountainous regions and in any area where iodine is periodically washed away by heavy rainfall or recurrent floods. People living in such areas are at risk, especially the unborn children. A number of staple foods like cassava, maize, bamboo shoots, sweet potato, lima beans and millet contain cyanogenic glucosides which can release large quantities of cyanide on hydrolysis. Cyanide is toxic and its metabolite, thiocyanate, is a goitrogen. With the exception of cassava, these glycosides are located largely in the inedible portions of the plant. In times of food shortages the inedible portions also may be consumed. Cassava, on the other hand, is cultivated extensively in developing countries and is an essential food item for more than 200 million people. The role of cassava in the causation of iodine deficiency disorders has been demonstrated in Zaire, Sarawak and elsewhere.

Table 5.15 Relationship of the diet and absorption of iron

	Absorption of iron from the diet
Less than 10% of calories from animal foods	10%
10–25% of calories from animal sources	15%
More than 25% of calories from animal sources	20%

Table 5.16 Recommended intake of iron

Age	Requirement (mg)	Animal foods as source of calories		
		<10%	10–25%	>25%
0.4 months	0.5	◄————————Breast feeding————————►		
5–12 months	1.0	10 mg	7 mg	5 mg
1–12 years	1.0	10 mg	7 mg	5 mg
13–16 years (males)	1.8	18 mg	12 mg	9 mg
13–16 years (females)	2.4	24 mg	18 mg	12 mg

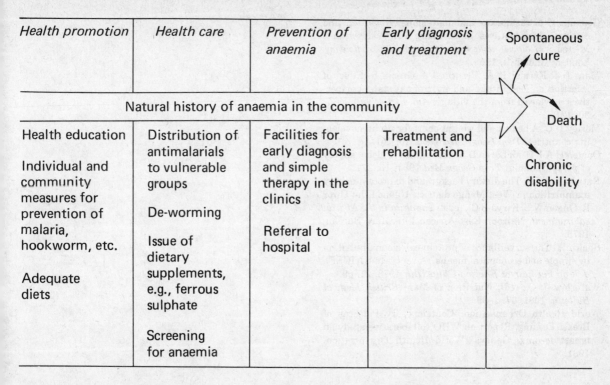

Health promotion	Health care	Prevention of anaemia	Early diagnosis and treatment	Spontaneous cure
Health education

Individual and community measures for prevention of malaria, hookworm, etc.

Adequate diets | Distribution of antimalarials to vulnerable groups

De-worming

Issue of dietary supplements, e.g., ferrous sulphate

Screening for anaemia | Facilities for early diagnosis and simple therapy in the clinics

Referral to hospital | Treatment and rehabilitation | Death

Chronic disability |

Natural history of anaemia in the community

Figure 5.17 Interventions for the prevention of anaemia

In pregnancy, iodine deficiency can cause spontaneous abortions, still-births and infant deaths. It interferes with brain development of the foetus and can result in the birth of brain-damaged babies. The condition is described as endemic cretinism and is characterised by mental deficiency, deaf mutism and spastic diplegia. There is also a less common myxoedematous type characterised by signs of hypothyroidism and dwarfism.

In childhood iodine deficiency can cause mental retardation, delayed motor development, growth failure or stunting, lack of energy, muscular disorders, as well as speech and hearing defects.

The biological importance of iodine is due to the fact that it is essential for thyroid hormone production.

The problems are preventable by making iodine available through iodised salt (at an estimated cost of five US cents per person per year) or iodised oil (slightly more expensive) or even iodised water. Using these intervention methods progress in the control of iodine deficiency disorders has been made in 40 countries. Potassium iodide and iodate are the most commonly used materials. Iodide is cheaper but iodate is more stable, particularly in warm and humid climates, or where there are significant

impurities in the local salt. Iodine is usually added to the salt in the ratio of between 1:10 000 and 1:50 000 depending on the average salt intake in the population. The minimum daily requirement of iodine is about 50ug and the recommended intake is 100–150 ug.

Iodised oil can be given orally or by intramuscular injection. The iodine is slowly released from the oil, and is removed from the circulation by the thyroid gland. Iodised oil provides adequate iodine for several years after its initial administration, and is an effective preventive as well as therapeutic measure for women in the child bearing age.

Further reading

Cameron M, Hofvander Y. *Manual on feeding infants and young children*, 2nd Ed. New York: United Nations, 1976.

Ebrahim G J. *Breast feeding: the biological option*, 2nd Ed. London: Macmillan, 1991.

Ebrahim G J. *Nutrition in Mother and Child Health*. London: Macmillan, 1983.

Gopalan C Kwashiorkor and marasmus. Evolution and distinguishing features. In: McCance R A, Widdowson E M (eds.) *Calorie deficiency and protein deficiency.* London: Churchill, 1968.

Mata L J, Kormal R A, Urrutia J J, Gracia B. Effect of infection on food intake and nutritional state: perspectives as viewed from the village. *Am J Clin Nutr* 1977; 30: 1215.

Morley D C. A health and weight chart for use in developing countries. *Trop Geogr Med* 1968: 20: 101.

Oomen H A P C, McLaren D S, Escapini A. A global survey of xerophthalmia. *Trop Geogr Med* 1964; 16: 271.

Rutishauser I H. The dietary background to protein-energy malnutrition in West Mengo district, Uganda. In: Owor R, Ongom V L, Kirya B G., (eds.) *The child in the African environment.* Nairobi: East African Literature Bureau, 1975.

Shakir A. The surveillance of protein-calorie malnutrition by simple and economical means. (A report to UNICEF). *J Trop Paediatr & Environ Child Hlth* 1978; 21: 69.

Waterlow J. C., (ed); Nutrition of Man. *British Medical Bulletin.* 1981; 37: 1–99.

World Health Organisation. Contemporary Patterns of Breast Feeding. Report on WHO collaborative study on breast feeding. Geneva: World Health Organisation, 1981.

6 *Growth and development*

Growth and development are the distinctive biological processes of childhood. Growth denotes an increase in the size of the organism which may be due to increase in the number of cells of tissues or increase in the size of each individual cell. Development indicates acquisition of function by the tissues or the organism as a whole. But there is much more to growth and development than is implied in such a definition. Since all mammalian species begin life as a single cell, there is a whole set of traffic in energy and information during growth, an ordered hierarchy of cell processes and a continuing r?????onship between structure and function. The ???? r functions of one phase set the stage for the ne?? phase, initiating it as well as controlling it.

The processes of growth and development begin at conception and continue throughout childhood and adolescence until maturity when the individual acquires reproductive functions. From the biological point of view the ability of the mature individual to produce germ cells and procreate is the equivalent of the process of growth and development in the young.

Very little is understood about the mechanisms controlling cellular growth in different organs. It is known that size of organ is adjusted to the functions they are called upon to perform. Therefore mechanisms regulating organ growth must be closely associated with those physiological functions which govern the activities of organs and tissues. In the case of visceral organs, function and growth are regulated by humoral factors like trophic hormones and blood chemistry. In other tissues such as bones and muscles, as well as some hollow organs such as the heart and blood vessels, mechanical factors, for example, stresses and strains are important. For some highly complex organs, for example, the liver, kidneys and lungs, growth control is not well understood.

It is now widely appreciated that with growth the composition of the body is changing as well as the shape. There is thus an age of chemical maturity just as there is sexual maturity. Each mammalian species reaches chemical maturity at a chronological time from conception peculiar to itself.

The growth and development of an individual represents the interaction between his genetic endowment and the physical and social environment, including nutrition. Because the genetic endowment of each individual is unique, each child has an individual growth process different from any other, though broad generalisations can be made for a family, or a community, or a racial group. Thus in a family all children may be tall or small; in a village all children may be short because of inadequate nutrition, and the children in Asia show a different growth potential compared to children in Africa. In each of the above groups, however, the individual child will have his own unique growth pattern within the broad generalisations stated.

Growth is not a uniformly continuous process but is characterised by two phases of rapid growth, each with a period of acceleration during which rapid increments occur, followed by a period of deceleration during which the increase in growth per unit of time is less than in the immediately preceding period. The onset and duration of each component of these two phases may vary from one child to another, depending upon his genetic composition and the effects of his environment, resulting in the wide variations seen in the size of the adult individual. These two phases of growth are better appreciated if the growth in an individual is charted by increments per unit of time (velocity curve) in addition to the traditional 'distance' curve (figure 6.1).

The first phase of rapid growth is in infancy and early childhood and the second phase occurs at puberty. During the intervening period growth takes place by smaller regular increments.

Within the general pattern of increase in height and weight along the lines mentioned above, different tissues of the body grow at different times. Thus, the central nervous system grows maximally during the first two years of life, whereas the reproductive system remains dormant until the onset of puberty

The Curve of Growth

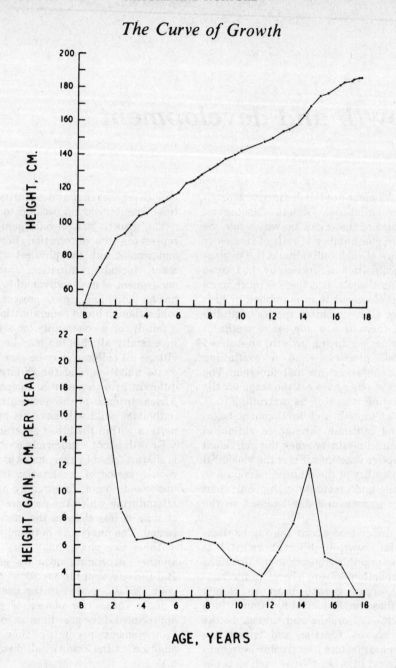

Figure 6.1 Distance and velocity curves of growth

when maximal growth takes place. The growth of the lymphoid system is in between (figure 6.2).

Experiments in laboratory animals have shown that in general the growth of organs such as the spleen, liver, pancreas and kidneys tends to follow the pattern of growth of the bony cage in which they are situated.

Because of the differential growth of the tissues in different parts of the body, changes in body proportions occur as growth proceeds giving rise to the characteristic appearances of the foetus, the infant, the young child and the adult.

Under normal circumstances the individual's growth follows a defined pattern enabling each child to achieve his own predetermined size at different times. If a growth disturbance occurs because of environmental stress like nutritional disorder or infection, this milestone in growth may not be reached, in which case, on recovery, the child usually undergoes a period of 'catch-up' growth (figure 6.3). During the period of 'catch-up' growth increments in growth may be twice the normal for the age period until such time as the lost ground has been regained, after which growth proceeds normally. Thus each brief illness is associated with a slowing of growth followed by a variable period of 'catch-up' growth during recovery. This compensatory mechanism enables the individual to overcome the effects of short periods of illness. However, if the

disturbance in growth is prolonged, for example, protein-calorie malnutrition or tuberculosis, or if it occurs at a very young age, for example, the early newborn period, the catch-up may not be total and an eventual stunting in height may be the end result.

Analysis of growth data collected over many years in the Western countries shows that there is a secular trend in growth. For the same age, children are taller and heavier than decades ago. This secular trend is also noticeable in the heights of the average adult as seen in the case of army recruits, and in the age of onset of menarche in girls. Improvements in living standards, in nutrition and control of environmental infections and parasitic diseases

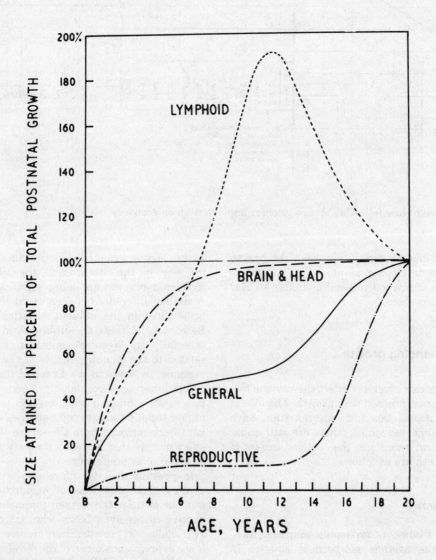

Figure 6.2 Different growth rates of body tissues

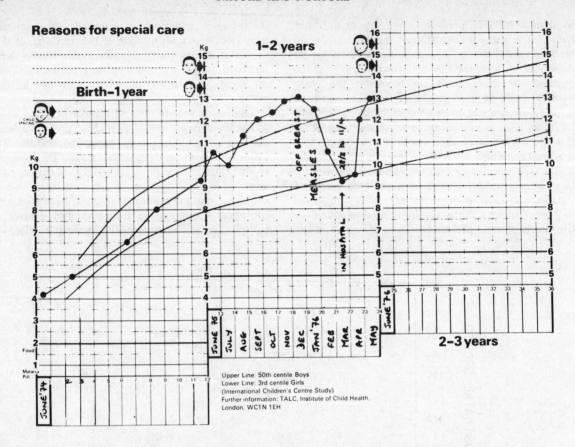

Figure 6.3   Weight loss following severe measles and catch-up on recovery

have no doubt contributed to this trend. As growth data from the developing countries become available, it will be of interest to see if a similar secular trend also occurs there.

Factors influencing growth

Several factors can adversely affect the various biological processes concerned with growth. The effects of some, such as infection and undernutrition, have been well documented whilst others are still under study. In clinical situations, the common causes of disturbed growth are as follows

Intrauterine growth

A number of studies in developing countries have shown that the average newborn is smaller in weight and shorter when compared to his counter-

part in Western countries. Social class has a marked influence on the size at birth, the babies of higher socio-economic groups being significantly heavier. A similar difference between social classes has also been noted in the affluent societies of the West. Besides social class, the difference in birth weight, especially in Western countries, appears to be related to the smoking habits of the mothers. For example, in Scotland it was found that 57 per cent of the lower socio-economic groups smoked during pregnancy compared with only 38 per cent in the higher social classes. In some studies, when the smokers were removed from the series, the social class effect disappeared, showing the very serious effects of smoking in pregnancy.

In peasant societies marriages occur early and usually about the time of menarche. In a large number of cases the woman commences her reproductive career even before she has completed her own adolescent growth. Short stature and its prevalence in pregnant women of the developing countries has been commented upon by several workers. In the majority of cases short stature is a consequence of stunting due to inadequate nutrition during childhood and adolescence. Thus, nutrition of the mother, and especially her nutritional status when she was a growing child, is an important factor with regard to intrauterine growth.

When mothers of the lower socio-economic group are given food supplements during pregnancy, there is significant improvement in the weight of the newborn. In a survey of dietary intake of pregnant women in Tanzania, it was found that to have a baby weighing more than 3.1 kg it was necessary that the mother should consume at least 50 g protein daily, and 40 per cent of the women in the survey ate less than this amount of protein. Energy deficiency was even more widespread and serious. To have a baby weighing 3.1 kg a mother had to consume 2200 calories per day and only 30 per cent of the women had as much. In a similar study in Guatemala, calorie intake was again found to be a more critical variable compared to protein.

The intrauterine growth of the foetus is affected by several maternal factors besides nutrition. For example, in babies who are born small-for-dates, the siblings and maternally-related near relatives have birth-weights smaller than the population mean. Similarly, in babies with a birth weight greater than the mean, a similar pedigree effect can be demonstrated. These observations indicate the influence of genetic constitution on intrauterine growth.

Various infections suffered during intrauterine life can affect the growth of the foetus. Congenital rubella, cytomegalovirus or syphilis affect foetal growth. Heavy malarial infection of the placenta also has a similar adverse effect. Chromosomal aberrations like Down's syndrome and congenital abnormalities in general tend to cause low birth weight.

It has been observed that the light-for-dates infants may continue to remain small and do not reach the average standards of normal for the community. The compensatory mechanism of 'catch-up growth' does not operate in the case of such babies. Thus the growth of the organism in intrauterine life may have some contribution to make to the overall pattern of growth after birth.

Social factors

In all countries, children in the upper socio-economic groups are taller and heavier than those in the lower. Adequate nutrition and a good standard of health, with relative freedom from intercurrent illnesses are the important contributory factors for the difference in growth.

Inadequate nutrition and ill-health occur concurrently with poverty, ignorance and poor environmental sanitation and the defective growth of children from such homes is due to the synergistic effect of all these factors. Considering that the vast majority of children in the rural areas of the developing world come from poor homes, the social as well as the biological factors need to be taken into account in programmes of growth promotion in such communities.

Nutrition

In the first few months of life breast milk provides adequate nutrition and most babies do well. A comparison of the weights and velocity of growth in African and Indian children with those of children in the United Kingdom shows very little difference (figure 6.4). Velocity of growth declines in the latter half of the first year and in the second year of life. Towards the end of the second year and in the third year the velocity of growth is again the same as that of children in affluent societies but the lost ground is never recovered. It has already been emphasised that 91 per cent of the deficit in height and 98 per cent of that in weight can be explained by the fall in growth velocity in the latter half of the first year and in the second year of life. Hence special attention to weaning practices and regular monitoring of growth during this critical period of growth is necessary.

Seasonal variations in growth, especially in relation to the onset of the rains, have been reported in several countries. The period immediately before the onset of the rainy season is often called 'the hungry months' and availability of food is an important factor. The increased incidence of malaria and lack of adequate mothering because everyone must work in the field to grow food, are other contributory factors. During this time the child is fed from a pot of gruel cooked in the morning before the mother goes to the family plot and left standing in a corner. Heavy bacterial growth has been demonstrated in such gruel and diarrhoeal episodes become frequent. Each such episode causes faltering of growth.

All illness leads to anorexia and there is decreased food intake. In addition many severe infections lead to a negative nitrogen balance due to a breakdown of lean body mass. In this respect the serious nature of measles has been reported from Nigeria and whooping cough from Guatemala. If the various illnesses are too close, one after the other, no catch-up of growth can possibly occur (figure 6.5). Even when episodes of illness are far apart, the diet may

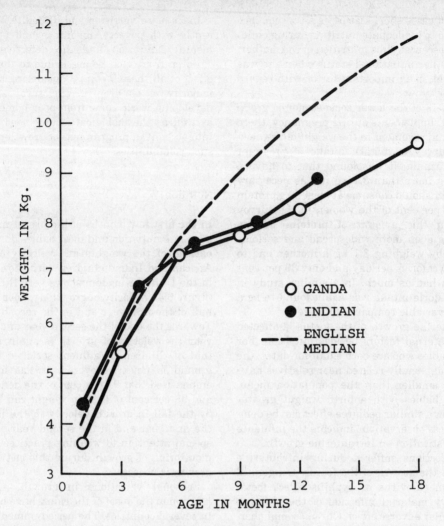

Figure 6.4 Growth in infancy. Note similar growth rates during early infancy in African, English and Indian children

be too poor to support the demands of a rapid 'catch-up'. Again, improvement of the weaning food, especially with regard to its energy content, is necessary to provide adequate support during the period of anorexia, and nourishment during convalescence.

Endocrine disturbances

Endocrine disturbances affecting secretions of growth hormones, thyroxine, corticosteroids and the sex hormones can cause aberrations of growth. Food nourishes the body in a manner that depends on the internal hormonal environment. Endocrine causes of growth disturbances do occur especially in areas

with goitre. However, the most serious cause is iatrogenic. Indiscriminate prescribing of corticosteriods and anabolic hormones in children can often lead to eventual stunting of growth.

Biological factors

There are sexual differences in growth so that in early life and during early school years boys tend to be taller and heavier than girls. The growth spurt of puberty occurs earlier in girls so that now girls become taller than boys. After the latter have experienced their pubertal growth spurt, they end up as taller adults compared to girls. Biological influence on growth is also seen in constitutional

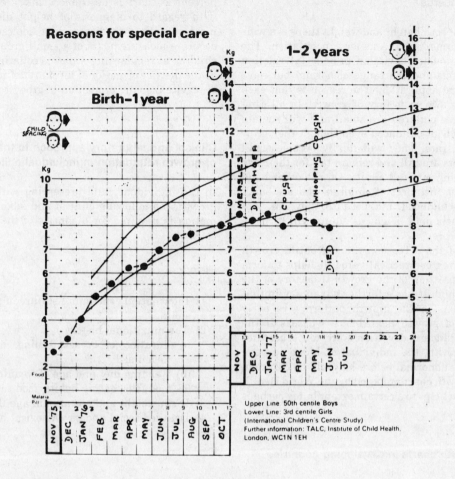

Figure 6.5 Failure of 'catch-up' when illness is recurrent

short stature, in family growth patterns, in age of menarche in girls and so on.

Measuring growth

Parameters of growth

The commonly used parameters are weight and height including the velocities of growth in both. In developing countries height measurement is not carried out as frequently as the measurement of weight with the result that one important disorder of growth and nutrition, namely, stunting, has gone unrecognised. Stunting in girls as an important

cause of foetal growth retardation has not received the attention it deserves until very recently. In rural Ecuador the average height of rural women is 146.5 cm and in Guatemala 50 per cent of rural women were found to be less than 143 cm (4ft 8in) in height.

Other parameters such as head and chest circumferences, mid-arm circumference and skin-fold thickness have been traditionally used for community surveys in child growth and nutrition. Of these, mid-arm circumference is now commonly recognised as a reliable index of lean body mass, especially in children under the age of five, and skin-fold thickness is an indicator of the energy stores of the body. Bone age and skeletal maturation provide valuable information in special circumstances like growth disorder in the individual.

Growth standards

In the case of both height and weight there is a wide range of 'normal' in the general population. The mean and standard deviation provide information on the average and the range of normal but have little practical application. The reason is that each child has its own trajectory of growth. In all communities some children are small and will remain small throughout childhood even though they grow at a normal rate. They will finally become small adults. Others are tall and remain tall for their age finally growing into tall adults. On the other hand there may be instances of children who are small throughout childhood, but because they are 'late maturers' their final height as adults will be more than their peers.

Because of these reasons the percentile growth chart is of greater practical value. It helps to form an early impression of the growth trajectory of the individual child. It has a further advantage in that any deviations in the growth pattern give early warning of a growth disturbance whereas if the mean and standard deviation were to be used for assessing growth, the individual child would have to be grossly abnormal before he could be detected. The new growth chart proposed by the World Health Organisation helps to a certain extent but is perhaps less accurate.

Use of growth charts in developing countries

Growth failure is a common condition in children in the developing countries. Its early detection by means of a suitable growth chart and institution of public health measures for the promotion of growth and the development of services are both highly desirable. Both these activities have been hampered by the lack of suitable growth charts. The promotion by WHO of an international growth chart (page 69) will help both from the practical angle of its wide scale adoption for use as well as by resolving the debate about the suitability or otherwise of a record based on cross-sectional data as compared to a percentile chart.

It is important to differentiate between growth charts for preventive-promotive use and those for diagnosis of growth disorders. In the first category fall the kind of weight charts first introduced by Morley in Nigeria and now adapted by several countries including the new WHO growth chart (see figures 6.3 and 6.4). In the individual case for the diagnosis of growth disorder, such a chart may be a help but will introduce some inaccuracies and a percentile chart is desirable. This is especially so with regard to diagnosis of height disorders and more so with such disorders at adolescence. Thus accurate measurements of a small group of normal children at regular intervals and collating such data at the district or national level are an integral part of services for the promotion of growth in children.

Clinical and laboratory approach to the diagnosis of growth retardation in individual children

In the individual child presenting with failure of growth, the following clinical and laboratory information is required for diagnosis of the underlying cause

History

(1) Information concerning stature of parents and siblings.
(2) The nutritional history:
    (a) duration of breast feeding, or the milk formula;
    (b) weaning diet and age of weaning;
    (c) food fads, eating habits, food taboos if any.
(3) Birth weight and gestational age if known.
(4) Detailed social and psychological history.

Evaluation

(1) Measurements of weight, height, head and chest circumferences and arm span. Serial measurements are more informative than a single reading.
(2) Comparisons of degree of retardation in weight and height and in bone age.
(3) Clinical examination directed towards identification of those diseases which are known to interfere with growth, for example, chronic lung disease; congenital cardiac defects; malabsorption syndromes; hepatic insufficiency; chronic renal disease; hypothyroidism; neurologic disease; metabolic illness.

Laboratory investigations

(1) Urine examination for pyuria, a fixed low specific gravity, constant alkaline pH.
(2) Stool examination for ova and parasites; faecal fat.

(3) If malabsorption is suspected, the following tests may help to confirm:
  (a) Complete blood count.
  (b) Serum iron, iron binding capacity; folic acid and vitamin B_{12} levels.
  (c) Sweat sodium.
  (d) Barium meal and follow through.
  (e) Antibodies against gliadin.
  (f) Jejunal biopsy.
(4) In girls with short stature a study of the buccal smear for chromatin. A karyotype, if facilities are available, in order to exclude Turner's syndrome.
(5) If endocrine disease is suspected, the following may help to confirm:
  (a) Fasting blood sugar, and glucose tolerance test.
  (b) Blood levels of T_3 T_4 and TSH if facilities are available.
  (c) X-ray of the skull for the pituitary fossa.
  (d) Urinary 17-ketosteroids and oxysteroids.

From the diagnostic point of view it is useful to bear in mind that growth in childhood can be conveniently divided into three component parts, each predominantly influenced by a different set of factors with a varying amount of overlap. These components of growth are as follows:

(i) Infancy

The very rapid growth of intrauterine life begins to decelerate after birth until the age of two years. Prenatal growth accounts for approximately one third of entire growth, to which the infantile component adds about 75 cm in length and 10 kg in weight. Prenatal and infantile components of growth are almost entirely dependent on nutrition. Growth defects in this period are usually due to problems related to supply, absorption or assimilation of nutrients. In the case of children born small for dates and children who have been nourished inadequately either before or after term, the failure to thrive may result in permanent stunting through loss of infantile contribution to growth. A detailed history with regard to pregnancy, and feeding since birth is helpful in arriving at a diagnosis.

Infective illness and associated feeding problems are also important reasons for growth faltering in this period. Chronic disease or other systemic illness are a third group of causes to be considered at this age.

(ii) Childhood

The childhood component from the age of about two years to puberty is largely dependent on growth hormone (GH), the receptors for which appear in the target tissues by this time. Nutritional deficiency and infective illness still play a major role, especially in developing countries. Systemic diseases which cause failure to thrive are usually sufficiently severe to draw attention by means of their characteristic symptoms rather than present merely as defective growth. A carefully taken history is important for excluding such illnesses. An exception to this general statement is renal tubular acidosis. Serum electrolytes and blood chemistries including calcium, magnesium and phosphorous levels are essential base line investigations.

The most reliable screening test of growth hormone secretion is the careful measurement of growth velocity. Tests of GH secretion are difficult to perform, and often more difficult to interpret. On the other hand measurement of growth velocity is cheap and easily available.

(iii) Puberty

The growth spurt at adolescence is determined by the secretion of the sex steroids. In girls growth velocity increases as soon as breast development starts, and is due to amplified GH response to the GH releasing hormone under the influence of oestrogens. By contrast testosterone in boys is a less effective promotor of GH, and has to be present in larger amounts. Hence the growth spurt of puberty occurs about two years later in boys.

Growth failure at this stage requires the careful assessment of puberty. In girls chromosomal abnormality, for example, Turner's syndrome, ranks high. In boys constitutional delay of growth is the most common cause. If pubertal signs do not match urgent investigation is needed. For example, breast development in girls in the absence of pubic hair, or large testes in boys with relatively small genitals indicate hypothyroidism. Conversely, small testes with advanced genitals and pubic hair suggest an extraneous source of testosterone, for example, Cushing's disease. It is useful to bear in mind that the normal harmony of pubertal signs and growth is the hallmark of constitutional delay. If constitutional delay in growth is the diagnosis and if there is emotional stress in the patient in spite of reassurance, a trial of treatment with an anabolic steroid like oxandrolone 1.25–2.5 mg daily for three to four months may induce the pubertal growth spurt in boys. In the case of girls who have constitutional delay of growth, oestrogen in small doses (for example ethinyl oestradiol 2 ug daily) may be administered to induce growth acceleration. When advance in signs of puberty has occurred the treatment may be stopped on the assumption that spontaneous puberty has started.

Promotion of growth in children

In the rural areas of the developing countries, it is not unusual to find 50 to 60 per cent of children in various stages of growth failure. The causes are mainly environmental, namely, the combined effects of inadequate nutrition and recurrent infection. The approach in such a situation has to be a simple system of growth supervision and health surveillance of children in order to detect those at risk and to bring the health and social resources in the community to bear on such children and their families. The emphasis has to shift from the hospital care of a few cases of disordered growth requiring bio-medical skills for diagnosis and management to a simplified system operated by auxiliary medical personnel aimed at providing a wide coverage of health supervision and selecting those who are not growing adequately. One such system which has proven its usefulness and has become popular is the under-fives' clinic. Crucial to this clinic is the weight chart based on local standards. For a child to benefit from such a system regular attendance at the clinic is essential, hence the clinic must also have a system of home visiting for the follow-up of non-attenders. Establishment of the under-fives' clinic in the rural areas and urban slums will be one major step towards promoting the growth and health of children.

As we have noted, the weaning and the immediate post-weaning period between the ages of four months to two years is critical. Reduced velocity of growth is common and is usually due to a reduction of energy intake besides the eroding influence of infectious illnesses on the lean body mass. Contaminated food causing diarrhoeal illness is another important factor. Awareness of these and other contributory factors in the community is essential so that they can be avoided.

The importance of energy density of the weanling's diet is an advance in our knowledge of paediatric nutrition. In all nutrition education the emphasis has been on the importance of protein, and energy is rarely, if ever, mentioned. Use of edible oils and fats and energy-containing foods such as groundnuts, soyabeans and sesame seeds needs to be emphasised for the preparation of weaning diets.

Another important advance has been in our understanding of the mid-arm circumference as a measure of the lean body mass. This is especially so in children under the age of five years but the relationship also holds true for adults. This then is a parameter of growth which parents, village health workers and even school children can apply for monitoring the growth of young children. A wider application of such techniques in the community will help to detect many early instances of growth failure.

Recurrent diarrhoea with its influence on appetite, the withholding of food by the parents, the malabsorption of nutrients from the gut and so on is an important cause of growth and nutritional disturbance. In recent years an important advance has been made in our understanding of the mechanisms underlying water and electrolyte absorption from the gut. Offering the child a sugar-electrolyte mixture at the onset of diarrhoea not only helps to maintain hydration but is more likely to lead to early recovery in gut function. The application of this knowledge in the home and the village will help avoid the adverse effects of diarrhoeal disease in children.

When the above techniques and knowledge are integrated with child care in the home and within the village it will be possible to evolve a rational approach to the promotion of growth in children. The under-fives' clinic then becomes both a support for such child care activities as well as a springboard for community health programmes.

Monitoring the growth of children by means of regular weighing *and* charting the weight on an appropriate growth chart is a useful way of sensitising the community for the promotion of growth in their children. Minor deviations from the normal or growth faltering can be detected early, and corrective action is taken through counselling or other interventions. Growth monitoring is one of the pillars of UNICEF's Child Survival Revolution; Oral Rehydration, Breast feeding and Immunisation are the other activities in this global programme.

Development

Growth implies increase in size, and development the acquisition of function. But development is more complex than can be described by such a simple definition. It is the process by which a single-celled zygote undergoes programmed changes over time to emerge as a completely formed individual. Genetic factors play a significant role. The remarkable constancy of steps along which development proceeds is the evidence for underlying genetic influences. Environmental influences are equally important. Every stage in development is the product of interactions between the genetic endowment and the environment. The subsequent stage then builds on the preceeding one, and so on. Genetic factors establish the limits of potential, but they are intricately interwoven with environmental experiences. Jointly they bring about the development of the individual.

Development has a great deal to do with the growth and maturation of the brain. Since the brain reaches 50 per cent of the mature weight by the age of six months and 90 per cent by the age of five years, the early years are crucial for development. A great deal of learning is involved, and the foundations for motor, social, linguistic and other learning skills are being laid during the early formative years. At the same time a great deal of acculturation takes place. Thus development is very much culture specific.

Development proceeds along a number of axes, for example, motor, cognitive, linguistic, social, and so on. An understanding of the usual sequence of development is essential in order to be able to diagnose deviations from the normal in time. After carefully observing the development of a large number of normal children several systems for developmental screening have been proposed like for example, the Denver Developmental Screening Test, and the Bayley Mental and Motor Scales. It is always important to bear in mind that all such scales are specific to the culture in which they were originally developed. They always need to be modified and adapted for the local situation.

On average 15 per cent of children will show a developmental problem, and in the case of about two per cent the problem will be a severe one. Suspicion should be aroused when any of the deficiencies shown in table 6.1 occur, and further careful assessment is indicated

Children growing up in disadvantaged circumstances are at risk of falling behind in one or other aspects of their development. Their home environment is very often deficient with inadequate parenting, and fewer opportunities for stimulation. As is often the case, material deprivation is associated with emotional and other difficulties. Disadvantaged children are also prone to frequent episodes of growth faltering because of poor nutrition and recurrent bouts of infection. Early intervention programmes in the form of play groups and nursery schools have been shown to ameliorate the adverse effects of disadvantage. The Head Start Programme in the United States and the Integrated Child Development Scheme in India are two examples of such national programmes.

Table 6.1 Indications for further evaluation

Age	Deficiency
3 months	No reaction to sudden noise
	Does not turn to the speaker
	Does not make eye contact when spoken to
	Does not make any sounds
	Does not raise the head when lying on the stomach
6 months	Does not respond to speech
	Does not respond to being played with
	No smile
	Does not reach out for a toy
1 year	No response to simple games
	Does not imitate speech
	Not standing on his own
	Does not say simple words like 'mama', 'dada'
18 months	Does not vocalise
	Is not moving about to explore
	Does not make eye contact
2 years	Does not name familiar objects or use simple phrases
	Is not noticing objects
	Is not moving about actively
	No eye contact
	Long periods of rocking or head banging
3 years	No speech
	Unaware of other people or children
	Does not play imitating adult activities
	Prolonged periods of repetitive behaviour

Further reading

Ebrahim G J. *Practical mother and child health in developing countries*, 4th Ed. London: Macmillan, 1991.

Gopalan C, Chatterjee M. *Use of growth charts for promoting child nutrition: a review of global experiences.* New Delhi: Nutrition Foundation of India 1985; special publication No. 2.

Morley D, Woodland M. *See how they grow.* London: Macmillan. 1979.

Tanner J M. *Foetus into man: physical growth from conception to maturity.* 2nd edition. Ware: Castlemead Publications. 1990.

7 Defence mechanisms

All living organisms have evolved body defences against invading microbes. In the larger animals, whenever bacteria or toxins gain entrance into the body, certain tissues or population of cells react to remove the intruder. Part of the reaction consists of production of a soluble protein carrying a specific pattern such that it can attach to the surface of the bacteria or the toxin molecule. This attachment facilitates ingestion and removal of the foreign substance by the scavenging cells of the body.

Invertebrates have some effective defences against bacteria yet no invertebrate has anything comparable to mammalian antibody – lymphocyte immune system. On the other hand, all vertebrates have circulating cells with the qualities of the lymphocyte and the capacity to produce antibodies. They are also capable of rejecting grafts from other individuals of the same species. Plasma cells make their first appearance in the fish and are well established in the amphibians, the reptiles, the birds and the mammals. In the evolution of the immune system the first immunoglobulin to appear is IgM in the monomeric form. Later, in the more evolved vertebrates it becomes a macromolecule. IgG appears relatively late in evolution. It may be present in some amphibians but is well established in reptiles, birds and mammals. The spleen and thymus occur in very early forms of vertebrates but lymph nodes are present only in mammals and then only in some and absent in others.

On entry into the body the antigen (which can be a virus, bacteria, parasite or foreign tissue cell, a fragment of some such structure, or a protein or a polysaccharide) moves along the lymphatics and the vascular channels where it is trapped by macrophages. Those macrophages deep within the lymph nodes are loaded with antigen. In the outer part of the lymph node there is a veritable web of fine strands of macrophage cytoplasm. This web traps antigen effectively. The trapped antigen attracts blast cells which begin to multiply and form collections of cells around the antigen. These are the germinal centres. The germinal centres put out lymphocytes which act as memory cells and develop further into antibody-forming cells.

A central feature of the body's defence mechanisms is the production of antibody by a specialised group of cells, the plasma cells. The plasma cells themselves spring from lymphocytes which have been sensitised by exposure to antigen. Each antibody has highly specific affinity with the particular antigen which stimulated its production. The various antibody molecules are surprisingly similar even though they possess an enormous range of specific combining power. If an individual has not been immunised he will still have a good concentration of immunoglobulin in his blood, usually about one per cent by weight. This material is made up of many thousands of antibodies against microorganisms he has encountered during his lifetime or against antigenic substances that accidentally enter the body through the gut, the respiratory tract or the skin.

The immune system

All the different mechanisms of immunity put together form a homeostatic and self-monitoring system whose task it is to maintain the integrity of the body substance. The cells and molecules of the immune system reach most tissues through the blood stream entering the tissues by penetrating through the walls of the capillaries. After travelling through the tissues they make their way back through the lymphatic system. The lymphatics collect the lymphocytes and antibodies along with other cells and molecules as well as the interstitial fluid which bathes all the body tissues, and pour their contents back into the blood stream by means of the thoracic duct. The lymphocytes, the main bulwark of defence, are found in high concentration in the lymph nodes and at other key sites of the immune system such as the bone marrow, the thymus and the spleen (figure 7.1).

Studies on the movements of the lymphocytes have shown that the stem cell in the yolk sac of the embryo later establishes itself in the foetal liver and spleen and, in later post-natal life, in the bone marrow. The lymphoid stem cells coming out of these sites of initial multiplication undergo differentiation by residing in the micro-environment provided by the thymus (T cells) and in the bursa of Fabricus or still unknown sites (B cells). T cells leave the thymus by the blood stream and later enter special regions of the lymph nodes and the spleen called the thymus dependent zones. In these sites as well as elsewhere in the body, the T cells participate in cell-mediated immunity.

The B cells carry a small amount of their specific antibody molecule on the surface of the cell membrane. These act as 'receptors' of the cell. When an antigen fits the receptor, the B lymphocyte is stimulated to produce the specific antibody and to undergo divisions which give rise to a large number of plasma cells. Some of the plasma cells produce

antibody and others carry the 'memory' of the antigen.

Not only is the T cell and B cell function interdependent and supportive of each other but there are also classes of lymphocytes which exert 'helper' or 'suppressor' effects.

The defence mechanisms of the body consist of general host defences as well as specific cellular and humoral systems which work together for the efficient disposal of antigen.

General host defences

Anatomic barriers

Body surface structures constitute physical barriers which prevent the invasion of body tissues by pathogenic microorganisms. Intact dermal, mucosal and endothelial surfaces protect underlying tissues. Specialised cell surfaces such as the ciliated epithelium of the bronchial mucosa help to clear

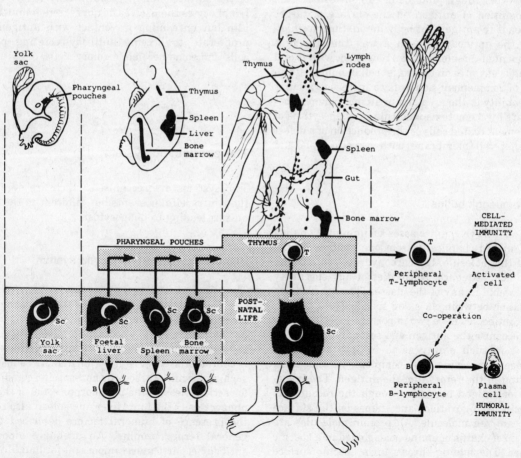

Figure 7.1   The immune system sc=stem cell

foreign particles from the respiratory tract. Endogenous body secretions, such as the acidity in the stomach or presence of lysozyme in tears and saliva, prevent the growth of microorganisms.

Humoral bactericidal systems

These have mechanisms similar to the immune haemolysis of erythrocytes as in Rhesus incompatibility. Such systems are useful for handling organisms of low virulence. For example, many nonpathogenic Gram negative bacilli are destroyed by small amounts of antibody and complement.

The complement system

A system of nine serum proteins interact sequentially to mediate some of the effects of the antigen-antibody reactions. The sequence of complement reaction is triggered by the union of complement fixing antibodies with soluble antigen or with other sites on the surface of the target cells like bacteria, erythrocytes, fungi, protozoa or tumour cells.

Recognition of antigen on the surface of target cells leads to antigen-antibody union. Such a union alters the antibody in such a way that the first component of complement can now react with it and with adjacent sites on the target cell membrane. The effect of complement action is to increase vascular permeability in the area and to attract polymorphonuclears by chemotaxis resulting in phagocytosis of complement coated cells or the production of a defect in target cell membrane with osmotic lysis and death.

The immunoglobulins

There are three main classes of immunoglobulins distinguished chemically from one another by the size of the molecule, the carbohydrate content and amino acid sequence. Antibodies of any specificity can be found in any of the classes. Thus there is no correlation between class and specificity.

The antibodies have two important functions. One is to recognise the antigen and secondly to combine with it in such a way as to initiate a chain of responses, involving the complement and cells, resulting in the removal of the antigen. The recognition of antigen happens through the recognition of specific configurations and shapes on the surface of the antigen molecule. All protein molecules are made up of chains of amino acids folded in a specific manner. The folding throws up a specific surface relief on the molecule. A change of just one amino acid in a polypeptide chain changes the surface pattern sufficiently to be recognised by the antibody molecule. In this way the immune system is able to check on mutant body cells that make mistakes in protein synthesis. It can also differentiate surface patterns of body cells from 'foreign' patterns. This recognition of pattern is an important step in dealing with foreign antigen.

Binding with antigen is dependent on a perfect fit between the shapes of the antigen and the specific antibody. Binding must change the state of the antibody in such a way as to 'turn on' its effector function. Protein molecules are known to alter their function and act as switches by changing their shape. It is believed that union with antigen causes rearrangement of the antibody molecule so that binding sites for complement fixing become exposed together with other sites for effector function.

The B-lymphocytes (figure 7.1) are an essential element in the antibody response to antigen. Between 20 and 30 per cent of peripheral lymphocytes can be identified as B-lymphocytes because of the surface immunoglobulin they carry. The B-lymphocytes themselves do not secrete immunoglobulin but on coming in contact with antigen they proliferate to become antibody-secreting plasma cells and some become 'memory' cells.

The phagocytic system

Two systems are recognised which are similar in their intracellular events but different in the mechanisms leading to phagocytosis.

Humoral mediated phagocytic system

The humoral mediated phagocytic system, of which the polymorphonuclears provide the best example is an effective defence against common pathogens like *Streptococcus, Pneumococcus, Staphylococcus, Hemophilus influenzae* and *Escherichia coli*. This system is characterised by the need for humoral substances such as specific antibody or non-specific complement for action. Besides the polymorphs some of the fixed phagocytes of the lung, liver and spleen also require the presence of humoral factors described by the general term 'opsonins'. An adequate amount of antibody is particularly important for handling pneumococci, streptococci, *Nisseria, H. influenzae,*

Pseudomonas, the *Candida* and many others. In most usual situations the capacity of antibody to facilitate phagocytosis is minimal and requires complement components and other humoral factors for enhancement. During an infective process antigen-antibody reaction, complement fixation, chemotaxis, lysis and the eventual ingestion of the organisms are all occurring simultaneously.

Hundreds of millions of polymorphs enter the blood stream from the marrow and leave the blood stream for the tissues each day. However, only a small percentage of the body's total population of polymorphs is in the blood stream at any one time. The circulating pool is only three to five per cent of the total polymorph population. Another five per cent are extravascular in tissues and up to 90 per cent are in the bone marrow waiting to be released. It is this large pool in the bone marrow which is the source of leucocytosis observed during acute infections.

Cell-mediated phagocytosis

The cell-mediated immune function is primarily responsible for host defence against those organisms which are capable of surviving and replicating within polymorphs. Examples of such organisms are the mycobacteria, fungi, many viruses and some bacteria. The cell-mediated immune function is also involved in graft versus host reactions and in cancer cell surveillance.

The essential element in cell-mediated immunity is the small lymphocyte derived from the stem cells of the bone marrow and processed by the thymus (T cells). The microorganisms which provoke cellular immune response are first recognised by large reticular macrophages in the lymph nodes. These cells carry IgM antibodies on their surface in a loosely attached form. The macrophages are capable of reacting with antigens which are common to a wide variety of microbial, animal and vegetable tissues. The macrophage-processed antigen provokes the small lymphocyte to react and give rise to effector cells and memory cells. The effector cells are capable of releasing cytotoxins, monocyte chemotactic factor and other mediators of inflammation. They induce an accumulation of monocytes which later become scavenger macrophages.

T lymphocytes comprise approximately 60 per cent of circulating blood lymphocytes. They are specifically committed and will respond only to that particular antigen to which they were previously exposed.

Humoral defences of the mucus membrane

Body secretions, especially those of the gut and the respiratory tract as well as the tears and the saliva, contain a specialised form of humoral defence. The gut and the respiratory tract are at the front line of defence since they are continually bombarded by antigens, infective organisms, atmospheric pollutants, dietary additives and similar other harmful agents. Their secretions contain a large amount of IgA produced by the plasma cells in the submucosa. Unlike serum IgA, that in the mucus secretions is made up of two molecules linked by a 'joining chain' and the 'secretory piece'. Both these are peptide chains and the latter allows the dimer of secretory IgA to pass through the lining cells of the mucus membrane. In the gut as well as the respiratory tract and elsewhere, the secretory IgA is capable of forming complexes with antigen and preventing their entry into the body. It is known that in the presence of lysosyme and complement, secretory IgA can kill bacteria. Viruses are neutralised without involving complement and resistance to virus infections is often closely associated with high levels of secretory IgA. For example, influenza virus neutralising IgA is found in high titres in the nasal washings of individuals infected with the influenza virus. Similarly, polio virus neutralising IgA is found in the intestinal secretions of infants following oral polio vaccine.

Dynamics of the immune response

A great deal has been learned about host mechanisms and how they operate. Foreign antigens are first recognised by macrophages, which ingest and process them after which one or more of the resulting peptides are presented on the surface for T cells to recognise. T cells recognise only those antigens which are presented by cells which share the same HLA type. On the surface of the macrophage the processed antigen is presented in intimate conjuction with one of their major histocompatibility complex (MHC) for T cells to recognise. The presenting peptides are recognised by means of specific T cell receptors, which can identify a three dimensional formation made up by the peptide – MHC complex. The formation thus recognised is referred to as an epitope. On recognition the T cell becomes irreversibly committed, discards other receptors, and begins to proliferate. It can now develop into a 'memory' cell which is quiescent but recognises the same antigen if re-exposed; or it becomes an 'effector' cell. The effector cells can either destroy the infecting agent (cytotoxic T cell or CD8) or help B cells to produce antibody (T helper cells or CD4). T cells also release soluble proteins (lymphokines) which recruit inflammatory cells to limit the spread of infection.

B lymphocytes have only one unique receptor on the surface. When a foreign antigen binds with the receptor the cell becomes activated. There is clonal proliferation and maturation to antibody forming plasma cells. Some of the activated B lymphocytes become 'memory' cells. They will mount an antibody response if the original antigen is met again.

Though antibody contributes to the recovery from infective illness, T cells are the main mechanism. In the absence of pronounced antigenic variation the neutralising antibody serves an important function. Together with complement and effector T cells it helps to lyse infected cells. In most cases antibody is sufficient to reduce the infection load from a subsequent challenge for the T cells to cope. However, antibody is very specific and reacts with just a few receptors on the surface of the infecting agent. If there is antigenic drift the antibody is ineffective. On the other hand for diphtheria and tetanus it is necessary to neutralise only the toxin, and a toxin specific antibody is effective.

Host immune response thus depends upon antigen presentation and lymphocyte differentiation. Different components of the immune response to antigenic challenge arise in time dependent fashion. Antibody secreting and memory B cells are present after exposure to antigen. The latter are continually being recruited by persisting antigen to form antibody secreting cells. Memory T cells arise later and persist. For activation they require further exposure to infection.

Infecting pathogens are often elusive targets for the host's defence mechanisms. Rapid multiplication with the possibility of exchange of genes, molecular switches as well as molecular mimicry allow them to evade the immune system of the host. Genetic drift is a common mechanism for a number of pathogens, the best examples being the influenza virus and HIV.

Altered host defences

The newborn

The foetus is capable of mounting an immune response to antigen challenge as early as the twentieth week of gestation. However, the immune response is not so well developed as in the adult, which explains the increased incidence, morbidity and mortality due to sepsis in neonatal life.

The newborn has a well developed humoral immune response at birth. With regard to T cell function, there is no general agreement. Earlier results indicating depressed cell-mediated immunity have now been shown to be due to deficient inflammatory response. There is evidence that the 'suppressor' T cell predominates which can explain depressed cell-mediated immunity as well as decreased antibody response. There is also clear evidence of depressed phagocyte function. In addition, quantitative deficiencies of a number of complement components have been found in cord and neonatal sera.

Besides the above laboratory data, both clinical and epidemiological observations confirm that an immunological gap exists during the newborn period. A mass of new research shows that in the normal situation this gap is filled by the immunological role of breast milk. Several factors have been identified in breast milk which confer immunological protection on the baby, for example

(1) The baby receives maternal antibodies in both the colostrum and mature milk. These antibodies are carried in the secretory IgA which constitutes a major proportion of the whey proteins of milk. Even in undernourished women the concentration of IgA is 340 mg per 100 ml in the colostrum and 136 mg per 100 ml in mature milk. Both IgG and IgM are also present in human milk.

The human placenta can transfer only IgG and the infant is born immunologically unprotected. Absence of IgA renders the infant defenceless against intestinal and respiratory infections during the early weeks of life and the relative lack of IgM reduces the resistance of the vascular space to infection and subsequent bacteraemia. In both these respects breast milk is the newborn's best protection.

(2) The effect of secretory IgA in discouraging the growth of E.coli in the newborn gut is supplemented by further protective substances in breast milk. Lactoferin, an iron-binding protein, works synergistically with antibodies as well as lysozyme and complement to suppress the growth of E.coli and promote instead the growth of lactobacillus.

(3) Secretory IgA also acts to reduce the entry of antigen through the gut wall of the newborn. There is both clinical and epidemiological evidence to show that in families with a strong tendency to atopic disease, breast feeding provides significant protection.

(4) Breast feeding also helps to avoid early exposure to cow's milk protein which carries a powerful allergic challenge for the newborn at a time when the immune mechanisms are not fully developed. Avoidance of cow's milk feeds is specially indicated in families with a strong history of allergy.

(5) Human milk is a live biological system with abundant numbers of cells averaging 1 to 2 x 10^6 leucocytes per ml. Of these, 85 per cent are monocytes or macrophages and 11 per cent are small lymphocytes with equal proportions of T and B cells. Functional tests have shown these cells to be capable of responding to mitogens and antigens and of phagocytosing bacteria. Milk lymphocytes are capable of responding to the Ki antigen of *E.coli* and this explains the extremely rare occurrence of *E.coli meningitis* in breast fed infants. The macrophages have also an active role and are known to confer protection from necrotising enterocolitis.

Nutritional status and host defence

Clinical and epidemiological observations reveal a high incidence of mortality and prolonged ill-health following infections in malnourished individuals. These observations have led to detailed study of the immune response in malnutrition.

It is well known that the central as well as the peripheral lymphoid organs of the immune system show evidence of gross and microscopic damage during malnutrition. For example, the thymus in four-month old healthy children weighs about 25 g but in malnourished children of comparable age the gland weighs less than 10 g and frequently 1 g. The histology of the thymus in malnutrition varies according to the degree of malnutrition. There is a progressive loss of cortico-medullary differentiation together with lymphocytic depletion, interstitial fibrosis and degenerative changes. Similar changes are noticeable in the peripheral lymphoid organs also. The spleen is small and has fewer and smaller germinal centres. The lymph nodes too lose their germinal centres. Such changes explain the very specific pattern of infection noticed during malnutrition. There is an increased tendency for Gram negative septicaemia, disseminated *Herpes simplex* infection, afebrile response to infection and the occurrence of gangrene instead of suppuration. This pattern is not very different from the one seen in newborns, the post-measles state, some reticuloses, patients on immunosuppressive agents and after burns. The severity of measles and whooping cough in poorly nourished communities is well known, and is largely due to the inability of the host to mount a strong immune response.

The antibody response in malnutrition

The serum levels of all immunoglobulin classes are often elevated in malnutrition. The proportion as well as absolute numbers of B-lymphocytes in blood is not altered. In general, the antibody response is normal but some vaccines fail to elicit a response and others not. The explanation is that some antigens are dependent on B cells only for antibody production and others require the presence of T cells as well in order to co-operate with B cells. It is the usual experience that those vaccines which are primarily B cell dependent produce adequate antibody responses in undernourished individuals. On the basis of clinical experience in children suffering from various forms of immunodeficiency diseases, the following immune mechanisms can be postulated for different microbial agents (table 7.1). The ability of malnourished individuals to withstand those infections where the main body defence mechanism is humoral tends to be reasonably good.

However, it is important to bear in mind that factors other than nutrition can influence the immune response. For example, it is well known that during infection with measles virus, the immune response is depressed. There is also laboratory and epidemiological evidence to suggest that a similar suppression of immune response occurs with malarial infection.

Table 7.1 Main body defence mechanisms against various pathogens

Main defence mechanisms	Pathogens
Humoral immune response	*Pneumococcus* *Hemophilus influenzae* *Streptococcus* *Meningococcus* *Pseudomonas aeruginosa* *Hepatitis virus* *Pneumocystis carinii*
Cellular immune response	*Rubella virus* *Varicella virus* *Vaccinia virus* *Cytomegalic virus* *Mycobacterium tuberculosis* *Mycobacterium leprae* *Candida albicans* *Histoplasma capsulatum*

Secretory IgA

Secretory IgA is reduced in mucus secretions during malnutrition. This would result in an impaired response with IgA antibody to viral antigens on mucosal surfaces. For example, oral polio vaccine is much less effective in developing countries compared to its effectiveness in the West. In addition to interference from other enteric viruses, reduced response of the mucosal surface may be a factor.

The gut flora undergo both qualitative and quantitative changes in malnourished subjects. Invasion of the proximal gut by microflora whose normal habitat is the distal small intestine, results in altered digestive function and a tendency to diarrhoea. Defective antigen clearing due to faulty secretory IgA mechanism secondary to malnutrition is thought to be the cause of the altered profile of the gut flora. When undernourished children are fed adequately, there is a return to normal.

Phagocyte function

Phagocyte function is severely affected in malnutrition. For example, in kwashiorkor, leucocytosis often fails to occur in the presence of infection. Moreover, the leucocytes in kwashiorkor show diminished phagocytic activity as well as decreased bactericidal capacity.

Cell-mediated immunity

Cell-mediated immunity is altered in malnutrition. A negative tuberculin test in the presence of infection with *M.tuberculosis* is a common occurrence in malnourished children. Laboratory studies in such children have revealed a significant reduction in the number of T-lymphocytes as well as impaired function. No improvement in cell function or number can be demonstrated even after four weeks of treatment. This suggests that prolonged nutritional rehabilitation may be necessary for the restoration of normal immune response. In clinical paediatric practice, prolonged observation and care of children recovering from malnutrition is essential. This is especially so with regard to children who suffered malnutrition in early life since experiments in laboratory animals suggest that early nutritional deprivation can lead to a permanent reduction in the number of T-lymphocytes. For example, it has been shown that infants who are born small for dates, presumably due to intrauterine malnutrition, show low levels of T-lymphocytes for several years (figure 7.2). Besides undernutrition of the mother, a common cause of low birth weight in the tropics is placental infection with malarial parasites. These observations provide a strong reason in favour of prophylaxis against malaria during pregnancy.

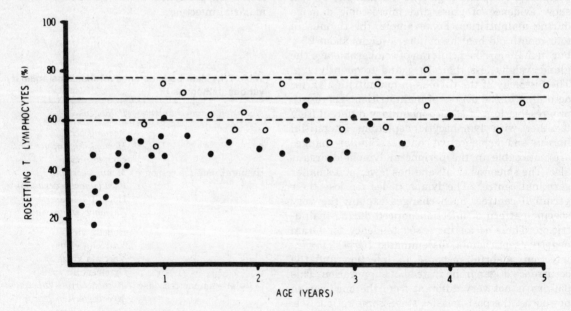

Figure 7.2   Cell-mediated immunity in small for date infants. O denotes infants with persistent growth retardation.   Source: R K Chandra; 1976

A common cause of depressed cell-mediated immunity is infection itself. Decreased cutaneous hypersensitivity to tuberculin in measles and after several viral vaccines is now well recorded, even in healthy children. Also in the case of measles it is known that malnourished children tend to excrete the virus in nasopharyngeal secretions, in skin flakes, and probably from other sources for a longer period compared to well-nourished children. In the case of measles, as also in many other infections, the immune response is dependent upon the host's nutritional status, the dose of the invading organisms, and their virulence.

Interaction of nutrition and infection

Malnutrition does not occur alone. In communities where nutritional deficiencies are common there also exists poor hygiene, over-crowding, insanitary living conditions, poverty and ignorance, all of which contribute to the prevalence of poor nutrition as well as infection. Sufficient clinical, epidemiological and laboratory data exist to indicate a synergism between infection and malnutrition. In severe bacterial infections such as tuberculosis and typhoid, the nitrogen loss in the urine can be as high as the equivalent of the nitrogen content of 2.3 kg of muscle. In severe pneumonia, the loss of vitamin A in the urine has been estimated at 1000 μg/day. Episodes of infections occurring in close proximity will not only prevent the recovery of the nutritional status of the host but also that of the immune mechanisms. Thus, not only do trivial infections become severe, but there is also an increased incidence of complications following common childhood infections such as whooping cough, measles and diarrhoea.

Intervention programmes
Immunisation

All vaccines do not have the same efficacy. Depending on the antigen, the adjuvant used, the care taken during storage and transport, as well as population coverage the efficacy of immunisation in the control of common infectious illnesses will vary. In the past decade a great deal of progress has been achieved in the developing world by the Expanded Programme of Immunisation (EPI). In 1974 when the programme commenced only five per cent of children under one year old in developing countries were immunised. By the end of the 1980s two-thirds of the child population aged less than one year in the developing world was immunised against the six main vaccine preventable diseases, namely poliomyelitis, diphtheria, whooping cough, tetanus, measles and tuberculosis.

In the more developed countries the target is now for the elimination of these diseases. In the Americas poliomyelitis has been brought under control, and in the European Region of the World Health Organisation the target is now to eliminate whooping cough, tetanus and poliomyelitis in the 1990s.

Experience with EPI has taught that the availability of vaccines is not enough and by itself does not make a programme. There should be channels for regular supply, facilities for adequate storage and transport carefully watched over by a supervisor. There should also exist an efficient system of surveillance to ensure that a sufficiently large number of children in the towns, villages and in the district as a whole are being immunised. The minimum target to aim for is 80 per cent. Even though for infections like measles the concept of herd immunity may not apply, a target of coverage is useful. There should also be periodic campaigns of mass vaccination in order to cover those children who may have been missed out because of non-attendance at the clinics. In addition, a programme of notification of all vaccine preventable diseases will help to identify new pockets of infections in the district. Mini campaigns can then be carried out in and around these pockets to isolate them and to protect all susceptibles in the neighbourhood.

The strategy of clinic based immunisation all the year round, however important for the protection of the attenders, may not be adequate for breaking the chain of transmission because it tends to leave enough susceptible children. This is what happened in the past in the developing world with regard to polio, measles and whooping cough. With EPI new strategies have evolved. In the case of *polio*, the strategy of annual vaccination in a short period of time of all children in a specified age group, regardless of the number of doses previously administered, has proved highly successful in Cuba (since 1962/63), in most of Brazil (since 1980), in the Dominican Republic (since 1983), in Paraguay (since 1985) and in Mexico (since 1986). For *measles* a slightly different approach has been evolved. It involves initial vaccination in a short period of time of all the children nine months of age to under five or ten years (depending on the age by which about 95 per cent of the reported cases occur) regardless of previous history of disease or vaccination, followed by subsequent annual campaigns for vaccinating the new generation of children. This strategy has been successfully used in Cuba (since 1986) and in the state of Sao Paulo in Brazil (since 1987).

The best vaccines are worthless without an adequate system of storage, delivery, coverage, surveillance and monitoring of incidence together with an aggressive approach for the containment of infectious disease.

Schedule of immunisation

There is a continuing debate about an effective schedule of immunisation for developing countries. The earlier schedules were based on the response to older vaccines. With further experience and improved vaccines it has become increasingly clear that if sufficient time (six to eight weeks) is allowed between doses and even longer time (four to six months) between the second and third dose, then a booster fourth dose is no longer necessary. Also, in the event of the schedule being interrupted, there is no need to start the series of injections all over again. In most cases immunity will have been achieved despite long intervals between doses.

Based on the above principles table 7.2 shows a recommended schedule of immunisation. The basic plan is to provide protection in the first year of life

Table 7.2 Recommended schedule of immunisation

Age or visit	Vaccine
Antenatal period	Tetanus toxoid to the mother (2 doses in the last trimester if not previously immunised. One dose if immunised.)
Birth	BCG; oral polio.
One month (or first visit)	Triple antigen (DPT); oral polio. (BCG if not previously immunised.)
Second month (or second visit)	Triple antigen; oral polio.
After nine months	Measles; triple antigen; polio.
Entry to school	BCG; diphtheria and tetanus; oral polio.

against those infections which are known to cause severe illness in early childhood, and to follow this up by booster immunisations.

Table 7.3 Rates of complications compared with adverse reactions

	Complication rates per 100 000 cases of the disease	Adverse reaction per 100 000 immunisations
BCG		
Disseminated BCG infection		<0.1
Osteitis/osteomyelitis		<0.1 – 30
Suppurative adenitis (<2 years old)		100 – 4300
Polio		
Paralytic polio		
-in vaccinee		0.1
-in close contact		0.02
Pertussis		
Permanent brain damage	600 – 2 000	0.2 – 0.6
Death	100 – 4 000	0.2
Encephlopathy	90 – 4 000	0.1 – 0.3
Convulsions	600 – 8 000	0.3 – 90
Shock	–	0.5 – 30
Measles		
Encephalitis	50 – 400	0.1
Subacute sclerosing panencephalitis	0.5 – 2.0	0.05 – 0.1
Convulsions	500 – 1 000	0.02 – 190
Deaths	10 – 10 000	0.02 – 0.3

The rates of adverse complications following immunisation compared with complication rates of disease if the immunisation is withheld are given in table 7.3.

With regard to the indications for immunisation WHO has made the following general recommendations.

(1) Use every contact as an opportunity for immunisation.

(2) BCG and OPV can safely and effectively be given to the newborn and DPT and OPV as early as 6 weeks of life (and even earlier if need be). In countries where measles poses a major threat before the first birthday, measles vaccine should ordinarily be given at the age of nine months.

(3) No vaccine is totally without adverse reactions, but the risks of serious complications from BCG, the triple vaccine, OPV and measles are much lower than the risks from natural diseases.

(4) The decision to withhold immunisation should be taken only after serious consideration of the potential consequences for the individual child and the community.

(5) It is particularly important to immunise children suffering from malnutrition. Low grade fever, mild respiratory infections or diarrhoea, and other minor illnesses should not be considered as contraindications to immunisation.

(6) Immunisation of children so ill as to require hospitalisation should be deferred for decision by more skilled personnel.

(7) The immunisation status of hospitalised children should be evaluated, and they should receive appropriate immunisation before discharge, or even before admission.

(8) A second or third DPT injection should not be given to a child who has suffered a severe adverse reaction to the previous dose. The pertussis component should be omitted, and diphtheria and tetanus immunisation completed.

(9) Diarrhoea should not be considered a contraindication to OPV, but to ensure full protection doses given to children with diarrhoea should not be counted as part of the series. The child should be given another dose at the first available opportunity.

Viability of vaccines

All vaccines are sensitive biological products which can be easily destroyed by adverse conditions of storage and transport. In addition, live vaccines are extremely sensitive to sunlight and other forms of ultraviolet light. During storage and transport temperatures between 3–7°C should be rigorously maintained and direct exposure to sunlight avoided.

It is not generally appreciated that even within the optimum temperature range of between 3–7°C, fluctuations of temperature can be harmful. The frequency of such fluctuations will depend upon the frequency with which the refrigerator is opened. Hence other items such as medicines, perishable foods, and cool drinks should not be stored in the same refrigerator as vaccines (figure 7.3). For the same reason, chest type refrigerators are better than the cupboard type for the storage of vaccines.

New vaccines

A number of innovative approaches are being used to develop more effective vaccines utilising the new knowledge about immune functions and genetics. For example, in some infections the immune response is evoked by one or more peptides in the epitope. In such instances synthetic peptides can be important starting points for vaccines. When the peptide is presented to the immune system together with epitopes for helper T cells and B cells in an appropriate configuration, a powerful immune response can be evoked in the case of some vaccines. In the case of *menigococci, pneumococci* and *H.influenzae* the epitopes contain carbohydrates as well as amino acids. Vaccines containing a polysaccharide as antigen are less effective in evoking T cell response in young children in whom macrophages are less competent at antigen presentation. A better response can be evoked when the polysaccharide is conjugated with a protein. Measles vaccine as currently employed in the EPI programme has been effective in lowering measles related mortality in developing countries. However, in sub-Saharan Africa up to a third of the cases occur in children below the age of nine months which is the recommended age of vaccination. Certain vaccine strains can generate antibody as early as four to six months of age, and vaccines made from these strains are likely to be recommended for countries where transmission occurs early in life. Another candidate for improvement is the pertussis vaccine. The current vaccine consists of *B.pertussis* cells that have been killed by heat or formalin. Up to 3000 different antigens have been identified in the vaccine. Many are toxic and cause serious side effects. The more important ones have been isolated and chemically purified. Pertussis toxin which is antigenically more important has been genetically modified and rendered less toxic. A number of acellular vaccines are

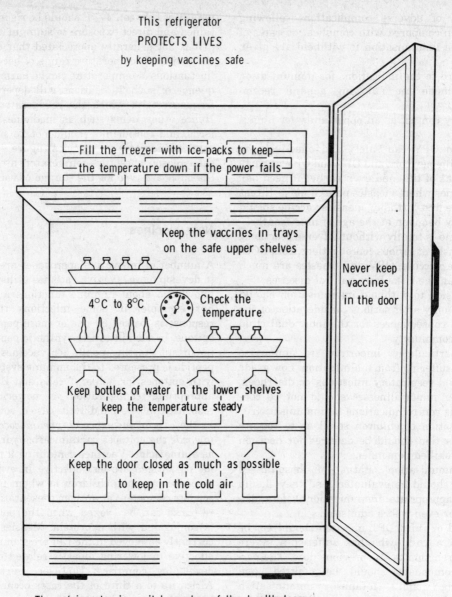

Figure 7.3 Storage of vaccines

undergoing trials, and a safe vaccine is expected to be on the market in the near future.

Genetically engineered recombinant vaccine against hepatitis B is now already on the market. Precisely targeted mutations within crucial genes of the infecting agent have been used to produce recombinant mutants which can become candidates for new vaccines, for example against enteric fever. Such mutant typhoid strains (for example Ty21a) can be used as vectors for the plasmid of *Shigella sonnei*. The hybrid strains express antigens against both *S.typhi* and *S.sonnei* on their surface, and are the starting point for a vaccine against both. Similar encouraging developments are reported with regard to *V.cholera*, *E.coli* and rotaviruses.

The experiences gained with the EPI programme and the social/political mobilisation achieved have been timely. The infrastructure, delivery systems and methodologies of evaluation will enable countries to benefit from the recent scientific advances. Exciting prospects lie ahead for the control of the major infectious diseases.

Service programmes

Urban and rural poverty is at the heart of the problem of infection in malnourished populations. It is obvious that health and nutrition interventions cannot relieve poverty nor change the structure of society. Health workers, however, need to recognise the facts of poverty and make sure that the actions and programmes they recommend will not aggravate poverty. In all interventions proposed, an element of improving the quality of life of the poor should be included. The law of inverse care operates in all societies and health workers need to ensure all the time that their services are reaching out to the poorest sections of society. To that effect the nutritional and welfare implications of the plans and strategies of various government and aid organisations should be kept constantly under review.

Effective interventions require an infrastructure designed to penetrate the ecosystem and the social and cultural life of the people. To deal with the synergism of malnutrition and infection, a synergism of services is necessary. Many services like surveillance of growth, immunisation, nutrition education, primary curative care, family planning, as well as some social services can be delivered through the under-fives' clinic described in chapter 6. Depending upon the health personnel available, such clinics can operate at varying grades of complexity ranging from the health-centre clinic operated by the auxiliary to the village clinic under the part-time health worker. But at each level the primary function of the clinic is to inculcate self-reliance in health and to improve the parents' understanding of the needs of children.

Early treatment

Early treatment of common illnesses brings about rapid improvement in appetite and thereby diminishes the effect of infection on nutritional status. This is especially so with regard to diarrhoeal dis-

ease. The contribution of diarrhoea to ill health in the child can be considerable. For example, in South India there were 22 episodes annually per child aged 6 to 11 months, and in Guatemala it is thought that children under two were ill with diarrhoea 10–14 per cent of the time. The success rate of treatment with oral rehydration is high, being in the range of 85 to 95 per cent, depending on the severity of diarrhoea.

The feeding of children during convalescence has not received enough attention. A sick child loses up to one to two per cent of body mass daily. It is more in measles, whooping cough and diarrhoea and less in respiratory infection. Such a loss must be recovered during convalescence. Early treatment, as mentioned above, will bring about improvement of appetite early and cut short the deterioration in nutritional status. Secondly, increased intake of calories during convalescence will initiate rapid catch-up growth. The normal pre-school child grows well at a calorie intake of 150 cal/kg daily. Just doubling the calorie intake by increasing the calorie density of the convalescent diet for a period of time equal to the duration of illness will expedite restoration of lean body mass.

In a community-orientated programme, self-reliance and increased awareness of health needs can be promoted in several ways. For example, it is known that up to 35 per cent of babies born in developing countries have low birth weights of less than 2500 g. Most of them are small in weight-for-age. A clear relationship has been shown in several studies between weight at birth and subsequent morbidity.

Maternal malnutrition, especially inadequate energy intake during the latter half of pregnancy, is largely responsible for retardation of foetal growth. With only a little increase of food intake, such as cooking an extra handful of rice daily, the energy needs of pregnancy and lactation can be met, and adequate growth of the foetus ensured.

Some of the simple interventions mentioned above are effective if there is good rapport between the providers of health care and the community. It requires regular contacts, consultation, ongoing dialogue and the setting up of programmes of primary health care. The providers of health care must appear to be continually concerned about the health of the people, especially the vulnerable groups. Just the provision of services or making health technology available is not enough. The continuing utilisation of health services by the maximum number and the development of appropriate interventions at the village level should become the main challenges in organising service programmes.

Further reading

Dudgeon J A. Immunising procedures in childhood. In:
Hull D. (ed.) *Recent advances in paediatrics* (5) Edinburgh and London: Churchill Livingstone, 1976.

Faulk W P, Mata L J, Edsall G. Effects of malnutrition on
the immune response in humans: a review. *Trop Dis
Bull* 1975; 72(2): 89.

Roitt I, Brostoff J, Male D. *Immunology*. London; Gower
Medical Publishing Ltd, 1985.

Section III

Infections and the Child in the Tropical Environment

8   *Measles*

Measles is a common infectious disease of childhood with a world-wide distribution. In the 1970s when vaccines were reaching only 10 to 20 per cent of the children in the developing world measles was claiming an estimated 5 million lives of children annually. The 1980s have witnessed an immunisation revolution in the developing world. Even though in many countries measles vaccine has been introduced only recently the spread of vaccination has been rapid on account of an efficient infrastructure for the Expanded Programme of Immunisation. Between 1980 and 1988 the immunisation rate against measles increased from 15 to 59 per cent in the developing world. The main reason for this remarkable improvement in rates is the massive immunisation programmes in densely populated countries like China, India, Pakistan, Indonesia, Nigeria and Brazil. However, a great deal still remains to be done.

Most global estimates in the late 1980s indicated that more than 1 million children a year were dying from acute measles. The actual number of deaths may be even higher. In addition, the impact of delayed mortality following measles infection is only now being realised. Many months after they contract measles children continue to suffer from higher levels of mortality and morbidity compared to those who have not had measles.

With a highly contagious disease like measles immunisation rates of even 80 per cent are not enough to contain epidemics. Continuous maintenance of immunisation to achieve rates in excess of 90 per cent are needed to break the chain of transmission (figures 8.1 and 8.2).

Because measles is an ubiquitous disease of children with no effective treatment, it has given rise to various beliefs and practices. Rural societies have recognised its seriousness since ancient times,

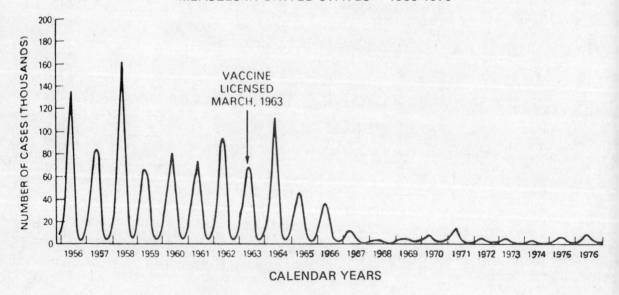

Figure 8.1   Measles in the United States

which is shown in several proverbs like 'Small-pox will make your children blind but measles will send them to the grave'. Because of various superstitions, children are often not brought for medical care and attention. For example, in Northern Nigeria it is believed that an injection given to the child with measles will lead to his death. The local method of treatment is to cover the child's body with chalk powder and to give him palm wine to drink. The latter may even be smuggled into a hospital by the parents. In India, the rash of measles is ascribed to the visitation of a goddess and the child may be hidden away lest the health workers come to know about him. Many societies consider the rash of measles to be due to 'heat' in the body, and so the various foods considered as 'hot' are not allowed in the diet.

Such traditional attitudes, combined with other factors like measles being a common illness of children, the general lack of vital statistics and the absence of therapeutic measures have led to insufficient understanding of the seriousness of the disease. With a good system of follow-up care and maintenance of records it should not be difficult to measure the contribution of measles to child morbidity in rural communities.

The severity of measles in developing countries as compared to its milder nature in Western countries is not due to a difference in the virulence of the virus but because of host factors. Thus, measles in expatriate European children and in higher socio-economic groups of the indigenous populations in developing countries is a mild disease no different from the type encountered in the West. In the other groups the high incidence of mortality is related to overcrowding and poor socio-economic circumstances.

Two other important host factors are the age of the child and his nutritional status. It is known that the younger the child, the more serious is the outcome. The age at which measles occurs in many tropical countries is often below 24 months and over 30 per cent of cases may occur before the age of one year in some regions. This contrasts with Britain, for example, where the mean age was 52 months before the vaccination programme in 1966. Most deaths from measles in developing countries occur in the second year when nutritional disorders in children are also common.

In the extended family systems of the developing countries exposure to infection occurs at an early

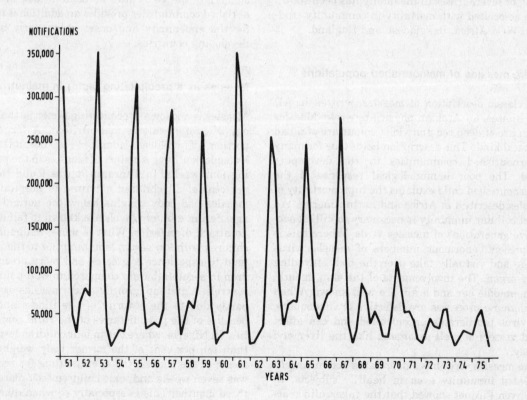

Figure 8.2   Measles in the UK

Table 8.1   Age of occurrence of measles

Country	Mean age of measles (months)
Ghana	24.7
Jordan	18.0
Nigeria, Eastern	21.5
Nigeria, Western	16.5
Tanzania, Zambia, Zimbabwe	29.7
Uganda, Kenya, Malawi	18.5
England and Wales	51.7

age (table 8.1). When infection is acquired before the age of six months the risk of mortality in the next five years tends to be three times more compared to children in whom the infection occurred after that age.

Normally the index case in the family is infected through a chance contact outside the home. The secondary cases are infected within the home through close and continuing contact with the index case, and thus receive a comparatively heavy dose of the virus. Intensive exposure to the index case because of overcrowding in the home can be a more important determinant of measles mortality. Clustering of several cases in the family has been shown to be associated with mortality in community studies in West Africa, Bangladesh and England.

Severe measles of malnourished populations

In a classic description of measles, written in AD 850, Rhazes, an Arabian physician, wrote 'Measles which are of deep red and violet colour are of a bad and fatal kind.' This description holds true for many undernourished communities in the developing world. The poor immunological response of the undernourished child explains the high mortality of measles described in Africa and Latin America. An intact cellular immunity is necessary to kill off successive generations of measles virus. Where this is not present, enormous numbers of measles virus invade and virtually take over the body, invading every organ. The involvements of the skin, mouth, lungs, middle ear and brain are well known. When the immune processes are defective or inadequate, the virus proliferates uncontrolled and can affect blood vessels as well as organs like the liver and kidney.

The measles virus has a depressing action on cell-mediated immunity even in healthy subjects. In 1908, von Pirquet showed that the tuberculin reaction became negative during an attack of measles.

Moniliasis, herpes and tuberculosis, infections normally controlled by cell-mediated immunity, are known to follow measles. More recent studies of lymphocyte function in measles have shown that T cells were depleted and up to 37 per cent of them carried the virus. Seven per cent of B cells also carried the virus but their numbers were not depleted. Such studies have led to the recognition of lymphocyte response in measles as an important prognostic sign. When children with measles show severe lymphopenia defined as an absolute lymphocyte count of less than 2000 per cu mm within two days of the appearance of the rash, the risks of death or progression to chronic chest disease are high. The persistence of such lymphopenia for at least a fortnight after onset of rash is also a reliable predictive sign of developing complications or mortality.

Giant cells carrying measles virus are excreted in the urine and can also be identified in nasal aspirates and stools during an acute attack of measles. In the well-nourished child these cells are found for up to about three days before and after the appearance of the rash. In severe measles, these cells are excreted for a fortnight or more. Malnourished children who tend to get severe measles also excrete the virus for a prolonged period. This prolonged persistence of the virus after an acute attack in malnourished communities provides an additional reason for the endemicity and onset at an early age in developing countries.

Measles as a precipitating factor in malnutrition

Measles is a known precipitating factor in the etiology of protein-calorie malnutrition. A large proportion of children admitted to hospital with kwashiorkor have a history of measles in the preceding four weeks. In Tanzania it was found that 60 per cent of all children admitted to hospital with measles had body weights below the normal average. Serum albumin levels are known to fall during an attack of measles. What is more, malnourished children with low serum albumin prior to the illness tend to experience a greater and more precipitate drop in serum albumin compared to well-nourished controls. Catch-up growth after measles is slow, partly due to the severity of the illness and also because of the poor dietaries of the rural communities. In Nigeria, where one in four children lost more than ten per cent of the former body weight as a result of the illness, the average time for recovery was seven weeks and some children took more than three months. This is especially so when diarrhoea is a complication of measles.

Table 8.2

	Day	Event
Exposure	0	Entry of virus in the upper respiratory tract
Incubation period	1	Multiplication in regional lymph node
		Primary viraemia
		Lodgement in viscera and multiplication there
		Secondary viraemia
Prodromata	10	
Rash	14	
Recovery phase	15–17	Appearance of antibody in the blood stream

Measles causes losses of vitamin A from the body. In endemic areas it is a common precipitating agent of blinding malnutrition.

Characteristics of the measles virus

Measles virus belongs to the group of paramyxo viruses characterised by an internal core of RNA and an outer envelope of glycoproteins and lipids. The glycoproteins are important in immune protection responses. The immune responses include haemagglutination antibody response (HA) and the fusion of cells to form multinucleated giant cells (F). The corresponding immune responses are haemagglutination inhibition as well as complement fixing antibody production.

Measles resembles very closely two animal viruses, namely, canine distemper and the rinderpest virus. Both of these cause illnesses in animals having similarities to measles in man. Other viruses of the myxo-virus group which cause illness in man are the influenza and the mumps viruses. However, virus variation does not occur in the case of measles as in influenza and in consequence no 'new' virus epidemics are known to occur. There are no natural reservoirs and the measles virus relies on a continuous supply of susceptible hosts for endemicity. Because of this, the incidence of measles in a community is governed by the immune status of the population. There is also no carrier state known with measles. Thus the pattern of infection is one of continuous endemic infection with periodic 'epidemics' every two or three years when a sufficient number of susceptibles builds up.

In the pathogenesis of measles the most interesting feature of the virus is its association with mononuclear leucocytes and lymphoid tissue in which the virus replicates and by which it is disseminated within the body.

The measles virus is highly contagious. The secondary attack rate in susceptible household contacts was 75–80 per cent in a multi-centre study in the United States. Clinical and epidemiologic evidence suggests that measles is transmitted by droplet infection from nasopharyngeal secretions and that the portal of entry is the mucosa of the respiratory tract. During the incubation period of 14 days a series of events occur in the body before the onset of the disease as indicated in table 8.2.

Clinical picture (figure 8.3)

In a typical case of unmodified measles the incubation period between contact and appearance of rash is approximately two weeks. The prodromal symptoms of coryza, conjunctivitis, nasal discharge, cough, fever and a red mouth precede the rash by three or four days and the koplik spots on the buccal mucosa by one to two days. During this period virus can be recovered from the blood, urine and especially the nasopharyngeal secretions.

The fever rises abruptly as the rash appears; the child becomes very ill and presents a picture of misery, with a hacking cough, irritable, unable to sleep and refusing all feeds.

The rash spreads over the rest of the body and in about two days reaches the feet. At this point the temperature drops and there is rapid improvement in the clinical condition of the child. The fading of the rash follows the same sequence as its appearance, leaving behind a brownish discolouration and desquamation, which may take about two weeks to disappear.

During the illness, cervical lymph nodes may be palpable or there may be splenomegaly. Gastrointestinal symptoms and sores in the mouth are additional problems in some cases.

Complications

The commonest complications occur in the respiratory tract. Of 171 children seen in the paediatric wards in Kampala, Uganda, 96 had diffuse pulmonary involvement described as bronchopneumonia, 19 had laryngotracheobronchitis and 15 had anatomically segmental lesions. A large proportion of

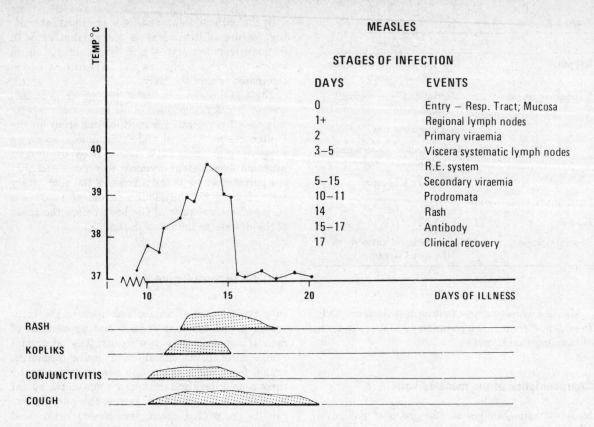

Figure 8.3 Natural history of measles

children suffering from measles will show radiological evidence of lung involvement in the form of interstitial pneumonia or bronchiolitis with air-trapping. Similar X-ray appearances have been described in other viral illnesses also and are largely due to viral pneumonitis during which giant cells are present in the lung parenchyma. In the uncomplicated case of measles there is complete resolution. Giant cell pneumonia has been described in children with altered immune states as in the case of malignancies or during treatment with immuno-suppressant drugs. This form of pneumonia is almost uniformly fatal.

Secondary bacterial infection of the lung is common and is responsible for almost half the mortality from measles. Such secondary infection is usually encountered when the patient is well on the way to recovery. A week to 10 days after the onset of the rash, fever returns, the coughing intensifies and X-ray of the chest shows consolidation. Energetic antibiotic management greatly improves the outlook.

Laryngotracheobronchitis is one of the most life-threatening complications of severe measles, made

worse by the lack of facilities for intensive care needed for such children. The management consists of providing humidity, intravenous and oral rehydration and provision of oxygen. Most of all these children need close observation to keep the airway clear.

Exacerbation of a latent tuberculous focus is a common complication. In such a situation the child does not completely recover after the attack of measles. There is weight loss, persistent cough and later on low-grade fever. Diagnosis is often difficult because the tuberculin test is invariably negative and the chest X-ray may be non-specific. This is a situation where a trial of therapy with anti-tuberculous drugs may be life-saving.

Nutritional problems arise during the illness as the intake of food is often difficult because of soreness of the mouth. The red mouth may reflect the rash of measles on the oral mucosa. On the other hand, it may be due to a superimposed *Candida* infection which is at times extensive and very painful. Similarly, *Herpes* infection can also occur causing painful and extensive ulcers on the tongue, the buccal mucosa and the palate. These bleed easily and there is usually a blood-stained thick mucoid discharge. These children tend to be extremely ill and the 'slimy mouth' of measles is a danger signal. The painful lesion and toxaemia interfere greatly with the child's ability to eat and contribute to his deteriorating nutrition.

Loss of specific nutrients, especially vitamin A, is common so that xerophthalmia and keratomalacia are often added complications. *Herpes* can also invade the eye in measles causing severe dendritic ulcers on the cornea and is another cause of blindness following severe measles.

Diarrhoea is a common accompanying symptom of severe measles. It may become severe enough to cause dehydration. Anorexia and abdominal discomfort will contribute to decreased intake of food. In some children protein-losing enteropathy has been described. All of this contributes to a rapid deterioration in the nutritional status of the child.

Neurological complications are rare but are extremely serious when they occur and always lead to neurological deficit. These are either in the form of a post-infectious encephalitis or a much slower process of sub-acute sclerosing panencephalitis.

In an analysis of clinical features most frequently associated with death the following were commonest: confluent or haemorrhagic rash; darkening of rash or desquamating in large plaques; signs of laryngeal obstruction; evidence of dehydration; diarrhoeal stools more than five per day; convulsions, or loss of consciousness; and weight below the tenth percentile. In children less than three months old, additional features like soreness of the mouth and dyspnoea were significant.

Management

Bed rest with antipyretics and sedatives to make the child more comfortable and an adequate fluid intake are the usual requirements. The nutrition should be maintained with frequent small feeds and a varied diet to stimulate a failing appetite. Antimicrobial therapy will be required to deal with superadded bacterial infections.

Regular twice daily toilet of the mouth and the eyes is necessary to prevent complications. Oral administration of multivites, especially vitamin A, will help to avoid xerophthalmia. Children with malaria parasites in the blood or intestinal parasites require treatment with antimalarials and the appropriate vermifuge.

Several studies have shown the beneficial effects of vitamin A 400000 i.u. in severe measles. Recovery from complications like pneumonia and diarrhoea is more rapid, the duration of illness is shorter and mortality rates are lower among children given vitamin A.

Measles vaccine

With the advent of the vaccine against measles, control and even eradication of the disease have become distinct possibilities.

The vaccines currently in use have been derived from the Edmonston strain of the virus. After several passages a vaccine containing a live attenuated measles virus causing the least number of reactions and an adequate immune response is now marketed.

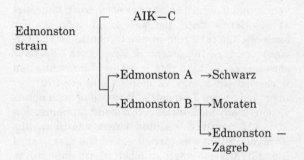

Other strains are:

Tanabe	Leningrad	Shanghai
↓	↓	↓
CAM — 70	Leningrad — 16	Shanghai — 191

The vaccine is presented as a freeze dried product and is administered as a single dose of 0.5 ml by deep subcutaneous injection. With the help of improved stabilisers a more robust vaccine has been marketed since 1979. Even then the recommended temperature range for storage and transport, as well as protection from exposure to light should be carefully observed.

In recent years vaccines from the Edmonston – Zagreb and AIK – C strains have been developed. These vaccines hold the promise of being more immunogenic and effective even when administered at less than the recommended age of nine months. This vaccine is not recommended at present. With the advent of the MMR (measles mumps rubella) vaccine the trend in the more developed countries is to use the combined vaccine.

Measles vaccine promotes both cellular and humoral immunity. Cell mediated immunity is difficult to measure and so seroconversion is assessed by the humoral immune response.

In developing countries seroconversion rates in excess of 90 per cent amongst children nine months of age and over have been reported. But in urban squatter communities intense transmission has been observed. Infants younger than nine months in age suffer measles as soon as maternally derived antibody wanes to non-protective levels. Hence the recommended age of vaccination is nine months.

In carefully supervised clinical trials it has been shown that between two and five per cent of children fail to develop an immune response and consequently there will always be a group of vaccinated children who will subsequently develop measles. The explanations for this failure of take can be: (1) the extreme lability of the vaccine; (2) interference from the maternally-derived antibody in the case of young infants. Such antibodies are known to persist at low levels until the age of 11 months. For example, the take rate at age 9 months in the UK was found to be 75 per cent. Studies in the USA have shown that the take rate is better if immunisation is carried out at age 12 months and even further improved at age 13 months. Because of such observations many authorities recommend immunisation at age 15 months or a second dose at age 15 months if immunisation was carried out in the first year of life. (3) A very small number of infants fail to develop antibody response in spite of all precautions. The above observations have important implications for immunisation programmes.

Further experience with vaccination against measles has shown that a coverage of 90 to 95 per cent vaccination is necessary to interrupt the regular occurrence of epidemics in a community. In developing countries where measles occurs at an early age, not more than 50 per cent of infants can be expected to be responsive to measles vaccine between the ages of 9 and 15 months. A substantial number will still be protected by maternal antibodies or would have already contracted the disease. Hence in a measles vaccination programme the aim will be to vaccinate all children between 9 and 15 months of age who have not yet suffered from the disease, and to maintain a continuing programme. Failure to do so will result in a rapid build-up of the number of susceptibles.

Recent experience with large scale vaccination programmes in Nigeria, Cameroun and Yemen has shown that the sero-conversion rate is much smaller than anticipated. In some cases only a third of the children immunised were protected. Part of the difficulty lies in unsatisfactory storage conditions and lack of protection of the vaccine from destruction during transport. For maximum effectiveness the following guidelines need to be strictly observed:

(1) All vaccines arriving in the country should be carefully supervised to ensure that they are stored, distributed and transported under the recommended temperature range.
(2) Within the district, transport from the base refrigerator to the clinic or the village should be by means of efficient cold boxes or storage bags which are protected from light.
(3) Reconstitution with the diluent should be made only after all the clients have been assembled. Once the dilution is made the vaccine should be used immediately.
(4) The vaccine is sensitive to both heat and light and also to heavy metals. Hence syringes with metallic plungers should be avoided for administration of the vaccine. Disposable syringes or those with glass plungers should be preferred.
(5) Any vaccine which is not used within six hours of dilution should be discarded. Hence to avoid wastage, vials with ten doses are to be preferred to those containing a large number of doses.
(6) A careful check on the efficacy of vaccination should be maintained. Even though sero-conversion provides an absolute proof, a much easier and effective method is a system of notification of the disease, especially in vaccinated children.

Following a nation-wide immunisation programme with adequate coverage a number of outbreaks of measles occurred in the United States in 1985 and again in 1986. Amongst the pre-school age children 14 per cent of the cases had been previously vaccinated. In the case of school age children the proportion was 60 per cent. Because of the persistence of outbreaks in highly vaccinated populations a two dose schedule is being recommended in the US, both with the MMR vaccine. The first dose is recommended to be given at 12 to 15 months, and the second dose at school entry. Further modifications may be required in the schedule of immunisations in the light of future experience.

Further reading

Aaby P, Bukh J, Kronberg D, Lisse I M, de Silva Mc. Delayed excess mortality after exposure to measles during the first six months of life. *Am J Epidemiol* 1990; 132:211–9.

Barret T. The molecular biology of the morbillivirus (measles) group. *Biochem Soc Symp* 1987;53:25–37.

Black F L. Measles active and passive immunity in a worldwide perspective. *Prog Med Virol* 1989;36:1–33.

Clinical trial of live measles vaccine given alone and live vaccine preceded by killed vaccine: Fourth report of the Medical Research Council by the Measles Subcommittee of the Committee on the Development of Vaccines and Immunisation Procedures. *Lancet* 1977, ii: 571.

Chalmers A K. *The health of Glasgow 1818–1925*. Glasgow: Bell and Bain, 1930.

Dudgeon J A. Measles and rubella vaccines. *Archs Dis Childh* 1977; 52: 907–11.

Fraser K B, Martin S J. *Measles virus and its biology*. London and New York: Academic Press, 1978.

McLean A R, Anderson R M. Measles in developing countries. I. Epidemiological parameters and patterns. *Epidemiol Infect* 1988;100:111–33.

II. The predicted impact of mass vaccination. *Epidemiol Infect* 1988;100:419–42.

Morgan E M, Rapp F. Measles virus and its associated diseases. *Bacteriological Reviews* 1977; 41: 636–52.

Morley D C. Measles in the developing world. *Proc R Soc Med* 1974;67: 1112–15.

Whittle H C, Bradley-Moore A, Fleming A, Greenwood B M. Effects of measles on the immune response of Nigerian children. *Archs Dis Childh* 1973;48:753.

9 *Whooping cough*

Whooping cough has a world-wide distribution and is seen in all crowded communities. It can occur at all ages but is most serious in the young infant and the elderly. Unlike those for measles, maternal antibodies for this disease are not transmitted to the foetus through the placenta so that the neonate has no immunity against whooping cough.

In a longitudinal study in rural Kenya, 918 cases were observed in a population of 24 000. The peak incidence was between December and January. The attack rate was highest during the first year of life at 15.8 per cent, and 90 per cent of cases occurred in children six years of age or younger. In the age group 0–15 years, pertussis accounted for 4.1 per cent of all deaths.

The prevalence of whooping cough as well as mortality have shown a marked decline in all countries of Western Europe and the USA. Nevertheless, as recently as 1948 pertussis remained a leading cause of death of children under 14 years of age in the USA.

In Guatemala, as in several other countries of South America, whooping cough is often a more severe disease than measles. Case fatality rates of up to 15 per cent have been recorded. Fatality was found to be particularly high among infants and pre-school children. Similarly in Nigeria the disease still carries a high mortality rate at 15 per cent. By contrast, the mortality rate of pertussis began to decline in many of the industrialised countries in the West around the beginning of this century despite a continued very high incidence rate. Improved nutrition and major changes in the demographic characteristics of the population are thought to be mainly responsible for this. In more recent years immunisation has played an important role in reducing the incidence of whooping cough. For example, in 1960 there were over 58 000 cases notified in England and Wales with 37 deaths. By 1975, there were 9000 notifications with 12 deaths. In more recent years the rates of immunisation have fallen in several countries for a variety of reasons, including complacency, and fears of major epidemics have been raised.

Age and mortality

Whooping cough is a serious disease of children at all ages. In addition to the complications of the disease process itself, the chronic and prolonged nature of the illness, the emotional and physical distress caused by paroxysms of coughing and the accompanying disturbances in nutrition and sleep combine to have adverse effects on the child's health. In infants particularly, whooping cough can give rise to a severe respiratory disturbance which is largely responsible for the high mortality of this age group. The case fatality rates in infants have been reported to be three times as high as those in older age groups.

In all developing countries, because of the extended family system and the general cultural life of the community, the risks of droplet infection tend to be high. This is much more so with diseases like whooping cough which have a high communicability rate. In some studies the risks of developing the illness have been found to be as high as 75–90 per cent in family exposures. In the rural society, because the infant accompanies the mother or the older sibling everywhere, infection tends to occur at an earlier age. Moreover, siblings often share the same bed or children may sleep together in one room or the same hut. The mean age of infection in studies from 17 developing countries was found to be between 1.7 to 3 years compared to between 4.4 and 5 years in some Western countries. It is not surprising that because of its incidence at an early age whooping cough is responsible for a high degree of mortality either directly or by causing severe nutritional upsets.

Etiology

The vast majority of cases are caused by *Bordetella pertussis* although *B. parapertussis* is an important agent in some areas of the world. These two bacterial species are exclusively human parasites. Rarely, cases have also been associated with *B.*

bronchiseptica which is a bacterial species normally enzootic in cats, rodents and other animals.

Pertussis is one of the most contagious of diseases. When introduced into isolated communities, attack rates of up to 98 per cent have been recorded. In most developing countries pertussis is highly endemic and can affect all ages. However, its high prevalence means that the infant and the young child are most at risk.

Infection with *B. pertussis* almost invariably produces symptomatic disease, most of which is typical pertussis. Many would doubt if the carrier state ever occurs. On gaining entry through droplet infection, the organisms can multiply only in association with the ciliated ephithelium of the respiratory tract. Here they cause a necrotising inflammation in the tracheo-bronchial mucus membranes. Toxins produced by *B. pertussis* paralyse the cilia of the respiratory ephithelium, thus interfering with the normal clearing mechanism of the lung. At the same time, the increased secretions and the severe inflammation cause stasis and accumulation of debris. There is bronchiolar obstruction and atelectasis followed by infection so that a diffuse bronchopneumonia is a common accompaniment of whooping cough.

Clinical picture

The incubation period varies between one to three weeks with a mean of seven days. The onset is insidious in the form of an upper respiratory infection and catarrh with little constitutional symptoms. After several days of this catarrhal stage a cough develops which is mainly nocturnal at first. It gradually increases in intensity becoming diurnal and is often followed by vomiting.

As the cough gets worse it becomes paroxysmal so that one explosive effort is followed by another without a break in between and the child struggles for breath. The face goes purple or cyanotic and with increasing anoxia the child is in severe distress. At the end of the paroxysms a deep breath is taken producing the 'whoop'. It is important to bear in mind that not all patients with pertussis whoop, nor do patients whoop in every paroxysm. It is generally true that of the patients experiencing a well-developed paroxysm, the majority will exhibit a whoop.

Two important characteristics of the cough of pertussis distinguish it from other causes of cough. Firstly in the absence of complications the patient is usually afebrile. In most series, fever has been reported in only 20 to 25 per cent of the cases. Secondly, at the termination of a paroxysm the patient will usually vomit.

The paroxysmal stage lasts several weeks after which the bouts of coughing become less severe and the child now enters the convalescent stage. The cough will persist for a long time during recovery, five to ten weeks being the average.

In the young infant this clinical pattern is altered because of lack of resistance and diagnosis becomes difficult. In the early catarrhal stage, there may be thick stringy mucus in the oropharynx causing difficulty with feeding; often a mother may be seen pulling out the mucus strands from the child's mouth with her fingers. As the cough develops it comes in paroxysms as in the older child but there may be very little 'whooping'; instead, apnoea and cyanosis are more commonly seen. Exhaustion from the physical effort, obstruction of the air passages by thick mucus and cyanosis cause spells of apnoea which may prove fatal. The small infant requires close observation for administration of oxygen and assistance with respiration during the apnoeic attacks.

Diagnosis

An individual is most infectious during the catarrhal stage when a definitive diagnosis is usually difficult. During an epidemic any child, who has not been protected by immunisation, and presents with heavy upper respiratory catarrh, should be considered to be infected. The lymphocytosis characteristic of whooping cough is usually not seen until the paroxysmal stage, so that in the early catarrhal stage the only means of making a definite diagnosis is by culture studies. The very young infant, the adult or the vaccinated child may not show the full blown picture and yet the nasal secretions may be full of organisms. In the paroxysmal stage blood examination shows leucocytosis with a high lymphocytic count which helps to make the diagnosis in an atypical case. Eosinophilia is also common, especially during convalescence.

Several conditions are known to cause a paroxysmal cough resembling pertussis, for example, pulmonary eosinophilia, lipoid pneumonia, endobronchial tuberculosis, aspirated foreign body or an allergic cough.

Complications

The commonest complication is produced by an

invasion of the damaged respiratory epithelium with secondary bacterial infection causing bronchopneumonia or pneumonia. Such an infection occurring in an atelectatic part of the lung may lead to bronchiectasis. Re-activation of a latent tuberculous focus is a relatively frequent complication. Severe bouts of coughing could cause pneumothorax or surgical emphysema.

Whooping cough invariably leads to debility and emaciation by interfering with the food intake of the child. Many patients lose up to five per cent or more of body weight and may need as long as two months to regain body weight. It is not uncommon to find a child suffering from pertussis develop oedema of the feet or other clinical signs of malnutrition. The constant straining effort in a child who is getting rapidly emaciated can lead to rectal prolapse or an inguinal hernia. Thus, the nutrition of the patient needs careful attention.

The most challenging complications are those concerning the central nervous system. In various series encephalopathy has been reported in 1.7 to 7 per cent of cases. This is a serious complication. Approximately one-third of the children who develop pertussis encephalopathy die and about half of the survivors are left with neurological deficits. Anoxia, cerebral haemorrhage or oedema, or a toxic effect of the organisms may all contribute to the involvement of the nervous system. The occurrence of fits during an attack of pertussis must be taken seriously. Signs of focal neurological damage like visual disturbances or hemiplegia may also be the first indication of an encephalopathy.

Management

By far the most important aspect of management is good nursing care and attention to feeding, maintenance of clear airway and water and electrolyte balance. Small feeds at frequent intervals are tolerated better. In the infant or child who has frequent spasms oral feeding is difficult, and gavage feeding with an in-dwelling nasogastric tube may be required. Gentle handling of the child is essential in order to avoid precipitating a spasm of coughing. In the small infant, administration of oxygen or stimulation of respiration may be needed during attacks of apnoea.

Whooping cough is often a frightening and sometimes a terrifying illness and sedation helps in allaying the child's anxiety. Phenobarbitone is probably as effective as anything. Also phenobarbitone in doses of 5–10 mg twice daily has been found useful in reducing the number of paroxysms of coughing.

Antibiotics may help in the early catarrhal stage but later on when the lung tissues show marked pathological changes they are of little use. Much of the mortality of whooping cough is due to bacterial complications and early experience with antibiotics showed their usefulness in reducing mortality to almost half of what it was in the pre-antibiotic days. In one carefully organised study on the use of chloramphenicol and Aureomycin (chlortetracycline) in pertussis it was found that there was no dramatic response to antibiotics as compared to placebo. However, some benefits from both the drugs was seen in patients in whom treatment was commenced within eight days of developing symptoms. Further studies have confirmed this limitation of chemotherapy in treating established cases of whooping cough. At present, on the basis of in vitro studies, erythromycin is considered the antibiotic of choice. It should be administered in the early catarrhal stage in a dose of 40 mg/kg body weight daily in divided doses six hourly.

A secondary consideration in the use of antibiotics is from the public health point of view. By inducing early bacteriological cure, transmission is interrupted. Here again the patient is more infective in the early stage of the illness and early institution of treatment will be more beneficial for controlling spread of the disease. Antibiotics may be useful in some instances for the protection of siblings in the household where pertussis has been confirmed. Secondary bacterial infection, especially in the lungs, is the usual cause of death in whooping cough. Here antibiotics are of doubtless value.

Protection by immunisation

The first vaccines from killed B. pertussis came into use in the late fifties and early studies showed that some batches gave satisfactory protection. There was a rapid decline in the incidence of pertussis in areas where vaccination was widely practised. But soon sporadic cases began to appear. In the UK where record keeping and epidemiologic surveillance is of a high standard, it was noted that the number of cases increased in 1963. Since then further studies showed a change in the serotype of the prevailing organisms. In one survey it was found that 56 per cent of the immunised children developed whooping cough after a household contact compared to 67 per cent in the unvaccinated group. Similar reports have continued to appear suggesting that immunisation is not universally successful. Nevertheless the introduction of the vaccine has coincided with a major decline in the incidence in the general population. On the other hand, the vaccine does not appear to be very effective in closed populations, for example, household contact or institutions. This may be due to the intensity of the infection. Protection from the vaccine is adequate for a chance infection in the general population and inadequate if repeated infection occurs within the household or the institution.

Another problem with the vaccine has been the frequency of side effects. Pertussis vaccine is a relatively crude preparation and contains the majority of the constituents of the organisms. Toxic substances do get extracted to some degree along with protective substances.

In recent years neurological complications were reported following the administration of pertussis vaccine. The resulting publicity led to a fall in the uptake of immunisation in several countries, followed by increase in the incidence of pertussis. Sweden, Japan and the UK experienced mini epidemics.

Experimental work on the different components of the organisms has shown that only a few are responsible for the majority of the biological effects. Of these pertussis toxin (PT) and a component of the cell wall – filamentous haemagglutinin (FHA) – are the most important. These two components form the basis of new a-cellular vaccines, currently in use in Japan and Sweden. In Sweden the protective efficacy of the a-cellular vaccine containing PT alone has been estimated to be 54 per cent, and that of the vaccine containing PT and FHA as 69 per cent. By comparison the efficacy of the whole cell vaccine was considered to be 80 per cent.

The National Childhood Encephalopathy study in the UK analysed the first recorded 1000 cases of neurological symptoms occurring within one week of administration of the whole cell pertussis vaccine. An attributable risk of 1 in 310 000 inoculations was reported by this study. The following highly relevant observations were also made by this study.

(1) No previously normal child suffered permanent injury with an onset less than 48 hours after vaccination.
(2) All normal children experiencing a febrile seizure after vaccination were normal on followup.
(3) There was no evidence that previously neurologically abnormal children had a greater risk of an adverse event within several days of vaccination.
(4) If all cases of Rey's syndrome and proven viral disease were excluded there was no statistical evidence of permanent brain damage, and no increase in death related to the vaccine.

A balanced assessment of all reports favours pertussis immunisation. This is particularly so with regard to the protection of young infants from severe morbidity as well as appreciable mortality. In the developing countries the benefits of vaccination against pertussis far outweigh the small risk of adverse reactions. Routine use of the vaccine in all children's clinics as well as in mass campaigns to reduce the number of susceptibles in the community is therefore recommended. A continuing surveillance is also important in view of the difficulties discussed above.

Since the rare neurological complications tend to be so serious, immunisation should be avoided in the following high risk groups.

(1) Children with existing disorders of the central nervous system.
(2) Children with a history of convulsions or a strong family history of seizures.
(3) Children with a history of cerebral irritation or fits in the neo-natal period.
(4) Children with developmental defects.
(5) Children who have had a severe local or general reaction to previous dose of the vaccine.
(6) Immunisation should be temporarily withheld if the child is unwell.

More recent studies on the efficacy of vaccination have shown that within affected families, immunised young children are less likely to suffer whooping cough and if infected it will be less severe compared to the unprotected. Those at maximal risk are children under the age of six months. For them, immunisation provides useful protection against a very severe disease.

Further reading

Anon. Treatment of whooping cough. (Editorial) *Br med J* 1970; 2: 619–20.

Anon. Whooping cough immunisation. (Editorial) *Br med J* 1977; 2: 5–6.

Anon. Whooping cough. (Editorial) *Br med J* 1978,; 1: 1007.

Department of Health and Social Security. *Whooping cough vaccination.* London: HMSO, 1 977.

Medical Research Council. Prevention of whooping cough by vaccination. *Br med J* 1951; 1: 1463.

Medical Research Council. Vaccination against whooping cough. *Br med J* 1956; 2: 454.

Medical Research Council. Vaccination against whooping cough. *Br med J* 1959; 1: 994.

Miller C L, Fletcher W B. Severity of notified whooping cough. *Br med J* 1976; 1: 117–19.

Olson L C. Pertussis. *Medicine*, Baltimore: 1975; 54: 427–65.

Voorhoeve A M, Muller A S, Schulper T W J, Mennetje W, Van Rens M. Agents affecting health of mother and child in a rural area of Kenya- IV. The epidemiology of pertussis. *Trop geogr Med* 1978; 30: 125–39.

Robinson R J. The whooping cough immunisation controversy. *Arch dis childh* 1981; 56: 577–580.

Report from the PHLS epidemiological Research Laboratory and 21 area health authorities. Efficacy of pertussis vaccination in England. *Br Med J* 1982; 285: 357–359.

10 *Poliomyelitis*

Poliomyelitis is an acute infectious disease caused by an enterovirus. It appears in sporadic or epidemic forms in the community during specific seasons when environmental conditions become suitable for the propagation of the virus. In temperate climates, summer and autumn are the two seasons in which infections most commonly occur. There are three antigenically distinct subtypes of the poliovirus designated as I, II and III. Infection in man from one subtype does not protect against the others. This is important to know from the point of view of immunisation, and the vaccine should be offered to even those who have suffered from poliomyelitis.

Sewage carries intestinal viruses nearly all the time and most sewage treatments do very little to reduce viral content in the effluent. As regards the water supply, the usual methods of treatment such as dilution, storage, flocculation and filtration all help to reduce the amount of virus in the water. However, poliovirus and coxsackie A2 and A9 are resistant to free chlorine. It is now known that during an epidemic, subclinical infection is far more common than clinically manifest illness. This means that even when there are sporadic cases in the community, the infection is widespread and the community water supply may be a route of low-level transmission of the disease.

In developing countries, poliomyelitis is mainly a disease of young children; for example, in those countries of tropical Africa for whom age-specific notifications of disease were available in the year 1963, 76 per cent of notified cases were in children below the age of five years. Since the introduction of the vaccines, the incidence of polio has fallen to insignificant proportions in North America, parts of Europe and several other countries. In the Americas poliomyelitis has now been brought under control, and global eradication of the disease during the 1990s is a distinct possibility.

The pattern of infection

From the epidemiological point of view, poliomyel-itis shows three phases – endemic, epidemic and post-vaccination. The endemic pattern is the most common in a large majority of developing countries. Here polio is a disease of infancy and virtually all children over four years of age are already exposed to the virus. Antibodies to all three types of the poliovirus are universally present in women of childbearing age. Passive immunity is transferred from mother to offspring and the majority of infants experience their first exposure to the virus whilst they are still protected by maternal antibodies or through immune agents in the mothers' milk.

As sanitary conditions improve, opportunities of infection at a young age become fewer. Increasing numbers of people encounter polio later in childhood or in adult life when infection is more likely to result in paralysis. The delay in the age of infection also leads to a build up of susceptibles in the population to a point where epidemics can occur. This was the pattern in Western Europe and North America during the fifties. Such a pattern may be emerging in many developing countries, especially in the cities. For example, in 1974 the observed prevalence of lameness in Ghana among school children was 7 per 1000 and the annual incidence was estimated to be at least 28 per 100 000 population, which is similar to that of Europe and the USA prior to the introduction of the vaccine. In almost all the cities of the developing world there are the septic fringes in the form of slums, shanty towns and inner city areas where the virus can be assumed to be circulating freely giving rise to immunising infections at an early age. On the other hand, in the more affluent sections enjoying better sanitation, there is a build up of susceptibles whose first contact with the polio virus is likely to occur in late childhood.

After the introduction of the killed vaccine in 1955 and of the live vaccine in 1960, a marked reduction in the incidence of poliomyelitis occurred in all countries of Europe and North America. In those countries where vaccination now reaches almost all the children, wild polioviruses are rarely identified. Almost all polioviruses isolated closely resemble the vaccine strains and are generally assumed to be vaccine progeny.

Transmission

Man is the sole reservoir of infection. Transmission occurs mainly through those who have an inapparent infection or through healthy carriers rather than by patients with acute illness. The period of highest communicability of naturally occurring paralytic poliomyelitis is more closely related to the presence of virus in the pharynx than to the excretion of virus in the faeces. This oral–oral route of virus dissemination is particularly important when sanitation is generally good.

Unlike temperate countries where most of the waves of enterovirus infections occur in summer and autumn, there is no clear cut seasonal incidence in the tropics. Besides, there is also a very high carrier rate of other enteroviruses. For example, in Mexico it was found that 70–80 per cent of young children were carriers of enteroviruses. In a longitudinal study of young children in Vellore, 35 per cent of all rectal swabs examined grew enteroviruses and the maximum positive rates were obtained in the months of June, July and August.

Poliovirus is always ready to spread and circulate among susceptibles if the opportunity arises. Unlike measles, the majority of infections are subclinical. It is estimated that 90–95 per cent of the infections are without any clinical symptoms and only 1–2 per cent of infections end up with paralysis. Thus whenever 'wild' polio virus spreads among susceptibles, there are bound to be some paralytic cases. The incidence of polio paralysis amongst children in a community thus gives a good indication of the prevalence of infection in that community. The risk of an epidemic increases as a population composed of unvaccinated infants, children and even young adults builds up.

Poliomyelitis virus is highly infectious. The intestinal tract of the infected person is an important source of infection besides transmission through droplets. This latter route, as we have seen, may be more important than oro-faecal transmission in some cases. The spread of the virus thus occurs not only through direct contact, but also through contamination of the infected individual's immediate environment. Since the majority of infected persons suffer no symptoms, or the illness may be too mild to be recognised, spread of infection in the community can be rapid. In general, exposure to poliovirus occurs early in life in many developing countries. In surveys carried out in several cities of India,

it was observed that by the age of six years, 85–90 per cent of children have developed antibodies.

During epidemics of poliomyelitis which swept through many Western countries during the fifties; two important observations were made. It was noted that when infant mortality falls below 75 per 1000 live births, the rates of polio paralysis rise above 3–4 per 1000. The reasons have been discussed above. This observation is true for communities with generally improving socio-economic conditions and living standards. Whether it also holds true for communities where a well-developed health programme provides good immunisation coverage of the susceptibles, remains to be seen. Certainly in Cuba, falls in infant mortality rates have not been accompanied by increasing incidence of paralysis. A second observation is concerning the incidence of clinical poliomyelitis in older children. It was found that when 20 per cent or more of paralytic cases are recorded in children over the age of ten years, an increased activity of the illness in the community should be suspected.

Pathogenesis

On entry through the oral route, the virus multiplies in the oropharynx and the lymphoid tissue of the intestinal tract from where it enters the blood stream causing viraemia. The prodromal phase corresponds with this early viraemia. In most natural infections, there is invasion and multiplication of the virus in lymphoid tissue followed by transient viraemia. If the infecting strain of the virus is highly invasive or if there is inadequate host resistance, the virus is then able to invade the nervous system (figure 10.1).

Several factors are known to predispose to severity of infection. Recent tonsillectomy enhances the chances of bulbar poliomyelitis. Intramuscular injections in a child incubating the disease may precipitate paralysis of the muscles into which the injection was administered. Administration of cortisone or heavy exertion during the incubation period are factors associated with large scale paralysis.

Once the invasion of the central nervous system occurs, the virus shows a predilection for specific areas. The anterior horn cells of the spinal cord are usually attacked especially in the cervical and lumbar regions. The motor nuclei in the mid-brain and medulla are also commonly involved and there may be involvement of the reticular formation or the nuclei of the roof of the cerebellum. Paralysis occurs when a critical number of motor neurones have been destroyed. After the onset of paralysis,

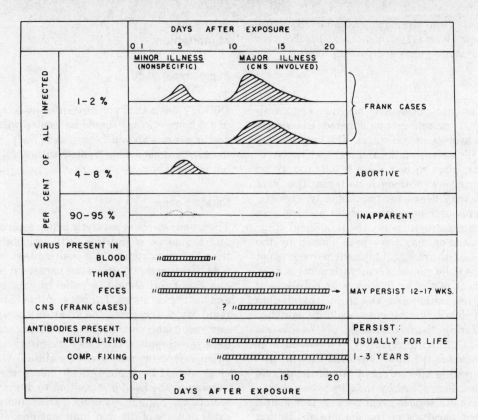

Figure 10.1 Natural history of poliovirus infection

some degree of regeneration and recovery is possible, but it is doubtful whether a muscle which has been completely paralysed will ever regain normal function. Muscles which have been severely but not completely paralysed at the end of the acute period may regain functional value in about 50 per cent of the cases; when the paralysis is light, the chances of complete recovery are 90 per cent. The maximum functional recovery takes place in the first year and a little more in the second year after the attack.

Clinical manifestations

The incubation period varies from one to three weeks, after which the illness takes any of the following forms

Inapparent infection

In crowded communities people in close contact with a person infected with the polio virus can receive the infection and the virus will be isolated from their stools or the oropharnyx. As a result of the infection antibody response occurs and this is the basis of the immunity prevalent in many communities living in unsanitary conditions.

Abortive infection

This may take any of the following forms

(1) Upper respiratory illness with mild fever, catarrh and cough.
(2) Gastro-intestinal symptoms of anorexia, nausea and vomiting.
(3) Fever with body aches and cramps.

In the case of all these three forms, polio may go undiagnosed except during an epidemic.

Non-paralytic illness

After a brief illness characterised by fever and upper respiratory or gastro-intestinal symptoms, involvement of the central nervous system becomes apparent because of signs of meningeal inflammation and headache. The illness may subside without any muscular involvement. Lumbar puncture during the acute stage of meningeal involvement may show lymphocytosis and raised protein.

Paralytic polio

The non-paralytic illness may progress and paralysis of various muscle groups is noted. Classically the disease evolves in two stages. The first stage of prodromal illness with fever and non-specific symptoms lasting three to four days is followed by an interval during which there is no fever. The fever rises again with headache, neck rigidity, restlessness and muscular pain followed by paralysis. In many cases of paralytic polio, the prodromal stage may be absent or may have been missed by the parents so that the classical biphasic pattern is not seen and the child presents only with paralysis.

Involvement of the vital centres or paralysis of muscles of respiration give rise to life-threatening situations. Hence the patient should be watched carefully during the acute stage of the disease especially if the disease is mainly in the thoracic or cervical portion of the cord. When the cervical portion of the cord is affected, paralysis of the deltoid muscle which is supplied by the same roots as the phrenic nerve is a serious event because it indicates an imminent paralysis of the diaphragm. Bulbar polio is the most serious form of the disease. Paralysis of the muscles of the pharynx, the larynx and the palate endanger life from aspiration pneumonia. Involvement of the centres of respiration and the cardiovascular centres in the mid-brain interferes with vital physiological functions. The patient develops anoxia as indicated by rapid shallow breathing. With further progress of the disease apnoeic spells occur, finally ending in respiratory paralysis.

Diagnosis

During an epidemic, any illness in a child should be suspect and strict bed rest should be enforced. In the sporadic form, polio has to be differentiated from other illnesses causing meningeal involvement, for example, bacterial meningitis, the aseptic meningitis syndrome caused by viruses, etc. Pain in the muscles and limbs may be severe enough to require differential diagnosis from rheumatic fever, osteomyelitis, crisis of sickle-cell anaemia, or scurvy.

Management

In prodromal stage

During epidemics of poliomyelitis any febrile illness of unknown etiology should be treated with bed rest and injections should be avoided. Body aches and muscle pain should be treated with analgesics and hot fomentation.

Paralytic stage

The management of paralytic polio requires bed rest and avoidance of exertion with immobilisation of the affected extremity in a position that would provide best functional use of the paralysed limb. Pain and discomfort should be relieved with analgesics and hot fomentations. The patient should be checked regularly to recognise and treat any complications and respiratory insufficiency with urgency. When paralysis threatens muscles of respiration or deglutition supportive measures to maintain vital physiology should be applied. Such measures would be nursing in the head low position to drain bronchial secretions, regular suction, tracheostomy if indicated and use of the iron lung machine.

In the ordinary case bed rest is essential for at least two weeks or until such time as there is no further spread of paralysis, after which physiotherapy may be started to avoid deformities in the affected limb and to maintain weak muscles in as good a functional order as possible.

Recovery of function occurs in many of the affected muscles over a period of two years. During this period a programme of regular supervision with physiotherapy, emotional support and rehabilitation to active life is necessary. The degree of incapacity determines the extent of return to normal life and the advice of an orthopaedic surgeon as well as the physiotherapist is necessary in planning rehabilitation.

Prevention

The availability of vaccine since 1959 has made the control of polio possible. In almost all countries in Europe and North America the incidence of polio has shown a dramatic decline since the commencement of nationwide immunisation programmes. The *killed vaccine* (IPV) has been used extensively in Sweden, Finland and Holland with great success. It produces high levels of circulating antibodies, first IgM and later of the IgG type. These antibodies are the main means by which the vaccine confers immunity. Controlled trials show that IPV protects against infection and the serological immunity is maintained for long periods. However, the immunity does tend to wane over a period of time. The development of poliomyelitis in people who have been immunised with IPV is rare. However, it is to be expected that the occasional person may respond less well than usual, and also that the concentration of antibodies will decline slowly after immunisation. There are recorded instances of individuals who suffered from poliomyelitis during adolescence in spite of receiving IPV in childhood.

Live vaccine (OPV) mimics the natural infection and is expected to confer the same quality of immunity. The best immunising component of the vaccine is the Type 2 strain which is known to produce viraemia in 90 per cent of susceptible children. OPV not only gives immunity to the individual but it also limits the spread of the wild virus in the community, by increasing local resistance in the gut to reinfection. Experience with OPV in many developing countries, however, has been disappointing. For example, in Singapore the sero-conversion rate after two doses of a trivalent vaccine was only 50 per cent. Similar results have been obtained in Nigeria and in Vellore, South India. Increasing the quantity of the virus in the vaccine or administering multiple doses of the vaccine over a period of four to six weeks has not improved the conversion rates. It has been suggested that in the tropics a high proportion of infants and young children are subject to a succession of intestinal infection which can prevent the vaccine virus from establishing itself in the gut, which is a prerequisite to the development of immunity. However, an epidemic in Kenya was averted by a national immunisation campaign using OPV.

In the EPI programme it is recommended that OPV should be given as early as possible – at birth or at the time of first contact with the health service. The second dose is given at six weeks of age, followed by two additional doses – one at the age of two to three months and another when the child is nine months old. Booster doses at 18 months and at school entry are also required. An interval of two months is desirable between the first two doses of OPV to ensure proper replication in the gut. Breast feeding is no contraindication for the administration of OPV, nor is a minor illness. However, it is advisable to withhold vaccination during serious illness.

OPV induces a systemic as well as local (mucosal) immune response. This immune response prevents both nervous system invasion and intestinal infection in subsequent encounters with the wild virus, and resembles naturally acquired immunity. In addition other viral antigenic determinants may be released in the gut after digestion by trypsin, and induce relevant mucosal immunity. In general the immunity with OPV is longer lasting compared to IPV. However, in endemic areas booster doses in the case of both are advisable.

Poliovirus is composed of 60 copies each of four protein subunits described as VP1, VP2, VP3 and VP4. Of these the first three constitute the major antigens which induce the production of neutralising antibody. VP4 plays no known role in antibody production.

When the vaccine strain of the virus in OPV is compared with the wild virus only discrete base substitution is found in the viral proteins. This implies that point mutations in VP1, VP2 and VP3 contribute to attenuation. When the vaccine is administered considerable change occurs in the vaccine virus while multiplying in the gut, and there is always a risk of attenuation diminishing and neurovirulence increasing.

On rare occasions OPV is known to cause paralytic polio in the recipients or their contacts. It has been estimated that for every five million doses of vaccine given, about one case of paralysis may be expected in a recipient and about two cases in contacts of vaccinated persons. Recent surveillance studies on poliovirus in Britain indicate that most strains causing disease in that country are vaccine strains. Even though the incidence of the disease has fallen remarkably since the introduction of the two vaccines, the virus in one form or another continues to persist. A continued high level of vaccination is an essential price for maintaining the present low incidence of the disease in all countries.

Further reading

Beale A J. Immunisation against poliomyelitis. *Br med Bull* 1969; 25: 148.

Brown, F. From Jenner to genes – the next generation of virus vaccines. *Biochem Soc Symp* 1987; 53: 75–84.

Cockburn W C. World problems in viral vaccines. *Br med Bull* 1969; 25: 2.

Cossart Y E. Evolution of poliovirus since introduction of attenuated vaccine. *Br med J* 1977; 1: 1621–3.

Metselaar D, *et al*. Poliomyelitis: epidemiology and prophylaxis. *Bull Wld Hlth Org* 1977; 55(6): 747–53.

Melnick J L. Advantages and disadvantages of killed and live poliomyelitis vaccines. *Bull Wld Hlth Org* 1978; 56: 21–38.

Ofosu-Ammah S, Kratzer J H, Nicholas D D. Is poliomyelitis a serious problem in developing countries? *Br med J* 1977; 1: 1012–14.

Public Health Service Advisory Committee on Immunisation Practices, Centre for Disease Control, U.S. Dept of Health Education and Welfare, Poliomyelitis prevention, *Ann intern Med* 1978; 88: 218–20.

Sabin A. Strategy for rapid elimination and continuing control of poliomyelitis and other vaccine preventable diseases of children in developing countries. *Brit Med J* 1986; 292 531–533.

11 *Diarrhoeal disease*

Diarrhoea (more than three watery stools per day) is one of the most common illnesses of children, especially of those living in the poverty → malnutrition → environmental contamination cycle. Together with respiratory infection it ranks as a major killer disease in the paediatric age group. It is also responsible for a large proportion of the work load of hospitals and health centres. In some countries children under the age of five may suffer as many as ten episodes of diarrhoea per year, and spend 15–20 per cent of their time with a diarrhoeal illness. About 30 per cent of paediatric bed occupancy in developing countries is for diarrhoea, placing a heavy burden on health facilities.

It is estimated that diarrhoea is responsible for about four million deaths each year largely amongst children less than two years old. Diarrhoea kills because of acute dehydration, as persistent diarrhoea (more than three watery stools per day continuing for two weeks or more), and as dysentery.

Most diarrhoeal episodes are acute, lasting no more than two weeks. About five per cent last longer. These are cases of persistent diarrhoea and can be responsible for as many as 25 to 30 per cent of all diarrhoea associated deaths. Diarrhoea is also an important cause of childhood malnutrition.

Diarrhoea is of course very serious in newborns and young infants who cannot tolerate even small upsets in fluid and electrolyte balance. It is rare in infants who are entirely breast fed and very common in those who are artificially fed, especially if the standards of hygiene are poor. Dirty bottles and teats with left-over milk provide excellent media for the growth of pathogens and are common causes of diarrhoea in such infants. In a study of 608 cases of diarrhoea reported from the gastroenteritis unit of the Queen Elizabeth Hospital for Children, London, only two were breast fed, compared with 14 per cent amongst matched controls in the community. Several studies have now shown that human milk has factors that specifically protect against diarrhoeal illness. It is the experience of many paediatric units in Western Europe that the incidence of severe dehydration and hypernatraemia has been drastically reduced whenever there is an increase in breast feeding in the community. The importance of breast milk was well demonstrated during an outbreak of *E. coli* gastroenteritis which affected several newborn units in Britain in the late sixties. The main lessons learnt then were that such outbreaks are most difficult to control, and secondly they can easily give rise to resistant strains. Such outbreaks are even more difficult to control in the health centres and smaller district hospitals of the developing world.

A challenge facing child health in all traditional societies is the present widespread decline in breast feeding. The small amount of health education carried out by the health personnel is no match for the large-scale commercial advertisements and sales drives of the baby food manufacturers. In urban areas, where women are increasingly taking up paid employment for socio-economic reasons, there has been a precipitous drop in breast feeding, for example, only 30 per cent of women attending a young child clinic in Kuala Lumpur were found to be breast feeding their babies.

Weanling diarrhoea

Repeated diarrhoeal episodes are common during the weaning period not only in man but also in several other mammals. In the insanitary conditions of rural homes and overcrowded tenements, the weanling ingests heavily contaminated food and is surrounded by contamination. The water supply is invariably polluted. For example, in Djakarta, Indonesia, samples of water and environmental surfaces in and around the General Hospital contained a very large number of microorganisms including enteric pathogens. In the Gambia, water obtained from village wells showed colony counts ranging from 2.6×10^2 to 4.0×10^{10} per ml of water. Faecal coliforms always exceeded 1600 per 100 ml of water.

By comparison, in many Western countries a water supply with a bacterial count in excess of 10 coliforms per 100 ml is considered unsuitable for consumption. Not surprisingly, the food of the weanling showed heavy contamination. As a rule, freshly cooked food was of an acceptable quality, but on keeping, within 30 minutes the bacterial counts reached a dangerous level. This chronic ingestion of pathogens in large amounts is accompanied by significant overgrowth of bacteria in the upper small intestine. It has been suggested that this abnormality is responsible for repeated episodes of diarrhoea in such children. Besides microbial pathogens, several intestinal parasites are known to cause chronic diarrhoea. Chief among these are *Giardia lamblia, Strongyloides stercoralis* and *Cryptosporidium*.

Stool culture gives a positive result in only about a third of the children with diarrhoea. Moreover, it is doubtful whether pathogens seen in the stools are indicative of those colonising and infecting the small bowel. In a prospective study amongst weanlings where monthly rectal swabs were taken for culture, it was found that a positive stool culture was obtained only a day or two before and after the episode of diarrhoea, and even though the symptoms persisted, culture of stools did not reveal pathogens.

Epidemiologic studies in several countries have emphasised the role of the nutritional status of the child as an important factor in the etiology of childhood diarrhoea. Diarrhoea is not only more frequent in children with poor nutritional status but also tends to be more severe. This was first demonstrated in a field study in Guatemala and later confirmed by similar studies in several other countries. For example, in a two-year longitudinal study in India it was shown that 60 per cent of undernourished children suffered from diarrhoeal disease as compared to 29 per cent of the normal. Moreover, the frequency and duration of diarrhoea increased with deterioration in the nutritional status.

It would thus appear that a vicious circle becomes established. During the process of weaning a deterioration of nutrition may occur which predisposes the child to diarrhoeal episodes. Unhygienic conditions lead to ingestion of contaminated foods and contribute further to gastro-intestinal upsets. When any loose motions occur, the parents restrict the diet of the child so that only clear fluids or thin gruels are offered and nutrition suffers even further. It is not surprising that diarrhoea is a major precipitating factor in malnutrition in the developing countries. A review of case histories of children brought to hospital for malnutrition often reveals several episodes of loose stools in the immediate past, each such episode leading to increasing deterioration of nutritional status, and this, in turn, predisposing to further episodes of diarrhoea.

The same unhygienic environment and food also give rise to heavy parasitic infestations in the child. Amoebiasis, giardiasis and strongyloides are known to be associated with loose stools. Heavy infestation with ascariasis and ankylostomiasis can also be contributory. All these factors, namely, chronic undernutrition, ingestion of contaminated food and water, and helminthic infestation, may be responsible for changes in intestinal mucosa leading to absorption difficulties and loose stools. Recent studies on American soldiers in Vietnam and Peace Corps volunteers in Pakistan have shown that many suffered from mild recurrent diarrhoea overseas. About 35–50 per cent developed structural changes in the intestinal epithelium characterised by blunting of the villi and abnormal d-xylose excretion tests. Such changes usually disappeared within a few months of returning home in most cases. Similar changes have been reported in intestinal biopsies in the indigenous population. It has been suggested that this so-called 'tropical intestine' is due to chronic invasion of the gut by bacteria, helminths and viruses together with the effects of undernutrition.

The role of pathogens

Bacterial agents can be identified with certainty in relatively few cases of diarrhoea. In several studies conducted in the United States and Western Europe during the last decade the mean isolation rate of pathogenic bacteria has been reported as 36 per cent with a range of 22 to 63 per cent. At least half cannot be diagnosed by the application of conventional bacteriological methods. On the other hand, there is enough epidemiologic evidence to implicate contaminated food and water as important etiologic factors. The social origins of the illness must be emphasised at the same time as the role of pathogens. Multiple hospital admissions, lower social class and various kinds of 'social problems' are common characteristics of affected children. Many of these factors will interfere with the care and protection of these children making them vulnerable to environmental agents.

The common organisms associated with diarrhoea are *E. coli, Shigella, Salmonella* and the enteric viruses. In recent years the roles of *Campylobacter, Yersinia* and *Vibrio parahaemolyticus* as well as of several Bacillus and Clostridial species in causing food-borne diarrhoeal illness has come to be better defined. Cholera is endemic in some countries from where small scale local epidemic spreads have occurred since the last major pandemic of the 1960s and 1970s. Cholera is considered separately, in chapter 16.

Escherichia coli

Diarrhoea due to *E. coli* is commonly seen in the bottle fed infant, in the weanling, and has been implicated in the traveller's diarrhoea. It is a global disease transmitted by the oro-faecal route affecting primarily the paediatric age group, though traveller's diarrhoea and 'acute non-vibrio cholera in the tropics' also affect adults. In the 1940s and 1950s there were a number of outbreaks of gastroenteritis throughout the world with a high mortality and a high rate of cross infection. *E. coli* gastroenteritis can be a trying disease when outbreaks occur in newborn nurseries where artificial feeding is the common practice. Epidemics are usually started by the admission of a carrier baby to such a unit. Mortality can be high and many of the survivors become carriers. In all nursery epidemics adequate laboratory facilities for the culture and sensitivity of the infecting organisms should be arranged because of the possibility of a resistant strain being the causal factor.

Striking advances have been made during the past decade in elucidating the ways in which *E. coli* cause diarrhoea. This has resulted in a reclassification of the organisms according to their pathogenic properties.

Pathogenic *E. coli* are usually described as enterotoxigenic (ETEC), enteropathogenic (EPEC), enteroinvasive, and enterohaemorrhagic. Each class falls within a fairly small and distinct category of O serogroups and O:H serotypes, bears distinct capsular (K) antigens, and possesses specific virulence properties.

Adhesion to receptors on the gut epithelium is a critical first step in causing infection. Most pathogenic *E. coli* carry surface proteins which interact with receptor sites on the enterocyte as *adhesins*, or promoters of intracellular invasion. In the case of enterotoxigenic strains the adhesins have proved to be projecting hair-like protein organelles or fimbriae on the surface of the bacteria. Some fimbrial adhesins are long rigid structures easy to visualise by electron microscopy. Others are thin flexible structures which are difficult to visualise. The genes encoding for the adherence factors are normally present in plasmids which control the expression of an outer membrane protein. The fimbriae as well as other properties of the *E. coli* including chemotaxis and motility determine whether or not a particular pathogen is swept away, colonises the mucus layer, or penetrates the mucus layer and glycocalyx to attach to the cell membrane. In the case of enteroinvasive *E. coli* large plasmids carry genes that encode for several outer membrane proteins which are involved in the invasion of the enterocyte.

After adhesion to or invasion of the enterocytes elaboration of exotoxins takes place. This is the next critical step in the pathogenesis of many *E. coli* infections. Enterotoxigenic *E. coli* (ETEC) produce heat-labile or heat-stable (or both) enterotoxins which increase net secretion in the small intestine. The enteropathogenic (EPEC), enteroinvasive (EIEC) and enterohaemorrhagic *E. coli* (EHEC) produce a cytotoxin resembling Shigella dysentery Type 1 (Shiga) toxin which can cause cell death. Some *E. coli* (0157) produce cytotoxins which are detected in vero cells (an African Green Monkey kidney line). These serotypes (VTEC) cause haemorrhagic colitis and have been implicated in the etiology of the haemolytic uraemic syndrome. Some *E. coli* show aggregative adherence as distinct from the other pathogenic serotypes. In animal models such EAggEC cause a distinct pathology. The enterocytes on the tips and sides of the villi are destroyed together with severe blunting of the villi. There is some evidence to show that EAggEC may be involved in the etiology of persistent diarrhoea.

Enterotoxigenic E. coli (ETEC) are an important cause of diarrhoea in infants and young children in developing countries, causing an average of two to three bouts of diarrhoea a year during the first two to three years of life. Human beings are the major reservoir of infection, and ETEC can be isolated in the faeces of symptomless human carriers.

The mechanism of disease is similar to that in the case of *V. cholera*. After adherence to the enterocyte ETEC elaborate a heat-labile (LT) or heat stable (ST) toxin, or both, resulting in watery diarrhoea.

Enteropathogenic E. coli (EPEC) have been usually implicated in diarrhoea outbreaks in nurseries. Close adherence to intestinal mucosa with destruction of microvilli is an important factor in the causation of diarrhoea.

Enteroinvasive E. coli (EIEC) Infected food handlers or contaminated water are the principal sources of infection. The colon is the main site of infection. Invasion of the enterocyte and intracellular multiplication in the colon lead to inflammation and ulceration of the mucosa. The invasive ability is related to a plasmid that encodes for several polypeptides on the outer membrane which are involved in invasiveness. There is very close antigenic resemblance between these polypeptides and those carried by *Shigella*.

Enterohaemorrhagic E. coli (EHEC) are associated with haemorrhagic colitis, and the haemolytic uraemic syndrome because of the verotoxins. Dairy cattle are the chief reservoir of the infection. Most outbreaks have been linked to the consumption of undercooked ground beef and unpasteurised milk.

Shigellosis

When ingested by man, *Shigella* can cause a spectrum of clinical illness from asymptomatic infection to diarrhoea without fever or severe illness manifested by blood and mucus in stool, high fever, toxaemia and convulsions in children. There are four groups of *Shigella* containing a total of 39 types. *S. dysenteriae* and *S. flexneri* serotypes are isolated most commonly in the tropics, while *S. sonnei* is the most frequently isolated type in temperate climates.

Following ingestion the organisms first proliferate in the upper regions of the small bowel, then penetrate the epithelial cells of the large intestine multiplying subsequently within the mucosa and also the lamina propria. This leads to an inflammatory response and the rapid destruction of areas of intestinal epithelium. The fundamental virulence characteristic of *Shigella* is its ability to invade epithelial cells and subsequently multiply therein. After invasion of the mucosa, the proliferating *Shigella* elaborate an enterotoxin which initiates the diarrhoea.

In developing countries more than half the episodes of diarrhoea with blood and mucus in the stool are caused by *Shigella*, with a high mortality rate. Furthermore, *Shigella* infection tends to be more severe in the developing world because of the more prevalent *Shigella dysenteriae* type 1.

In the past two decades major epidemics of *Shigella* dysentery have been reported from Bangladesh, Burma, Guatemala, India, Rwanda, Thailand, Vietnam and Zaire. The predominant types have been *S. dysenteriae type 1* 1 and *S. flexneri*. The former causes a more severe disease. The other varieties like *S. boydi* and *S. sonnei* are more common in temperate countries and usually give rise to a febrile self limiting watery diarrhoea. These differences in the predominant types explain the marked difference in clinical presentation. Poor nutrition or immunocompetence are also important factors.

The clinical case passes large numbers of organisms (10^5–10^8/g faeces) in the stool. Even healthy carriers have 10^2 organisms/g of faeces. Only a small number are needed for infection. In adult volunteers infection could be established with just 10 *Shigella*. Thus, person to person transmission within the family through handling of food is a common pattern of spread.

Shigellosis is now widely prevalent in the urban squatter communities of several countries where overcrowding, poor levels of personal hygiene, inadequate water supplies and poor sanitation allow person to person spread facilitated by the small inoculum required for infection. Since many squatter families are involved in the food trade, cooking snacks at home and selling them on street corners, spread of *Shigella* infection into the larger community occurs from time to time. During epidemics both water and food-borne spread has been recorded. *Shigella* are hardy organisms. In experimental studies viable organisms have been recovered from water maintained at room temperature for six months. A disturbing factor is that most *SHIGELLA* infections are now resistant to the common antibiotics. The recent epidemics recorded in Central America and South-east Asia were caused by resistant organisms. The resistance which is mediated by plasmid DNA is transferable to other gut microflora.

The ability to invade enterocytes, intracellular multiplication and cell to cell spread is controlled by genes present in the chromosomes as well as those carried by plasmids. Cytotoxins are produced by various *Shigella* species. *Shigella* toxins cause net fluid secretion in the intestine. They also cause systemic effects, the most serious being the haemolytic uraemic syndrome and toxic megacolon both of which are principally associated with *S. dysenteriae* type 1 infection. High fever, malaise and occasionally seizures associated with shigellosis can be ascribed to the systemic effects of the toxins. The predominant site of mucosal invasion and ulceration is the terminal ileum and the length of the colon. Here there are micro ulcers through which red blood cells and plasma protein leak into the bowel lumen.

In the tropics shigellosis has its peak attack rates in toddlers and pre-school children. In community studies in Guatemala and India, *Shigella* have been cultured from rectal swabs in infants as young as two or three months old. It is believed that repeated clinical and sub-clinical infections in childhood make the individual resistant to the prevalent strain. However, introduction of a new serotype can result in high attack rates. Outbreaks of *Shigella* have been described from Central America, Somalia and Bangladesh in recent years. In particular a pandemic occurred in Central America during 1968–70 where in Guatemala alone there were 12 000 deaths.

Salmonellosis

Man is the only host and reservoir of *Salmonella typhi*, the agent for typhoid fever. For most of the other *Salmonellae* the main hosts are cattle and other farm animals, who carry them in their intestinal tract and associated organs. They usually cause little disease among their hosts but are excreted in large numbers in their faeces. The effluent from infected animals and man is an important source of contamination of water and the food chain. Some stereotypes are adapted to certain animal species in whom they are more virulent than in others. But almost all stereotypes cause illness in man. Infection occurs when there is close contact between man and cattle, as is the case in most rural societies. Packaged raw meat, poultry and dairy products are frequently contaminated with *Salmonellae* and must be properly cooked to avoid food-borne illness. Infection can also occur through eggs and there have been reports of epidemics occurring through commercial egg powder.

Vertical transmission can occur in poultry via transovarian infection of eggs. Meat can become contaminated at any stage during slaughter, dressing and preparation of cuts of meat for sale. In some countries it has been estimated that a large proportion of eggs, almost half the chicken and about one to two per cent of lamb carcasses are contaminated with salmonella. Hence thorough cooking of eggs and meats, and pasteurisation or boiling of milk is strongly recommended.

Like *Shigellae*, the virulence of *Salmonellae* is due to their ability to invade epithelial cells of the intestinal mucosa. Strains associated with diarrhoea and dysentery affect both the large and the small bowel but typically remain localised in the bowel wall. In contrast, *S. typhi* and *paratyphi* cause generalised systemic infections involving the entire reticulo-endothelial system, and bacteraemia is a cardinal feature of enteric fevers.

The principal symptoms of infection are diarrhoea, mild fever, abdominal pain with nausea and vomiting. Headache and malaise with prostration may also occur. Symptoms usually occur between 12 and 36 hours after infection and usually last from two to five days. Illness is generally more severe in the very young, in whom the infective dose can be as low as 10 to 100 cells.

Although the acute stage passes rapidly the carrier state can last for more than three months.

There is no evidence to show that the commonly used antimicrobial drugs exert any significant bactericidal action upon Salmonella gastroenteritis in man. There is usually no shortening of illness and the length of time the organisms persist in the intestinal tract remains unaffected.

Other bacterial causes of diarrhoea

Campylobacter enteritis

Two closely related species are responsible for pathogenesis namely *C. jejuni* (80–90 per cent of infections) and *C. coli*. The organisms have a spiral shape which facilitates 'cork-screw' entry into the mucus membrane. The Campylobacter produce a cholera-like enterotoxin and one or more cytotoxins. The clinical and histological features of resulting enterocolitis are indistinguishable from *Salmonella* or *Shigella* infection.

The average incubation period is three days, and most patients recover within a week. Reactive arthritis (about one per cent of patients) and more rarely peripheral polyneuropathy can occur as complications.

Campylobacters are present in almost all surface water, which can be an important source of infection. Domestic animals and foods of animal origin including milk are other sources. Poultry are an important source, and studies in several countries have shown that *Campylobacter* can be grown from most poultry meat sold in shops. Hence the single most effective measure of control would be the control of infection in poultry. As battery farming becomes more common in developing countries, usually as cottage industry, special measure of control of *Campylobacter* infection and education of the producers will be increasingly necessary.

Yersinia enterocolitica

Y. enterocolitica was recognised as a food-borne pathogen in the mid-1970s. Pigs are regarded as major reservoirs of infection, and contaminated pork has been found to be the common source of most outbreaks.

Most clinical isolates of *Y. enterocolitica* produce a heat-stable enterotoxin similar to that of *E. coli*. The virulence of the organism is related to a plasmid that encodes for several virulence-related antigens.

Vibrio parahaemolyticus

Diarrhoea due to *V. parahaemolyticus* is almost always associated with the consumption of contaminated seafood and shellfish, especially when consumed raw.

The pathogenecity is not adequately known, but there is a strong correlation between clinical illness and the production of a thermostable haemolysin by the organism.

Bacillus cereus

Two distinct forms of abdominal symptoms have been described, namely the 'diarrhoeal syndrome' (associated with protein foods, vegetables, sauces and puddings) and the 'emetic syndrome' (associated with starchy foods, particularly rice). *B. cereus* is widespread and occurs in most raw foods, especially in some spices and cereals. The spores survive cooking and lack of proper refrigeration of meals after cooking would allow the spores to germinate and multiply in the food.

Most strains of *B. cereus* can form toxins. The diarrhoeal enterotoxin is heat labile, whereas the emetic toxin is highly stable. Freshly cooked food eaten hot is safe, but if the food is allowed to cool and maintained at temperatures between 10°C and 60°C, spores which have survived cooking can germinate and the resulting bacteria multiply in the food. Hence food should be maintained at a temperature above 60°C, or cooled rapidly to a temperature below 10°C to reduce bacterial growth.

Clostridium perfringens

There are five types of strains A-E, according to the extracellular toxins. Type A strains cause gas gangrene and are also responsible for all infectious diarrhoea in humans. Most outbreaks are associated with meat and poultry served in restaurants, institutions, schools and refectories.

Symptoms occur within 24 hours of eating contaminated food, and consist of diarrhoea with severe cramps. The symptoms are due primarily to an enterotoxin which is released at the time of sporulation of ingested bacteria.

Very rarely, type C strains cause food-borne infection which results in necrotic enteritis. It is now largely reported in Papua New Guinea and Indo-China, especially Vietnam. The disease is due largely to a toxin which can be normally inactivated by proteolytic enzymes in the intestine. If the production of the enzymes is low because of poor nutrition or due to inhibitors present in the diet the risk of illness is greatly increased.

Clostridium perfringens are usually present in the soil. Type A strains occur widely in raw and processed foods but the numbers are too low to cause infection. Types B, C, D and E are found in domestic animals. *C. perfringens* are also part of the normal faecal flora of most individuals.

In all outbreaks the main cause is failure to refrigerate previously cooked food. Spores on raw foods like meat can survive cooking. After heat activation they germinate when a suitable temperature is reached during cooking. All cooked foods should be kept at above 60°C or cooled within two to three hours to less than 10°C to prevent food poisoning.

Staphylococcal food poisoning.

Unhygienic handling of food is the chief cause. Healthy individuals carry *S. aureus* to the extent of 20–50 per cent. The nose is the main site of multiplication, and staphylococci are also found on the skin. Milk is usually infected because of mastitis in cows. Staphylococcal enterotoxin is heat resistant so that even if the end-product is heat processed, it can still cause symptoms if the ingredients (for example, milk or cream) were contaminated.

The staphylococcal enterotoxins are a group of seven distinct protein molecules, the production of which depends on various environmental factors. All the seven enterotoxins can withstand heat and proteolytic digestion. Unlike the enterotoxins of *E. coli*, the staphylococcal enterotoxins do not exert their effect by stimulation of adenylate cyclase activity, but probably act through stimulation of vagal and sympathetic nerves in the gut.

Viral gastroenteritis

Bacterial pathogens can be isolated from the stools of 20 to 50 per cent of children suffering from diarrhoea. All those with negative stool culture were thought to be suffering from 'viral gastroenteritis'. As techniques for isolation of viruses developed, it was shown that adenovirus and echovirus could be cultured from the stools of some children with diarrhoea.

Over one hundred viruses are excreted in human faeces including poliovirus, echoviruses, coxsackieviruses, hepatitis A virus and certain adenovirus types. More than one million virus particles may be excreted per gram of faeces and high concentrations of virus particles have been reported in raw sewage. Many are able to survive for prolonged periods in soil (25–125 days), in water (up to 168 days) and also in sea water (2–130 days). Several studies have shown that human viruses adsorbed on soil are infectious for animals and in tissue culture.

Three categories of viruses are recognised as medically important causes of diarrhoea in children, viz. rotavirus, enteric adenovirus and a miscellaneous group of 20 – 35 nm diameter viruses (including Norwalk like agents, calciviruses, astroviruses, and other small round viruses) (table 11.1). Of these *Rotaviruses* are the most important viral agent causing significant diarrhoea in children. Children under two years are most affected though diarrhoeal symptoms have been described in children within the age range of neonatal period to five years. The reports of neonatal infections are specially challenging. For example, in Sydney, Australia, 49 per cent of 628 neonates were shedding rotavirus and of these more than a quarter had diarrhoea. Transmission in nurseries is probably by

Table 11.1 Viruses that cause diarrhoea

	Rotavirus	Norwalk-like viruses	Enteric adenoviruses
Age group commonly affected (months)	6–24	Older children	6–24
Incubation period (days)	1–3	1–2	1–3
Duration of illness	3–7 days	12–24 hrs	3–7 days
Mode of transmission	Feacal-oral	Feacal-oral Food borne	Feacal-oral
Vaccine	Being tested	No	No

environmental spread from the milk kitchen, especially if artificial feeding is the rule. Like many other gut infections, breast feeding is known to protect against rotavirus diarrhoea.

The rotavirus is made up of a double stranded RNA with inner and outer capsids. The various proteins of the rotaviruses allow them to be classified into groups, subgroups and serogroups. There are four serotypes of human rotavirus. Infection with any one serotype causes a high level of immunity to that serotype, and partial protection against the other serotypes. A number of enzyme immunoassays (ELISA) and latex agglutination tests have been commercially produced on the basis of this knowledge. Latex kits are rapid and do not require expensive equipment, but are not as sensitive as ELISA.

Rotavirus characteristically invades the mucosa of the proximal small intestine, but in severe cases infection can be detected along the entire length of the intestine, and even the whole gastro-intestinal tract. The virus characteristically invades the villus epithelium, causing injury to the enterocyte.

The spread is by the person-to-person route within the family unit or an institution, and also by the faeco-oral route in communities. Rotavirus is a hardy virus and can remain viable for as long as six months on any objects, furniture, walls and floors.

Rotavirus diarrhoea occurs in all age groups with the peak in children 6 to 24 months old. Characteristically there are sporadic episodes rather than large outbreaks except in institutions, for example, day care centres. A number of studies indicate that between 15 to 50 per cent of cases of diarrhoea in developing countries may be due to the rotavirus. The onset is usually abrupt with explosive watery diarrhoea and vomiting. Low grade fever is also common. Dehydration occurs in about 40 to 80 per cent of the cases but is usually mild/moderate.

Repeated infections are common. Usually only the first rotavirus infection causes significant illness. It has been estimated that in many developing countries about one third of children under the age of two years experience an episode of rotavirus diarrhoea.

Intestinal parasites

Some parasites cause acute diarrhoea, abrupt in onset and lasting for a few days as in the case of amoebiasis and girardiasis. However, most diarrhoeal disease of parasitic origin is chronic or recurrent following an acute onset as in the case of strongyloidiasis and trichuriasis as well as in some cases of amoebiasis and giardiasis.

In recent years cryptosporidium has come to be recognised as an important cause of diarrhoea in infants in developing countries. After the first year of life infection is usually asymptomatic except in the case of children rendered immunodeficient because of undernutrition or infective illness. In such cases the diarrhoea becomes persistent and is accompanied by wasting.

Intestinal parasites are further considered in chapter 21.

The pathophysiology of diarrhoea

The intestinal epithelium separates its secretory and absorptive functions. The cells arising in the crypts of the villi are secretory. As they move towards the villous tip they acquire absorptive functions. Finally when they have reached the tip they get discarded into the lumen to be replaced by younger cells.

In the small intestine Na⁺ is absorbed coupled with other nutrients, mainly sugars like glucose and galactose, but also amino acids. One molecule of glucose carries with it one of Na⁺ across the brush border. At the brush border there are also polypeptides and amino acids resulting from the digestion of food. Their absorption is also coupled with that of Na⁺. In the absence of luminal nutrients the principal mechanism for the absorption of Na⁺ is by a coupled extrusion of H⁺ into the lumen.

Water is driven by local osmotic gradients. Once the ingested food and fluid have reached osmotic equilibrium all subsequent movements of fluid, nutrients and electrolytes are isosmotic with plasma. Thus the mucosa of the small intestine is the chief mechanism for the equilibration of fluid and electrolytes between the contents of the small intestine and plasma.

Micro-organisms disrupt the absorptive physiology of the small intestine in one or more of the following ways.

Enterotoxin production (See figures 11.1a and 11.1b)

Early work on cholera toxin has greatly helped our understanding of how toxins act. For example, cholera toxin stimulates intracellular adenylate cyclase in the mucosal cells of the small intestine. This results in an increased level of cyclic AMP, which inhibits influx of Na⁺ and Cl⁻ into the villous cell and actively stimulates the secretion of Na⁺ and Cl⁻ by the crypt cells. In each affected enterocyte these changes remain permanent. Recovery depends on the shedding of the affected cells and their replacement by normal cells migrating from the crypt to the villi. If such a process of regeneration of cells is depressed, for example in malnutrition, the diarrhoea is prolonged.

Toxigenic strains of *E. coli* (ETEC) elaborate at least two distinct enterotoxins (heat labile and heat stable toxins) which induce active fluid secretion without injuring enterocytes. The heat labile toxin is immunologically similar to cholera toxin, and has the same mechanism of action. The ability to produce toxins can be passed between organisms through plasmids in the same manner as resistance factor is transmitted between enteric organisms.

Enterotoxins may be ingested preformed as in the case of *Staphylococcus aureus*. Toxins may arise in food during storage after cooking as in the case of *Bacillus cereus*, or in the gut during sporulation after ingestion of bacteria as in the case of *Clostridium perfringens*.

The clinical hallmark of toxigenic diarrhoea is that it is non-inflammatory, large in volume, very watery, and the patient is usually afebrile.

Enterocyte injury

Rotavirus and Norwalk like virus cause diarrhoea by injury to the enterocyte with early sloughing of mature cells and their replacement by functionally immature crypt enterocytes. There is loss of brush border disaccharidases and monosaccharide carriers with the loss of villous cells.

In infection with *Giardia lamblia* there is enterocyte injury with flattening of villi and inflammation in the submucosa. Another protozoon, *Cryptosporidium*, binds to enterocytes and causes self limiting diarrhoea. In the case of both these parasites the immunodeficient host shows marked villous damage with plasma cell reaction in lamina propria.

The clinical picture is of non-inflammatory diarrhoea or malabsorptive stools in a patient with mild fever.

Mucosal invasion

This occurs usually in the colon but also occasionally in the ileum. There is associated inflammation, mucus production and bleeding, with the typical symptoms of dysentery.

Shigella also cause secretory diarrhoea with high fever, prostration and a large volume of watery stools.

In *Salmonella* infection there is a varying degree of small bowel and colonic involvement with mucosal penetration into the lamina propria and an inflammatory reaction.

Some strains of *E. coli* cause mucosal injury by invasion, specific adhesion, or cell injury mediated by a shigella like toxin.

Entamoeba histolytica have a lytic effect on tissues resulting in mucosal ulceration and accumulations of necrotic material under the mucosa.

The clinical picture

Three types of clinical presentation are described, each reflecting different pathogenesis and requiring different approaches to management. These are acute watery diarrhoea, persistent diarrhoea and dysentery.

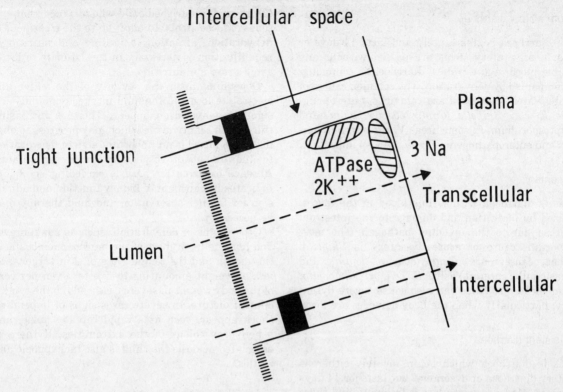

Figure 11.1a Absorption of water and electrolytes is by active as well as the passive route. Passive absorption is through the tight junction between enterocytes. Active absorption is through the enterocyte and is energy dependent. Sodium and glucose are absorbed jointly utilising a carrier mechanism at the brush border

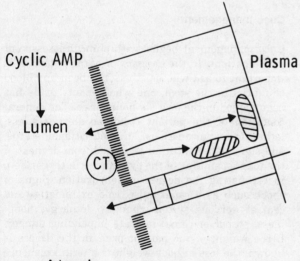

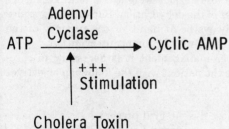

Figure 11.1b Cholera toxin stimulates adenyl cyclase which results in the formation of cyclic AMP. In experimental animals the presence of cholera toxin or cyclic AMP in the lumen results in the reversal of flow in salt and water causing profuse diarrhoea

Acute watery diarrhoea

The diarrhoea begins acutely and lasts 14 days or less. Loose watery stools are passed without any visible blood. Acute watery diarrhoea is commonly accompanied by dehydration. The common causes of acute watery diarrhoea are rotavirus, enterotoxigenic E. coli, Shigella, Campylobacter jejuni, and cryptosporidium. In some areas V. cholera, Salmonella and enteropathogenic E. coli are also important.

Dysentery

This is diarrhoea with visible blood in the faeces, caused by ulceration and damage to the intestinal mucosa due to the invading pathogen. The most important cause of acute dysentery is Shigella. Other causes are Campylobacter jejuni, and occasionally enteroinvasive E. coli or Salmonella. Entamoeba histolytica can also cause severe dysentery, particularly when the body defences are low.

Persistent diarrhoea

This is diarrhoea which begins acutely either as watery diarrhoea or dysentery, but lasts for 14 days or more. Marked weight loss is frequent, and there is also an ever present risk of dehydration. No single pathogen has been implicated, but it is likely that enteroadherent E. coli, Shigella and Cryptosporidium play a greater role than other pathogens. In endemic areas gut helminths may have a significant role. Persistent diarrhoea must be distinguished from chronic diarrhoea of non-infectious origin as in various malabsorption syndromes.

In acute watery diarrhoea, the onset can be explosive, with high fever and signs of toxicity, especially in young infants. There are only a few loose motions initially and it is only when watery diarrhoea supervenes that the true nature of the illness is realised. Alternatively, the onset may be gradual, with refusal of feeds, vomiting and loose stools. There is mild pyrexia, but later, as dehydration supervenes, the temperatures rises and signs of toxicity appear. If urgent measures are not undertaken, the child rapidly goes downhill with dehydration and shock.

In the mild and moderate cases there may be a few loose stools with or without mucus, occasional vomiting and refusal to feed. The older the child and the better his state of nutrition, the less severe is the illness.

Two kinds of children present special problems in diagnosis and management: (1) the overweight 'chubby' baby in whom dehydration is difficult to detect and the progress of the illness is rapid and (2) the undernourished child who has recurrent episodes of loose stools. In addition to the treatment of dehydration, attention to feeding and nutritional rehabilitation is necessary in the latter in order to avoid gross malnutrition.

Depending upon the severity of the water and electrolyte loss and the fluid intake, symptoms and signs of dehydration appear. There is increasing thirst with scanty urine which may progress to oliguria. The latter is an important sign of dehydration to inquire about, especially in young infants. Absence of urine for periods exceeding six hours indicates impairment of kidney function and admission for further observation and fluid therapy may be necessary.

Other signs of dehydration, such as sunken eyes and fontanelle, dryness of the mucous membrane of the mouth and the tongue, loss of skin turgor, and loss of weight amounting to five to seven per cent of the body weight in severe cases, add to the typical clinical picture. In severe cases signs of impending shock appear, such as a rapid thready pulse, and ashen grey colour of the extremities. If there is associated acidosis the child is also tachypnoeic and restless.

Case management

Case management begins with clinical assessment of the patient. In the assessment of the patient it is important to ask whether there has been any blood or mucus in the stool, and whether any urine has been passed in the past six hours or so. The general condition of the patient (whether alert, restless, lethargic or unconscious), the nutritional status, and signs of dehydration as judged from dryness of the tongue, sinking of the eyes and skin turgor help in estimating the degree of dehydration. Signs of shock such as a rapid pulse, cold extremeties and central nervous system changes (lethargy, floppiness, stupor or coma) indicate impending danger. If the weight of the patient prior to the illness is known, the loss in body weight is a useful measure of the extent of the dehydration. But weighing scales may not always be at hand, or the urgency of the situation may demand prompt intervention.

For proper management it is necessary to carefully assess the patient with the following objectives in mind

(1) Diagnose dysentery if present.
(2) Diagnose persistent diarrhoea if present.
(3) Estimate the degree of dehydration.

(4) Determine the nutritional status by means of dietary history and anthropometry.

(5) Diagnose the presence of any concurrent illness.

(6) Assess the immunisation status.

The most urgent aspect of management is the replacement of water and electrolytes. The main objectives of such therapy are: to replace the accumulated deficits; to provide for the continuing losses; to provide for maintenance; and to correct specific biochemical imbalances, for example, acidosis or alkalosis, hypernatraemia or hypokalaemia.

It is important to bear in mind that dehydration begins with the onset of the first diarrhoeal stool. In fact the moment normal absorptive functions of the enterocytes are disturbed and there is a net outward flux of water and electrolytes from enterocytes into the gut lumen, dehydration begins. Clinical signs of dehydration occur only after losses exceed five per cent of body weight. In other words,

fully one half of the maximum fluid deficit compatible with life may occur without any of the clinically recognisable signs of dehydration (figure 11.2). When fluid deficit exceeds five per cent, clinical signs like tachycardia, decreased skin turgor, oliguria, hypotension and severe thirst begin to appear. When the deficit equals about ten per cent body weight, shock occurs. In infants and small children where physiological reserves are poor, shock many ensue rapidly with relatively small losses, and a life-threatening situation arises within a few hours of the onset of diarrhoea.

In *severe dehydration* (altered consciousness; shock; oliguria or anuria; clinical signs of severe dehydration) initial support for the circulation is needed using a multiple electrolyte solution. A variety of solutions have been used but Ringer's lactate 100ml/kg is the most popular.

Ringer's lactate is administered intravenously at the rate of 30ml/kg in one hour for infants and 30 minutes for the older child, followed by 70ml/kg in

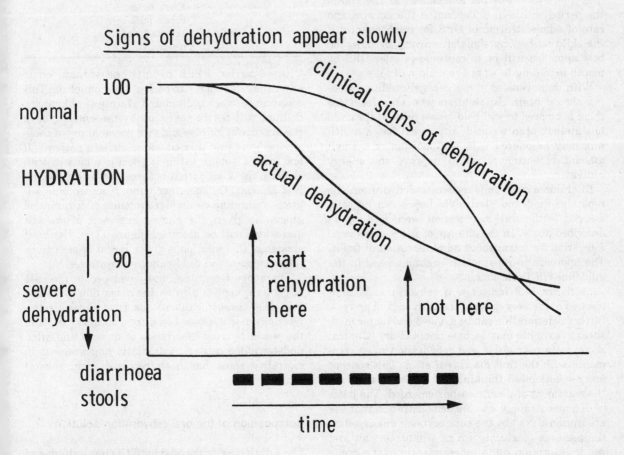

Figure 11.2 The need for early hydration

five hours for infants and two and a half hours for the older child. Hourly assessment of the child's condition during intravenous therapy is needed, followed by a thorough final assessment of the level of dehydration at the end. An appreciable improvement in the general condition, level of consciousness, blood pressure and peripheral pulse indicates recovery from shock. Now repair of fluid and electrolyte losses may be undertaken by the oral route. In emergency situations and when facilities for intravenous treatment are not available Ringer's lactate, or half strength Darrow's solution, or the oral rehydration solution may be given by the nasogastric route at the rate of 20ml/kg per hour for six hours.

Intravenous administration of fluids is for the treatment of shock. It is dangerous and even uneconomical to try to replace all the fluid and electrolyte losses by the intravenous route. Oral rehydration using a sugar-electrolyte solution (ORS, see below) is the more physiologically efficient approach. Depending upon the child's state of hydration 70–80 ml/kg of the fluid is administered by mouth in the first four hours. Further assessment at the end of the period will help to determine the amount and rate of administration of ORS for maintenance. If the child is showing signs of recovery by now, the best approach will be to continue to offer ORS by mouth according to what the child will take.

With improvement in the general condition feeding should begin. In children who are breast fed there is no need to withhold breast milk. If the child has already been weaned, any cereal based multi-mix may be offered with the addition of a small amount of butter or oil to improve the energy content.

In children with mild/moderate dehydration the repair of fluid and electrolyte losses can be commenced with oral rehydration and feeding as described above. In the absense of shock there is no indication for intravenous administration of fluids. The approach to rehydration is summarised in the guidelines in Table 11.2.

As figure 11.2 indicates, if rehydration is commenced at the very onset of the pathological process, further deterioration can be avoided and heroic measures to save life may become unnecessary. Clinical signs are a poor guide and rehydration must commence with the first diarrhoeal stool. This concept has revolutionised thinking and a new strategy for the treatment of diarrhoea has emerged. The basis of this new strategy was the demonstration that the absorption of Na^+ by the enterocytes is enhanced by the presence of glucose which stimulates salt and water absorption quite independently of the cyclic AMP. The brush-border of the enterocyte uses a

Table 11.2 Guidelines for the management of diarrhoea

	Amount to be given	Time required
Severe dehydration (shock; hypotension; weak or absent radial pulse)	Ringer's lactate 100 ml/kg i.v.	30ml/kg in ½ to 1 hour remainder in 3 to 5 hours
	oral rehydration to commence as soon as patient is able to drink.	
Moderate dehydration	ORS 70–80ml/kg by mouth. Offer breast milk and multi-mixes.	In 4 hours
Mild or no dehydration	ORS by mouth 50–100 ml/stool if age <2 years	500ml/day if <2 years
	100–200 ml/stool if age >2 years	1 000ml/day if >2 years
	Extra fluids breast milk as accepted, and usual diet.	

'glucose-carrier' which permits one sodium ion to enter the cell along with each glucose molecule. This coupling between sodium and glucose is obligatory. Sodium will not be taken up by the enterocyte in the absence of glucose and vice versa. Many of these studies were first carried out on cholera patients. If one litre of isotonic saline is given to a patient with cholera, the stool output is increased by an equivalent amount. On the other hand, if an isotonic solution containing equimolar amounts of sodium and glucose is given, the glucose and most of the salt and water will be absorbed (figure 11.3). Hence, if enough of this solution is given, faecal losses can be fully replaced and fluid balance maintained.

The above reasoning, first developed in the case of cholera, applies also to diarrhoea due to *E. coli* and other toxogenic diarrhoeas. Oral sugar-electrolyte solutions are now being used in many parts of the world to treat diarrhoeas of diverse and often undetermined causes. A dramatic improvement in mortality rates has been reported from several countries.

Composition of the oral rehydration solution

The solution recommended by WHO has sodium and glucose in equimolar proportions, is isotonic with

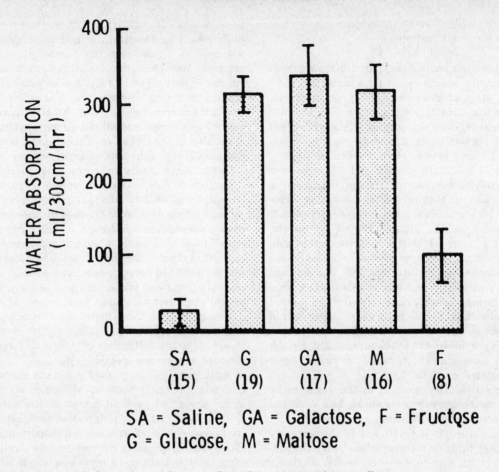

Figure 11.3 Improved absorption with sugar-electrolyte mixture given orally

plasma and contains sufficient potassium and bicarbonate to replace the losses in stools (table 11.3).

Glucose-electrolyte solution with the above composition is obtained by adding to one litre of water the following

Sodium chloride	3.5g
Sodium bicarbonate or	2.5g
Sodium citrate	2.9g
Potassium chloride	1.5g
Glucose	20.0g

Oral rehydration has markedly reduced the need for intravenous therapy so that infants and young children with diarrhoea can be adequately treated at the level of the health centre and sub-centre. In one study on the efficacy of oral rehydration it was found that in hospital admissions (and these represent only a small proportion of all diarrhoea cases) approximately ten per cent will require additional intravenous therapy. However, if oral rehydration

Table 11.3 Electrolyte content of stool in watery diarrhoea compared to composition of oral glucose–electrolyte solution (m eq/litre)

	Na	K	Cl	HCO_3
Cholera stool				
Adults	140	13	104	44
Children (5 years)	101	27	92	32
Diarrhoea				
Children (5 years)	56	25	55	14
Oral glucose/ electrolyte solution	90	20	80	30
Normal plasma	142	4.5	105	25

is commenced at the very onset of diarrhoea, before clinical signs of dehydration occur, almost every patient can be successfully treated by this method only.

The need for simplification

Once the scientific basis of oral rehydration was well established, the search began for simplification. In the rural areas of many developing countries glucose is not available. If found it is five to eight times more expensive than ordinary cane sugar. Several controlled studies using a sucrose-electrolyte solution have shown it to be equally efficacious.

Sucrose is split into glucose and fructose by a specific brush-border enzyme. Absorption of fructose is not coupled to that of sodium and it provides relatively little stimulation for the absorption of salt and water. It is the glucose released from the hydrolysis of cane sugar which is the active substance. The amount of sugar necessary for oral rehydration is twice that of glucose namely, 40g per litre of water. Analysis of mucosal biopsies taken from children during the acute phase of diarrhoea showed that although lactase was reduced in 75 per cent of the specimens, sucrase was reduced in only 18 per cent. This provides further encouragement for the use of the cheaper and more widely available sugar in oral rehydration fluid.

Having settled the question of the sugar to be used, the next step was to establish how essential was the presence of potassium and bicarbonate in the mixture. Clearly if treatment is started early before kidney function is compromised, then the kidneys should be able to compensate for whatever metabolic acidosis and potassium deficiency is present. Moreover, potassium can be supplied in the oral fluid in the form of fruit juices (lemon, orange or other citrus fruit). Trials with the more simplified solution containing just sugar and salt with or without added fruit juice have shown that such a solution is equally efficacious for the early mild/moderate type of dehydration.

The magnitude of potassium deficit in moderate/severe dehydration secondary to acute diarrhoea is approximately 10–12 mmol/kg, and tends to be more if there is co-existing malnutrition. Potassium rich foods should be continued for at least a week after diarrhoea has stopped.

Table 11.4 lists some common sources of potassium from locally available foods.

Cereal-based oral rehydration solution – super ORS

The demonstration that cane sugar when used in twice the amount can replace glucose has been an important development. The lesson learnt is that the digestive enzymes are not affected much in acute diarrhoea. Rice-based oral rehydration solution is not only as effective as the parent glucose-based solution, but there is also a reduction in stool volume in most cases. A variety of cereals have been studied including wheat, maize and millet as well as plantain and starchy roots. All have performed as well as glucose, and all reduce stool volume substantially. In the cereal-based solution for oral rehydration 50–80g of the cooked cereal replaces glucose.

In the early studies of cotransport mechanisms a number of substances like amino acids, di- and tripeptides as well as other compounds were shown to have effects similar to those of glucose and each used independent pathways. These compounds stimulate the transport of sodium additively to glucose. This observation has stimulated a search for a super-ORS. In fact the cereal-based solution has several advantages to recommend it as a super-ORS. Cereal grain is available in most homes, and is the mainstay of the local dietaries. Secondly, when digested the protein and starch of the cereal are presented to the epithelium of the gut as large polymers of sugars and peptides. Because of the low osmotic power of large food polymers there is no immediate osmotic penalty. Molecules of glucose, amino acids and peptides get presented to the gut epithelium in step-wise progression as digestion proceeds, each using a specific cotransport pathway. Cereal-based solutions provide two to three times more calories than the glucose-electrolyte solution. With improvement in the diarrhoea the quantity of cereal can be increased to provide more calories. Other foods, for example lentils may be added to make the intake more nourishing.

It is also likely that by presenting a protein substrate to the gut epithelium (all cereals are eight to ten per cent protein) the cereal-based solution supports rapid turnover of cells in the villi resulting

Table 11.4 Potassium content of some common foods

	Potassium content (mmol/100g)
Banana	9.0
Papaya	6.0
Avocado	10.3
Spinach	12.3
Pumpkin	8.0
Mango	4.9
Coconut water	8.0
Orange juice	4.6
Lemon juice	3.6
Grapefruit	4.2
Tomato juice	5.8

in their earlier shedding and loss of the toxin attached to them. Cereal-based therapy will also encourage early offering of food to the patient and thereby avoid malnutrition. In the coming years the use of cereal-ORS as a home-based solution, for example, rice gruel in China, is likely to establish itself as a super-ORS for the early treatment of diarrhoea. Similarly early institution of feeding with breast milk in infants and the staple cereal in the older child together with sugar or glucose-electrolyte solution will achieve the same purpose.

Taking oral rehydration into the village home

The child with diarrhoea and dehydration may not be brought for medical care early enough. Obviously the key to success is to educate the mother so that oral rehydration can commence early. The simplified formula for the rehydration fluid should make this possible but still one problem remains: How important is it to measure the exact amounts of the ingredients? In the poor home, sugar is a luxury, and always in short supply. There is every likelihood that solutions containing less sugar and excess salt may be administered giving rise to hypernatraemia. Several studies have shown that when mothers are left to prepare the mixtures using their hands to measure out the ingredients large errors in concentration can occur. On the other hand, in rural health programmes with resident village health workers, who are regularly supervised, mothers were able to carry out oral rehydration successfully at home.

The World Health Organisation has proposed the packaging of measured amounts of the ingredients and distributing them widely. This obviously will be expensive and in some cases the cost has been calculated to be several times the annual per caput expenditure on health. Moreover in many developing countries only 20 per cent of the rural population is in continuing contact with the health service. Hence the distribution of such packets will be ineffective if they are given out through the health institutions. Perhaps the key to the dilemma lies in some rethinking about diarrhoea and dehydration. It is a state of *fluid-electrolyte malnutrition* and the replacement of the losses should assume priority. We should stop thinking of oral rehydration as a medical procedure. Just as the key role of the mother in the treatment of protein-energy malnutrition is now well established, we must now make her the central figure in treating fluid-electrolyte malnutrition. It is the mother who must take the responsibility for early rapid replacement of salt

and water – the two vital nutrients in this form of malnutrition. Properly supported through education and encouraged by the presence of village health workers, many mothers are able to achieve this. The target is to give the child one glassful of the rehydrating fluid for every diarrhoeal stool. Each such glassful of fluid should contain a fistful of sugar and a pinch of salt. Measuring spoons, if available, may be used instead of the hand, but in their absence or in the absence of sealed packets, oral rehydration should still continue.

Nutrition and the child with diarrhoea

It is well known that malnutrition and diarrhoea go hand-in-hand. It is common knowledge that children recovering in hospital from severe diarrhoea show deterioration of nutritional status. This is partly due to the catabolic effect of the diarrhoeal illness and partly because of the time-hallowed tradition of 'resting the gut'. Added to this are the prolonged anorexia and nausea which are the common accompanying features of diarrhoea as well as the cultural practice of offering the child only liquid diet during a diarrhoeal illness. The final outcome is a marked nutritional insult.

With oral rehydration recovery is quick and there is a rapid return of appetite. Instead of the illness being drawn out over a period of a week or so, it is now a matter of days before the child is able to take solids. In breast fed infants there is no need to withhold the mother's milk. Even if the infant is not breast fed, early feeding with full strength milk is the rule and only in rare instances is there any difficulty because of lactose intolerance. These observations have further simplified the management of diarrhoea. In fact, with oral rehydration to correct fluid-electrolyte malnutrition and early feeding to avoid protein-energy malnutrition, rapid return to full nutritional status is the rule.

Diarrhoea tends to be more severe as well as more recurrent in undernourished children. On recovery, many of them need nutritional rehabilitation. A period of stay in a nutrition rehabilitation unit will also be useful for training the mother and improving her knowledge of child care.

Management of dysentery

Dysentery is a serious illness. About 15 per cent of all diarrhoeal episodes in children in some countries are associated with blood and mucus in the stool and 25 per cent of all diarrhoeal deaths occur in such children. Dysentery is particularly serious when it occurs in young children who have not been breast fed, or are undernourished, or following measles. Diarrhoeal episodes which commence as dysentery are also more likely to become persistent.

The most common cause of dysentery in developing countries is infection by *Shigella*, especially *S. dysenteriae* type 1 and *S. flexneri*. *Campylobacter, Salmonella* and enteroinvasive *E. coli* are also occasional causes of dysentery. In endemic areas *Entamoeba histolytica* can be a common cause.

A variety of potentially fatal complications can occur in dysentery, especially when caused by *Shigella*. These include convulsions, toxic megacolon, intestinal perforation, septicaemia, haemolytic uraemic syndrome, and prolonged hyponatraemia. Rapid deterioration of the nutritional status is a common sequela of dysentery.

Children with dysentery should be presumed to have shigellosis and treated as such pending results of stool culture or isolation of *E. histolytica* on stool microscopy. This is because *Shigella* are responsible for 60 per cent of all dysentery and almost all fatal cases. Early treatment of shigellosis with an appropriate antibiotic shortens the duration of the illness and reduces the risk of complications. Unfortunately in many places resistant strains have emerged, hence care in the selection of antibiotics is necessary. Cotrimoxazole (120mg–480mg depending on age, 12 hourly) is the first choice. Ampicillin (25mg/kg, every six hours) is effective in some areas. For organisms resistant to these antibiotics Ciprofloxacin (125–500mg, twice daily) may be needed. Antibiotic treatment should be continued for five days.

Dysentery due to *Campylobacter* is usually mild and self limiting. The occasional case may need treatment with Erythromycin (125mg–250mg, six hourly) or Ciprofloxacin.

Dysentery due to *Entamoeba histolytica* responds well to Metronidazole (10mg/kg every eight hours) for five days.

The management with regard to fluids for the dehydration, and feeding is the same as in acute diarrhoea.

Management of persistent diarrhoea

Up to 20 per cent of acute diarrhoeal episodes may become persistent with marked deterioration of nutritional status and intolerance of food, especially disaccharides, cow's milk protein and wheat. The mortality tends to be high, being as much as 30 to 50 per cent of all diarrhoea associated deaths. No single microbial cause has been detected though *Shigella* and enteroadherent *E. coli* are commonly found associated with persistent diarrhoea. *Cryptosporidium* is also an important causative agent in severely undernourished or immunodeficient individuals.

Persistent diarrhoea is associated with extensive pathology in the bowel. Flattening of the villi with marked reduction in the disaccharidase enzymes and bacterial overgrowth are common findings. It would appear that in some cases of acute diarrhoea the illness becomes prolonged because of either failure of intestinal mucosa to heal rapidly, or there is continuing injury to the intestinal epithelium. One reason for failure to heal rapidly may be undernutrition, or a deficiency of micronutrients. Continuing mucosal injury may be due to adherent or invading pathogens. Dietary constituents like lactose, proteins or antigens triggering immune mechanisms can also cause minor injury.

Five risk factors have been identified with regard to persistent diarrhoea. *Age* is a particularly important risk factor. The peak incidence is in the first year of life, and the chances of an acute attack becoming persistent are also greatest in that age group. *Animal milk* especially when fed by the bottle is often a precipitating factor. The risk of persistent diarrhoea is greatest in the first month of introduction of animal milk. *Impaired immune function* either primary or secondary to malnutrition often accompanies persistent diarrhoea. *Previous infection* either as diarrhoea, dysentery or measles is often a significant factor in the evolution of the disease. In such a case there may be an element of suppression of the immune system besides the direct effect of enteric infection on the gut epithelium. *Inappropriate management of acute diarrhoea* with antimotility drugs or antibiotics, or prolonged starvation can be significant factors.

Persistent diarrhoea is largely a nutritional disorder. Its management is based on the twin principles of maintaining hydration and nutrition while intestinal damage is repaired. It is important to continue feeding the patient using the following guidelines
(1) Never stop breast feeding.
(2) Use multi-mixes to provide complementary protein sources.
(3) Cereals are preferred as sources of carbohydrates to avoid hyperosmolarity and problems with lactose intolerance.
(4) Edible vegetable fats are useful to improve energy density and are well tolerated.

(5) Adequate amounts of vitamins and minerals (for example zinc and magnesium) should be included in the diet because of their role in the regeneration of the damaged gut.

Intestinal parasites, for example giardiasis, need treatment. Antibiotics are indicated when repeat stool cultures persistently show the same pathogens. A number of reports in the literature describe marked improvement after the administration of pooled colostrum or breast milk.

Further reading

Avery M E, Snyder J D. Oral therapy for acute diarrhoea. The underused simple solution. *New Eng J Med* 1990; 323: 891–893.

Candy D C A, McNeish A S. Human Escherichia coli diarrhoea. *Arch dis childh* 1984; 59: 395–396.

Cravioto A, Tello A, Navarro A, Ruiz J *et al.* Association of E. coli HEp–2 adherence pattern with type and duration of diarrhoea. *Lancet* 1991; 337: 262–64.

Ebrahim G J. Oral rehydration therapy in the 1990s. *J Trop Ped* 1989; 35: 209–210.

Ebrahim G J. Persistent diarrhoea. *J Trop Ped* 1990; 36: 50–51.

Field M, Rao M C, Chang E B. Intestinal electrolyte transport and diarrhoeal disease. *New Eng J Med* 1989; 321: 800–806, 879–883.

Keusch G T, Bennish M T. Shigellosis: recent progress, persisting problems and research issues. *Ped Inf Dis J* 1989; 8: 713–719.

Macfarlane P I, Miller V. Human milk in the management of protracted diarrhoea in infancy. *Arch dis childh* 1984; 59: 260–5.

Saha K, Dua N, Chopra K. Use of human colostrum in the management of chronic infantile diarrhoea due to enteropathogenic E. coli infection with associated parasite infestation and undernutrition. *J Trop Ped* 1990; 36: 247–250.

W.H.O. Scientific Working Group. Escherichia coli diarrhoea. *Bull Wld Hlth Org* 1980; 58: 23–36.

W.H.O. *The rational use of drugs in the management of acute diarrhoea in children.* Geneva: World Health Organisation, 1990.

W.H.O. *The treatment and prevention of acute diarrhoea. Practical guidelines.* 2nd. edition. Geneva: World Health Organisation, 1989.

12 Typhoid and paratyphoid (Salmonellosis)

The Salmonellae are Gram-negative aerobic rods with flagellae and grow readily on simple culture media. They are primarily pathogens of animals but can be transmitted to man, in whom they can cause disease. The very young and the elderly are particularly susceptible to *Salmonella* infection, which can be fatal in these age groups. The domestic fowl is the largest single source of *Salmonella* and the meat may be a cause of infection in man. Duck and hen eggs can become infected either in the oviduct, but more likely through the shell after the eggs have been laid, due to infection in the nesting box. Domestic animals such as cattle, sheep and pigs are important reservoirs of infection and the meat may become contaminated during slaughtering or in its various stages of preparation for marketing.

Many of the Salmonellae are important pathogens of animals, as their names suggest. For example, *S. typhimurium* is responsible for 'mouse typhoid' and *S. cholerasuis* causes cholera-like disease in hogs. Man is infected in most cases either accidentally or through close contact with animals or because of poor hygiene. While a few of the Salmonellae, out of 1500, are host-specific, most strains are able to interchange their hosts and can occur anywhere. *S. typhimurium* is geographically the most widespread and *S. dublin* the most common in cattle.

Salmonella typhi and *paratyphi* differ from the other Salmonellae in that they do not normally infect animals and are primarily human pathogens. Hence typhoid and paratyphoid fevers have always a human source of infection. Furthermore, they give rise to septicaemic illnesses, whereas the other Salmonellae mainly cause gastro-intestinal symptoms.

Certain disease processes render the individual susceptible to *Salmonella* infections. Thus, children with sickle cell anaemia are unusually susceptible to *Salmonella* infection, so that *Salmonella* osteomyelitis is a common complication of the disease. A high incidence of *Salmonella* infections has also been reported in liver cirrhosis, lupus erythematosus, leukaemia and lymphoma, and with schistosomiasis.

Typhoid fever

The ultimate source of infection with *S. typhi* is a patient or a chronic carrier. Individuals suffering from typhoid fever excrete the organisms in their urine and faeces for several weeks. The typhoid bacillus can survive for weeks in water, dust or dried sewage. Water contaminated with *S. typhi* has been a known source of epidemics of typhoid fever in many countries; milk adulterated with contaminated water has also been known to give rise to epidemics. Flies have been implicated in the transmission of infection to foods. Oysters and shell-fish from contaminated water have also caused outbreaks of the disease. However, in communities with high endemicity the infection is spread by direct contact, through the faeco-oral route, within families and neighbourhoods as well as in schools.

After an attack of typhoid fever some individuals become chronic carriers. The organisms persist in their biliary tract without giving rise to symptoms and are passed in the faeces for a year or more. Instances of life-long carriage have been recorded but in the majority of cases carriage is limited. Such individuals constitute an important part of the reservoir of infection in the community and become the source of future outbreaks, especially when they happen to be in a trade requiring handling of foods.

Water is an important vehicle for the transmission of infection. Improvement of water supply bears a direct relationship to a fall in the incidence rate in most countries. For example, typhoid has become rare in all countries which have good standards of hygiene and a well-developed sanitation

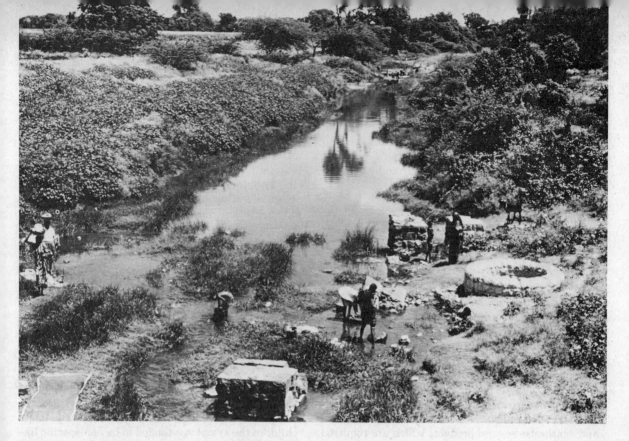

Figure 12.1   Pollution of water – rural India

Figure 12.2   Street vendors

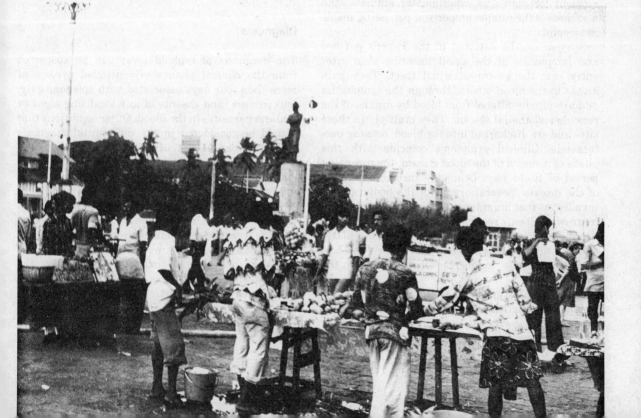

system. However, even in such countries constant vigilance is necessary. The introduction of infection in a relatively non-immune population can cause high morbidity and mortality. Modern means of travel and the popularity of package tours abroad have increased the risks of introducing infection in such societies. Similarly, the importing of foods which may have been processed and handled abroad can be a source of epidemics.

Pathogenesis

The development of disease after ingestion of *Salmonella* is influenced by the number and the virulence of the organisms, and by a variety of host factors. In most experimental infections 10^6–10^9 organisms must be ingested to cause symptomatic infection. But with unusually virulent organisms or in patients with reduced resistance symptomatic infection may result from smaller numbers of organisms. The *Salmonella* are intracellular pathogens, and synthesise several products which are required for entry and survival in the intracellular environment, in addition to factors necessary for existence in the gastro-intestinal tract and in the external environment. All *S. typhi* strains do not contain the virulence (vi) antigen. Vi carrying strains are more virulent for man and experimental animals, and also possess the unique property of persisting inside neutrophils.

S. typhi can be detected in the Peyer's patches and lymphatics of the small intestine soon after entry into the gastro-intestinal tract. They gain access to the blood stream through the lymphatics and are rapidly filtered from blood by organs of the reticulo-endothelial system. They multiply in these sites and are discharged into the blood, causing bacteraemia. Clinical symptoms coincide with this phase of invasion of the blood stream, the preceding period of 10–14 days being the incubation period of the disease. Several organs of the body may be invaded, so that organisms can be found in the bone marrow, spleen, respiratory secretions and the urine. Infection of the biliary tract occurs regularly and the multiplication of the *S. typhi* in the bile leads to a large number of them entering the intestines.

Infection of Peyer's patches and the lymphoid tissues of the small intestine is responsible for some of the well-known complications of typhoid fever like ulceration with bleeding and perforation.

Symptoms

The symptoms develop insidiously after an incubation period of 10 to 14 days. Fever and headache are common. Many children presenting with pyrexia of unknown origin turn out to be suffering from enteric fever. Because of the non-specific nature of the symptoms there is not uncommonly a delay in diagnosis of up to a week or more. Confusion and disorientation may be present from the onset or appear later as the disease process advances. The spleen is enlarged in more than half the cases. In one large study of over a 1000 cases in East Africa, fever and abdominal symptoms like pain and loose stools were present in almost 80 per cent of the cases. Headache occurred in approximately half and confusion was present in 20 per cent of the patients.

In adults, diarrhoea is a relatively late feature of typhoid fever, but in children diarrhoea and vomiting are common presenting features. In one series of 150 cases of typhoid fever in children reported from Nigeria, it was observed that in children over the age of five years the presenting features of the illness resembled those in adults, but in younger children the symptoms tended to be non-specific like fever, convulsions, diarrhoea and vomiting. Many children presented with anaemia without any fever, and after receiving blood transfusion developed fever with rigors which led to the diagnosis of the true nature of their illness.

Diagnosis

The diagnosis of typhoid fever can be suspected from the clinical picture of continued pyrexia of more than four days associated with splenomegaly, leukopaenia, and absence of any localising signs or malaria parasites in the blood. Other conditions that should be considered in the differential diagnosis are infections of the urinary tract, tuberculosis, infection by other Salmonellae, mycoplasma pneumoniae infection and, rarely, collagen diseases or a malignancy.

The diagnosis is confirmed by culturing *S. typhi* from the blood, urine or faeces. It has been observed that *S. typhi* can be isolated from blood in 90 per cent of cases in the first week and in 50 per cent of the cases in the second and third weeks. After the third week of illness, the Widal reaction is commonly used as a diagnostic indicator. More recently it has been observed that H antibodies may not be detected in 15 per cent of patients even with bateriologically proven typhoid fever. Similarly, O antibodies may not be detected in 41 per cent of proven cases. These observations throw doubt on the usefulness of the Widal test. Moreover, relapses are known to occur despite high antibody titres.

S. typhi may be cultured from the stools in the first few weeks of the illness. Those who continue to excrete the organisms for more than one year are likely to become chronic carriers. The biliary tract is infected in all chronic carriers who may excrete up to 10^6–10^9 bacilli/ml of bile.

Management

The patient should be admitted to hospital where safe disposal of the excreta is possible and facilities are available for isolation and barrier nursing. Intravenous fluids are required for the treatment of dehydration, which is frequent. Chloramphenicol is effective against *S. typhi* and is given in doses of 50 mg/kg body weight, reducing to 25 mg/kg when the fever has subsided, after which it is continued for two weeks or more. A safe nutritious diet and vitamin supplements to maintain the nutrition are also important.

In patients treated with chloramphenicol a relapse rate of between 10 and 20 per cent has been reported. There is also the likelihood of a three per cent rate of chronic carriage, and in rare instances, aplastic anaemia. For these reasons and because of the emergence of resistance to chloramphenicol, other antibiotics have been tried. Ampicillin (200 mg/kg/day) is effective but not superior to chloramphenicol. Moreover resistance to ampicillin has been reported from several countries. The same applies to cotrimoxazole. In the case of multi-resistant organisms third generation cephalosporins (for example cefotaxime) have been successfully tried with relapse rates of between one and six per cent in different studies.

Prevention

The current inactivated *S. typhi* whole cell parenteral vaccines confer useful protection against typhoid fever, but cause systemic and local reactions. Inactivated preparations of *S. typhi* administered orally give little or no protection. At present a live vaccine made from an attenuated strain of *S. typhi* (Ty21a) is undergoing trials with encouraging results. The level of protection appears to be influenced by the formulation, the number of doses, and the immunisation schedule. The level of protection reported in different trials varies from 65 per cent

for at least five years (Chile) to 96 per cent over three years' surveillance (Egypt). Another approach has been to administer purified vi antigen parenterally. Trials with the vi antigen vaccine have shown protection rates of 72 per cent at 17 months (Nepal), and 64 per cent at 21 months (South Africa). The immunogenicity of the vi antigen, which is a polysaccharide, can be further enhanced by conjugation with a carrier protein like tetanus toxoid.

Early diagnosis and isolation of the patient in the hospital is important in eliminating a source of infection in the community. During epidemics, regular supervision of the source of water supply and disinfection of wells in the rural community should be carried out. In communities with repeated outbreaks of enteric fever a search should be mounted for chronic carriers, especially amongst those who handle and sell foods, and in particular those who run small kiosks or sell home-cooked snacks in public places.

Four types of epidemiological patterns have been described with regard to typhoid fever as follows

(1) Communities with an appalling state of hygiene and sanitation (for example many rural communities in developing countries).
   – *S. typhi* probably very prevalent. Infection is usually acquired in infancy and early childhood, and goes unrecognised or is mild.
(2) Communities where hygiene and sanitation are poor.
   – *S. typhi* infection is common, and typhoid fever is particularly frequent in children.
(3) Communities where hygiene and sanitation are a mixture of primitive and modern (for example most cities in developing countries).
   – outbreaks of typhoid fever repeatedly occur and involve all age groups.
(4) Hygiene excellent.
   – *S. typhi* are rare and infection is related largely to tourism, imported foods or because of carriers or defects in the sewage system.

Further reading

Anon. Typhoid and its serology. (Editorial). *Br Med J* 1978; 1: 390.

Ashcroft M T, Singh B, Nicholson C C, *et al.* A seven year field trial of two typhoid vaccines in Guyana. *Lancet* 1967; ii: 1056–9.

Duggan M B, Beyer L. Enteric fever in young Yoruba children. *Arch Dis Childh* 1975; 50: 67.

Levine M M, Ferreccio C, Black R E, Chilean Typhoid
    Committee, Germanier R. Large scale field trial of Ty21a
    live oral vaccine in enteric coated capsule formulation.
    Lancet 1987; i: 1049–52.

Mulligan T O. Typhoid fever in young children. *Br med J*
    1971; 4: 665–7.

Wahdan M H, Serie C, Cerisior Y, Sallam S, Germanier
    R. A controlled field trial of live S. typhi strain Ty21a
    oral vaccine against typhoid; three year results. *J Infect
    Dis* 1982; 145: 292–96.

13 *Viral hepatitis*

The general term viral hepatitis refers to infection of the liver caused by two main types of viruses viz. type A and type B (HAV and HBV). More recently other agents have been identified which cause forms of hepatitis which are clinically and pathologically similar. These are the delta virus (HDV) and the virus of non-A non-B hepatitis (HCV and HEV). Clinical observations, epidemiological studies and volunteer experiments have helped to clarify our understanding of the natural history of different types of hepatitis. In recent years developments in molecular biology, combined with refined serological methods and the use of electron microscopy have helped our understanding of the structure of the different agents causing hepatitis, as well as the natural history of the illness. Other viruses which can occasionally cause hepatitis are the Epstein-Barr virus, cytomegalovirus, varicella, herpes simplex, rubella and the Coxsackie virus. In the case of these viruses hepatitis occurs as part of a multisystem infection.

The causative viruses in both type A and type B hepatitis are stable. They are capable of resisting heat at 56°C for 30 minutes to 1 hour, chlorine in the normal concentration used for sterilising water supplies and several disinfectants. The two diseases cannot be distinguished by clinical criteria and in many ways even their epidemiological characteristics overlap. The classical mode of transmission for hepatitis A (infective hepatitis) is the oral route due to infected food and water and for hepatitis B (serum homologous jaundice) is by the parenteral route due to infected blood.

Hepatitis A (infective hepatitis)

The virus was identified in 1972 using immune electronmicroscopy. Virus-like particles in stool filtrates from patients with acute infective hepatitis were described and infection was successfully transmitted to laboratory animals. The virus is found in the faeces for only a few days after the onset of jaundice. Antibody in the blood can be detected shortly after and may persist for many years. As yet there is no evidence that chronic liver disease may develop after hepatitis A virus infection.

Infective hepatitis has many epidemiologic similarities with poliomyelitis. Both are enteric infections associated with viraemia followed by localisation in one system. It has been observed that the older the patient the more likely is the localisation to occur. Asymptomatic infections are common in both, and infective hepatitis in children under the age of three is seldom recognised without laboratory tests. Such undetected cases may be important sources of infection in the community.

Most cases of infective hepatitis occur after contact with infected patients, and infection occurs readily in conditions of poor sanitation and overcrowding as in the slums and shanty towns of many of the cities of the developing world. However, several epidemics and outbreaks have been described as a result of contaminated water, food or milk. For example, a massive outbreak occurred in New Delhi in 1955–56 when over 29 000 cases were reported out of the city's population of two million and despite what must have been a high level of immunity in the population. This outbreak was traced to the contamination of the city's water supply with sewage following heavy rains. It was noticed during this outbreak that the virus was able to survive in water containing the usual bactericidal concentration of chlorine. In the USA, 66 waterborne outbreaks were reported during 1946–71 and another 13 during 1971–4.

In many epidemics, however, the usual mode of transmission observed is by person to person spread within families. Thus, during an outbreak in Bristol in 1960–62 it was found that the highest attack rates were in children aged five to nine years. Spread occurred largely in families, as shown by the fact that 37 per cent of 2107 patients were members of a family with one or more other cases. The disease occurred in the case of 10.3 per cent of adults and

39.6 per cent of children in contact with cases in the home. Data from several countries show that during an outbreak the attack rates among children are far higher than those in adults. In several epidemics it has been observed that parents and adults in a family are often infected by the children who develop the disease first.

Food-borne infections due to oysters and clams from sewage-contaminated waters or by food handlers have also been reported. Such outbreaks tend to be explosive, affecting several households in the community simultaneously, as compared to the ones where transmission occurs from person to person.

In developing countries the pattern of infection is one of chronic endemicity. Poor sanitation, unhygienic habits, lack of sewage disposal and large extended families living in overcrowded homes are major contributory factors in the transmission of infection. On this background of chronic endemicity may be super-imposed outbreaks of the disease usually taking place during fairs and religious festivals when large numbers of people congregate.

There is no known carrier state. Maintenance of hepatitis A in the population is through person-to-person spread. Transmission of infection takes place during an incubation period when virus shedding is at its maximum. In recent years day care centres have been identified as potential sources of infection in the community. This is particularly so in the case of day care centres with a high proportion of non toilet-trained children. Hepatitis A causes minor or unnoticed illness in children and young adults. On a world-wide scale fewer than five per cent of cases are recognised clinically.

Hepatitis B (serum homologous jaundice)

Hepatitis B ranks as the ninth major cause of death worldwide close behind chronic pulmonary disease, and only just being overtaken by human immunodeficiency virus. It is one of the most important chronic viral infections in Asia and Africa, and is rapidly becoming so in Latin America. Upwards of 10 per cent of the population in parts of Asia and Africa may carry chronic hepatitis B infection. They maintain a pool of virus that ensures a high incidence of

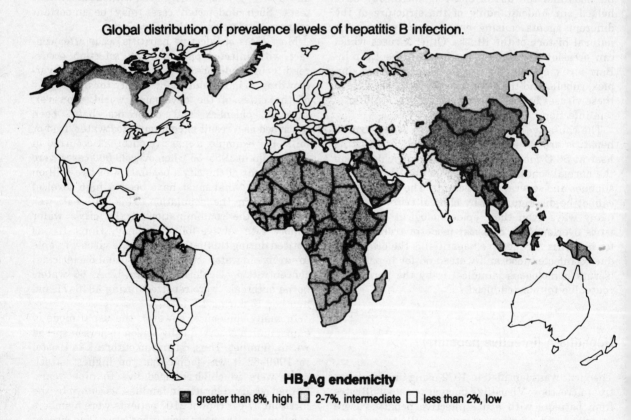

Global distribution of prevalence levels of hepatitis B infection.

HB$_s$Ag endemicity

■ greater than 8%, high ☐ 2-7%, intermediate ☐ less than 2%, low

Figure 13.1   Global prevalence of hepatitis B infection

new infections. Intermediate levels of hepatitis B are in Eastern Europe, Middle East and Latin America. North America, Western Europe and Australia are areas of low endemicity with carrier rates of <1 per cent (figure 13.1).

A specific antigen is detectable in the blood during the late stages of the incubation period and the acute phase of hepatitis. This antigen has been variously described as the Australia antigen, the SH antigen or hepatitis associated antigen. The discovery of this Australia antigen and its relation to serum hepatitis has greatly helped our understanding of the epidemiology and the natural history of the disease. Exposure to the hepatitis B virus can lead to any of the following events.

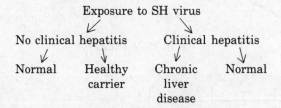

It has now been shown that the virus of hepatitis B possesses at least three separate antigens. There is a surface antigen now known as hepatitis B surface antigen (HBsAg), a core antigen now called hepatitis B core antigen (HBcAg) and the e antigen (HBeAg).

HBsAg is on the surface of the virus and several types have been identified, implying thereby the virus subtypes. It is thought that infection by one subtype of the virus may fail to confer immunity against infection by other subtypes. After an infection with hepatitis B virus HBsAg may be present in the blood for a month before the onset of symptoms. It persists for two to three months and occasionally for more than a year after clinical recovery.

Antibody response to the core antigen, HBcAg, is known to occur early in the illness. The antibody has a relatively short lifetime and hence its detection is evidence of recent infection and virus replication.

Presence of HBeAg indicates infectivity. Hence blood samples positive for Australia antigen (HBsAg) as well as containing the e antigen (HBeAg) are highly infectious. In the carrier state after an illness its presence indicates chronic active hepatitis and is an indication of poor prognosis. After an infection HBeAg like HBsAg is detectable

in the blood for two to five months and even longer. On recovery, after the various antigens have disappeared from the blood stream, anti-HBc and anti-HBs are known to persist for more than seven years and anti-HBe for up to two years.

The epidemiology of hepatitis B resembles HIV infection. The classical way of transmission of the infection is through blood transfusion or contaminated syringes and needles. A high incidence of carrier rate is found amongst drug users. Mixing of blood or body secretions through intimate physical contact, for example amongst sexual partners, is also a source of infection. Vertical transmission from an infected mother to her infant is a well-known source of transmission. It is likely that transmission by other routes, for example scarification, tattooing or similar rituals, may be more important in some societies.

Cell-mediated immunity plays an important role in clearing the infective agent from the blood stream. It has been known that immunologic deficiency predisposes to a carrier state of the Australia antigen. This type of carrier differs from 'healthy' carriers in being more susceptible to chronic liver disease which can be mild or subclinical and overshadowed by the primary disease like leprosy or the use of cytotoxic drugs.

Clinical features

Infection by either of the two viruses can be mild and go unnoticed (abortive form); on the other hand, there may be an illness of varying degrees of severity from anicteric hepatitis to acute hepatic necrosis.

Anicteric hepatitis

The symptoms are non-specific. Malaise, loss of appetite or vomiting, and fever are the usual presenting symptoms. The diagnosis is suspected if there is a history of contact with a patient suffering from hepatitis or during epidemics. Presence of bilirubin in the urine or alteration of serum enzyme levels may provide confirmatory evidence. In an epidemic, such anicteric cases will outnumber those with detectable jaundice.

In hepatitis A about two-thirds of those with symptoms go on to develop jaundice (figure 13.2). A small percentage of those may have fulminant hepatitis with a fatality rate of one per cent.

In hepatitis B sub-clinical infection is more common. About 25 to 30 per cent develop symptoms, and one per cent go on to have fulminant hepatitis

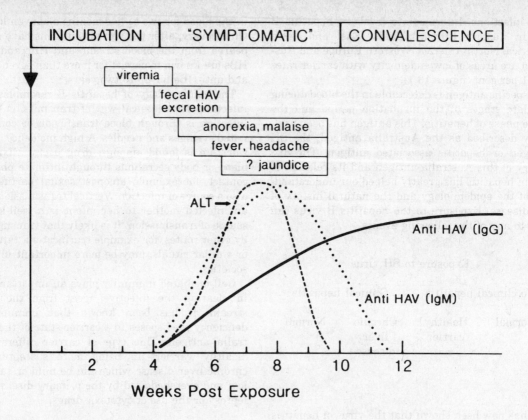

Figure 13.2   Phases of hepatitis A infection

(figure 13.3). Amongst adults and older children between three per cent and ten per cent become chronic carriers (figure 13.4). The carrier rate is higher at about 20 per cent in younger children. Babies born to HBeAg positive mothers are at very high risk of infection. The estimated risk of chronic hepatitis B infection in such newborns is between 66 and 93 per cent. As many as 40 per cent of the 200 million carriers worldwide may have been infected at birth.

The icteric form

Prodromal symptoms of anorexia, nausea, abdominal discomfort and fever gradually increase in severity and jaundice appears. The liver is palpable and tender. Fever subsides within a few days of onset of jaundice. After about a fortnight of increasing severity, the jaundice begins to clear gradually and serum bilirubin levels return to normal in about six to eight weeks. Convalescence may last a few weeks to months; in some cases malaise and gastro-intestinal symptoms persist for several months.

The fulminant form

It is not uncommon to see this form of hepatitis in developing countries where malnutrition and anaemia are common and cause poor resistance to infection. In addition, the child may have been subjected to dietary restrictions at home, or been administered indigenous medicines, some of which may be hepatotoxic. The clinical picture is one of massive acute necrosis of the liver with deep jaundice, mental changes like apathy or irritability progressing to disturbances of consciousness and death. With supportive treatment, recovery is possible, but the prognosis in general is poor.

Hepatitis caused by the delta virus

Transmission occurs by the parenteral route, and is generally associated with blood transfusion or administration of blood derived products. The delta virus is a defective RNA virus which requires the presence of hepatitis B virus to cause infection. The

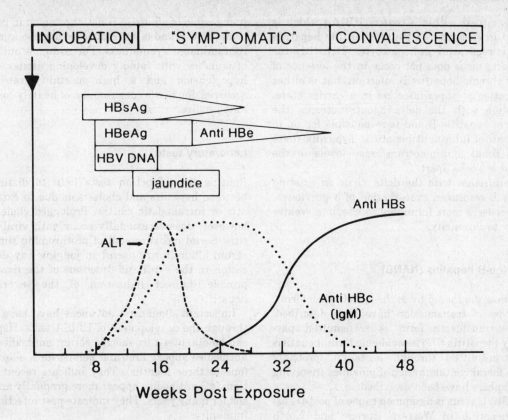

Figure 13.3   Phases of hepatitis B infection

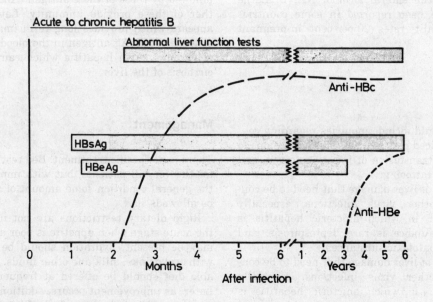

Figure 13.4   Acute to chronic hepatitis B

virus is encased within a coat of HBsAg which is produced in excessive amounts when the hepatitis B virus is replicating in hepatocytes. Hepatitis due to the delta virus does not occur in the absence of acute or chronic hepatitis B infection, but is either a co-infection or super-infection in a carrier state. Co-infection with the delta agent increases the severity of hepatitis B and is responsible for up to 30 per cent of fulminant hepatitis. Typically there are two peaks of aminotransferase levels in the blood a few weeks apart.

Super-infection with the delta virus on existing hepatitis B results in exacerbation of a previously stable disease, a more fulminant course, or a greater tendency to chronicity.

Non-A Non-B hepatitis (NANB)

This form is diagnosed by exclusion of other forms. Two modes of transmission have been described. The post-transfusion form is transmitted parenterally (hepatitis C). The epidemic form (hepatitis E) is transmitted through ingestion, probably through faecal contamination. Epidemics involving large numbers have been described.

Hepatitis C virus is a common cause of post-transfusion hepatitis in Western Europe and North America. In about 20 per cent of chronic cases gradual progression to cirrhosis of the liver occurs.

More than half of acute viral hepatitis in some developing countries is not hepatitis A or B, and is thought to be the enteral form of NANB. Large epidemics have been reported in some countries with high mortality rates (20 per cent) in pregnant women.

Diagnosis

The history should include inquiries regarding contact with jaundiced patients, previous admissions to hospital, blood transfusion or injections given, and scarification or tattooing.

Other causes of liver damage that need to be considered are: other virus infections, especially glandular fever in which anicteric hepatitis is common but jaundice is rare; leptospirosis; and ingestion of hepatotoxic substances.

Other causes of liver damage that need to be considered are: other virus infections, especially glandular fever in which anicteric hepatitis is common but jaundice is rare; leptospirosis; and ingestion of hepato-toxic substances. Hepatitis due

to ingestion of aflatoxin is not uncommon in peasant communities and is not restricted to consumption of contaminated groundnuts. For example outbreaks of jaundice with rapidly developing ascites, portal hypertension and a high mortality rate have occurred due to the consumption of heavily contaminated maize.

Laboratory tests

Routine liver function tests help to distinguish between hepatitis and cholestasis due to extrahepatic or intrahepatic causes. Prolonged cholestasis, however, does occasionally occur with viral hepatitis. Serial measurement of prothrombin time and serum albumin are useful in judging any deterioration in the synthesis functions of the liver, and provide indirect indication of the severity of hepatitis.

Important diagnostic advances have been made through the development of ELISA tests. Hepatitis can be diagnosed by specific serum antibodies. IgM antibodies appear first and persist for a short time (one to three months). They indicate recent infection. IgG antibodies appear more gradually and persist for many years. They indicate past infection and immunity.

Early in acute hepatitis B, the surface antigen (HBsAg) and the e antigen (HBeAg) appear in the serum (figure 13.5). During the course of the illness antibodies to the core antigen (Anti-HBc) appear followed by those of the e antigen (Anti-HBe). Neither of these provide immunity. Later anti-HBs appears which provides long term immunity. Persistence of HBeAg antigen in the blood is a marker of chronic active hepatitis which can progress to cirrhosis of the liver.

Management

There is no specific treatment. Bed rest is necessary for the very ill patients, but with improvement in the general condition some amount of activity may be allowed.

Rigid dietary restrictions are not necessary. In the acute stage when appetite is poor and vomiting may be present, hydration should be maintained with oral drinks, milk and other fluids. A soft palatable diet should be offered at frequent intervals. Later, as improvement occurs, additions to the diet may be made with protein foods. Restriction of protein is not justified except in those cases which show

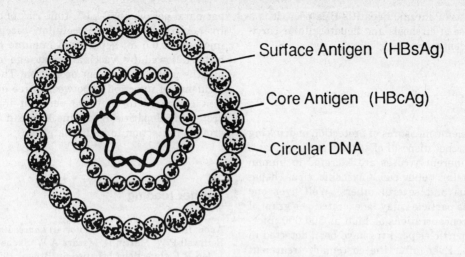

Surface Antigen (HBsAg)

Core Antigen (HBcAg)

Circular DNA

THE HEPATITIS B VIRUS

Figure 13.5 Structure of hepatitis B virus

evidence of fulminant hepatitis and liver failure.

Associated anaemia or parasitic infestation may require treatment. Vitamin supplements, especially of the B complex group, may be given if deficiency is suspected.

Sequelae

Complete recovery occurs in the majority of the cases in children. Very few progress to the chronic stage of hepatitis with malaise, ill-health and raised amino transferase levels. Chronicity is suggested by raised levels of gamma globulin and prolonged prothrombin time within three weeks of onset of apparent acute infectious hepatitis. Recurrence of jaundice after clearing is another clinical indicator of chronic liver disease. Presence of arthralgia, erythema nodosum, gastro-intestinal symptoms, acne and finger clubbing should arouse suspicion of chronicity and there should be regular follow-up of such patients.

The frequency of chronic liver disease after type A hepatitis is usually stated to be one case or two out of every thousand. In undernourished communities this may be higher but in the absence of specific diagnostic tests the true frequency is difficult to assess. Moreover, many cases are anicteric and an even larger proportion are not seen by the health services. With hepatitis B infection, persistent hepatitis is more commonly recognised and in some outbreaks it is reported to be as high as 50 per cent.

Chronic persistent hepatitis

Chronic persistent hepatitis is defined as continuing clinical or biochemical evidence of hepatic dysfunction for longer than six months. It normally follows hepatitis B or NANB infection.

This can be insidious and clinically non-apparent. Malaise is the predominant symptom. There may be hepatomegaly of varying degree. Histologically, the necrosis of liver cells is not extensive and there is no evidence of cirrhosis. The process is self-limiting and in almost all cases the prognosis is good. A needle biopsy may be required to distinguish it from the *chronic aggressive form of hepatitis* in which there is gross disturbance of liver function and apart from hepatosplenomegaly there is evidence of involvement of other systems. Histology shows extensive necrosis.

Reactivation of disease can occur in a previously stable form of chronic hepatitis because of

(1) Spontaneous reactivation or due to immune suppression.
(2) Superinfection with the delta virus.
(3) Liver injury by any cause other than virus infection.

The prognosis of chronic hepatitis B is poor. It is a leading cause of cirrhosis and hepatocellular carcinoma in endemic areas.

Prevention

General hygienic measures of protection of drinking water and proper disposal of sewage are important. Over 100 different viruses are excreted in human faeces including poliovirus, Coxsackie virus, hepatitis A virus and several others. Well over one million virus particles may be excreted per gram of faeces and concentrations as high as 500 000 infectious virus particles per litre have been detected in raw sewage. Even after the customary treatment and chlorination, sufficient numbers of virus particles survive. Hence hepatitis A is an ever present danger in areas where raw sewage is used as a fertiliser.

Gamma globulin in a dose of 0.1 ml/kg has been shown to provide individual protection and may be offered to household contacts if possible. Field studies of inactivated vaccines have shown that they are safe, well tolerated and effective.

With regard to hepatitis B, in endemic areas vertical transmission from an infected mother to her infant in the perinatal period is a common mode of infection. The estimated risk of chronic hepatitis B infection among such infants is in the range of 66 to 93 per cent. Moreover individuals infected in the perinatal period stand a life-time risk of death from liver cirrhosis or hepatocellular carcinoma. An injection of 0.5 ml hepatitis B immune globulin at birth followed by vaccination at age one to six months provides excellent protection. The observed incidence of infection is between three and ten per cent compared to 66 to 93 per cent in those not protected. Hepatitis B vaccine also can be used to provide protection to high risk groups.

Further reading

Anon. Infective hepatitis. (Editorial) *Lancet* 1968; i: 79–80.

Bothwell P W, Martin D, Macara A W, Skone J F, Wofinden R C. Infectious hepatitis in Bristol 1959–1962. *Br med J* 1963; 2: 1613–16.

Heathcote J, Sherlock S. Spread of acute type B hepatitis in London. *Lancet* 1973; i: 1468–70.

Krishnamachari K, Bhat R, Nagarajan V, Tilak T B G. Hepatitis due to aflatoxicosis. *Lancet* 1975; i: 1061–63.

Krugman S, Overby L, Muchahwar I K, Ling C M, Frosner G G, Deinhardt F. Viral hepatitis type B: studies on natural history and prevention re-examined. *New Engl J Med* 1979; 300: 101–6.

Shinhaj P, Cohen J, *et al*. Transmission of hepatitis type B from healthy HBsAg positive mothers. *Br med J* 1975; 1: 10–11.

Hoofnagle J H. Chronic hepatitis B. *New Eng J Med* 1990; 323: 337–9.

Zuckerman A J. (Ed). Viral hepatitis. *Brit Med Bulletin* 1990; 46: 301–558.

14 Tuberculosis

Tuberculosis is one of the most prevalent communicable diseases in developing countries being responsible for chronic morbidity and a high mortality. Nearly 3 million people die annually from tuberculosis. It is estimated that there are 8 million new cases of tuberculosis every year. Nearly half of them are infectious. Thus there is a large reservoir of active cases of tuberculosis (estimated to be 20 million) globally, and nearly a third of the world's inhabitants have come into contact with the infection. About 10–20 per cent of all tuberculous disease is in children, most of whom may have acquired their infection from a sputum positive adult.

The countries with the largest number of deaths from tuberculosis are Bangladesh, Brazil, China, India, Indonesia, Nigeria, Pakistan, the Philippines and Vietnam (table 14.1). But the *rates* of the disease are highest in sub-Saharan Africa. In some East and Central African countries the reported cases of tuberculosis have almost doubled in recent years. One of the reasons for this increase is infection with the Human Immunodeficiency Virus (HIV). In HIV infection latent tuberculosis becomes active. Conversely in tuberculosis HIV rapidly progresses to the acquired immunodeficiency syndrome (AIDS).

In a disease like tuberculosis, characterised by a prolonged latent period and chronicity, the extent of the problem in the community is best measured by two indices – prevalence of tuberculin sensitivity in children and the prevalence of infection proven bacteriologically by examination of the sputum. According to the World Health Organisation, tuberculosis is to be considered a public health problem if the prevalence of infection is more than one per cent among children up to age 14.

In many of the more developed countries there has been a marked decline in the prevalence of tuberculosis (figure 14.1). Mortality from tuberculosis has fallen at the rate of about three per cent annually during the first two decades of this century. The fall accelerated to about five and a half per cent annually in the 1920s and 1930s as a result of rapid improvements in socio-economic conditions and hygiene. The risk of infection also declined in a parallel manner. After the 1950s the development and use of chemotherapy further accelerated the risk of tubercular infection by about 10–14 per cent annually. An annual decrease in the risk of infection at the rate of 14 per cent can halve the problem in five years, as indeed has been the experience in most countries of Western Europe. This improvement has been brought about by a combination of several factors, namely

(1) Reduction in the size of the reservoir of infection by
    (a) active notification and case-finding in adult cases in combination with effective chemotherapy;
    (b) safe milk supply.
(2) BCG vaccination of children.
(3) Improved knowledge of the natural history of primary infection and epidemiology so that both BCG and chemotherapy are used to the best advantage.
(4) Improved socio-economic circumstances and a general awareness of the disease amongst the population.

By comparison the decrease in the annual risk of infection in the less developed countries has been

Table 14.1 Global rates of tuberculosis (WHO 1990)

Region	People infected (millions)	New cases (millions)	Deaths ('000)
Africa	171	1.3	656
Latin America	117	0.564	220
Eastern Mediterranean	52	0.572	163
South-east Asia	426	2.48	932
West Pacific	574	2.5	894
Industrialised countries	382	0.4	42

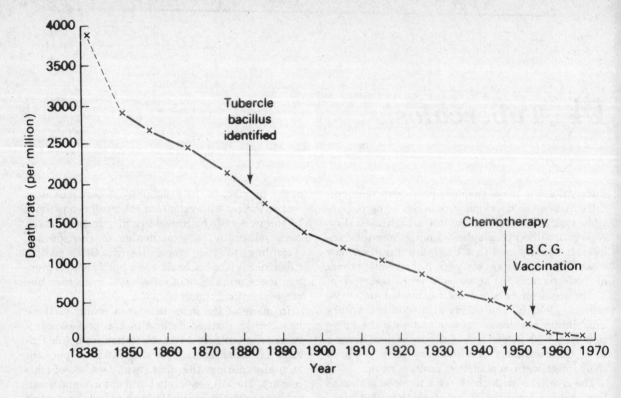

Figure 14.1   Respiratory tuberculosis death rates – England and Wales

much slower, being five to ten per cent per year in Latin America, six to seven per cent in some Asian countries and zero to three per cent in sub-Saharan Africa.

The tools for the control of tuberculosis are the same for both the less and the more developed countries, but the quality of these tools and the extent of their application differ markedly. In most developing countries case finding is less efficient, transportation is enormously difficult and chemotherapy does not always produce a satisfactory outcome because of high drop out rates. The result is that only a fraction of active cases of tuberculosis are being diagnosed, and amongst those diagnosed only a fraction are being cured on the standard regimens hitherto in vogue.

Natural history of childhood tubercle

In children, infection may be acquired from an 'open case' of tuberculosis in an adult or from a bovine source through infected milk. The course of events that may follow will depend upon the resistance of

the host, the virulence of the organisms and the size of dose received. In a large number of cases, the body is able to overcome the invading bacilli and the primary infection may even pass unnoticed, the only indication of such an infection being a positive reaction to tuberculin. In those cases where the bacilli are able to establish themselves and multiply, disease occurs. It is difficult to know precisely in what percentage of children who have been exposed to infection tuberculous disease occurs. In England and Wales, during several investigations carried out by the Medical Research Council in connection with the efficacy of BCG vaccine, the rates shown in table 14.2 were noted.

In the individual child who has been exposed to the infection, the following host factors may determine whether disease will occur: (1) the age of the child, the occurrence of disease being more common the younger the child; (2) the state of nutrition – poor nutrition predisposes to illness (in addition, a focus of tuberculosis in the body may flare up into active disease when there is deterioration of the nutritional status of the body); (3) intercurrent illness such as measles or whooping cough, and (4) the heaviness of the infection. Of these, perhaps the age of the child is the single most important factor. In a tuberculosis survey of children in Bombay, it was found that amongst those with positive tuberculin test, active disease was present in all under the age of one year; this risk fell to 75 per cent in the age group four to five years. Before the days of chemotherapy it was estimated that 15–20 per cent of children infected in the first year of life would develop miliary spread or meningitis within two years and about seven per cent would develop a lesion in a bone or a joint; this risk of dissemination is much less after the age of five years. Such findings still apply to many of the rural areas of developing countries where adequate health services have not yet evolved.

A second important influence is that of the nutritional status of the infected host, and the incidence as well as severity of intercurrent infections. The clinical picture of childhood tuberculosis in many of the affluent societies of the West is very different from that seen in the tropics. Thus, the involvement of regional lymph nodes, the amount of caseation at the site of infection, spread to other body organs including the nervous system, as well as the frequency of primary cavitation are more commonly observed in the tropics. Hence there are marked differences between the classical description in Western text books and what is observed in clinical practice in the tropics. Many of these differences can be explained on the basis of poor nutrition and intercurrent infections affecting the immune responses of the host. For example, hypersensitivity phenomena such as erythema nodosum and phlyctenular conjunctivitis are rare in developing countries. There is also a decreased response to tuberculin so that diagnosis often becomes difficult.

Pathology

When tubercle bacilli enter the body for the first time, they produce a small focus of infection at the site of entry and travel along the lymphatics to the draining lymph nodes which become inflamed. In a larger number of cases, the primary focus is caused by inhalation of bacilli and as such is situated in the lung, with enlarged bronchial and para-tracheal lymph nodes on the same side. In those cases where infection is derived from drinking infected milk, the primary focus may be in the tonsils, with enlargement of the cervical glands. These two components, namely, the primary focus and the draining lymph node, together constitute what is known as the primary complex (figure 14.2a and b). The primary complex is in marked contrast to the body's reaction to tubercle bacilli on subsequent exposures, for example, in adult tuberculosis. Here, because the tissues have been sensitised to tuberculoproteins during the early infection, a marked reaction occurs in the form of caseation, breakdown of tissue and fibrosis at the site of infection with little reaction in lymph nodes.

During the early stage of the primary complex, before hypersensitivity develops, at least a few bacilli probably reach the blood stream, either directly from the primary focus or by way of regional nodes. Not all will cause foci of tuberculous disease where they lodge. Some may do so, but ultimately die, and others progress at varying rates into foci of active disease. Such foci may regress and heal completely, or they may remain quiescent but contain viable bacilli. The results of such 'seeding' is determined by: (1) dose of bacilli implanted in an

Table 14.2 Response to tuberculin test and later development of tuberculosis

	Participants	First 2½ years		Second 2½ years		Beyond 5 years	
		Total	Annual incidence	Total	Annual incidence	Total	Annual incidence
Negative to 100 TU (unvaccinated)	13 300	66	1.98	87	2.62	30	1.38
Positive to 3 TU (15 mm or more)	7 200	63	3.50	30	1.67	10	0.88
Positive to 3 TU (5–14 mm)	8 800	17	0.77	18	0.82	6	0.44
Negative to 3 TU, positive to 100 TU	6 600	12	0.73	18	1.09	8	0.76

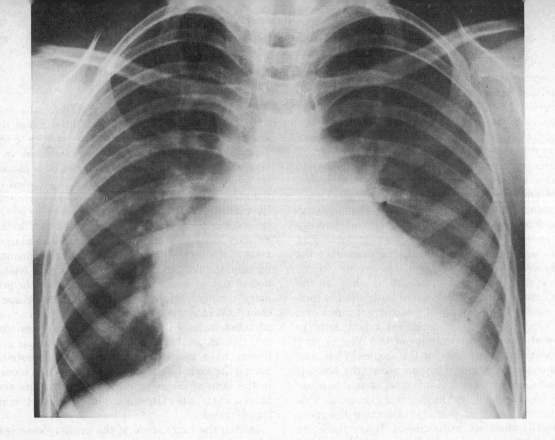

Figure 14.2a   Primary complex

Figure 14.2b   Primary complex – note enlarged paratracheal gland

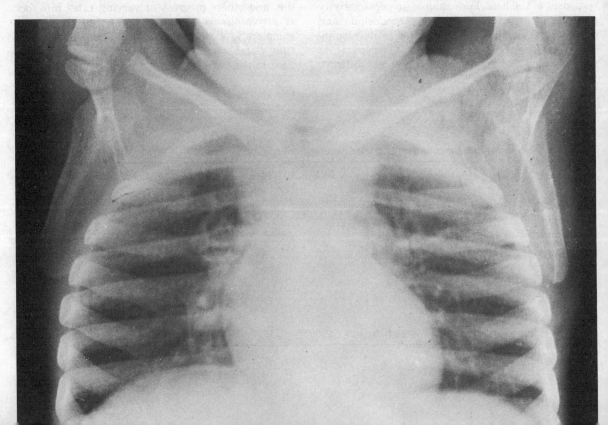

area; (2) hypersensitivity in the host as a result of the primary focus; (3) factors of inherent and acquired immunity and (4) local differences in organ susceptibility. When acute generalised miliary tuberculosis occurs, it is usually the result of a single hemic dissemination of a large number of tubercle bacilli.

Before the advent of chemotherapy it was found that after exposure to infection and development of the primary complex, most complications and 90 per cent of deaths occurred within one year of first diagnosis. Late complications, for example, in the meninges, in the skeletal system or in the kidney, are in most instances due to a reactivation of foci caused by 'seeding' from the primary infection.

On the basis of hypersensitivity and using the tuberculin test, any group of people can be subdivided into tuberculin reactors and non-reactors. The reactors are those who at some time in the past have been infected by tubercle bacilli and who still harbour those bacilli in their bodies. In most developing countries where tuberculosis is widespread, a large proportion of a population are tuberculin positive, and what is more important, many become so at an early age. The prevalence of a positive tuberculin test in the youngest age groups is generally considered to be a good measure of the amount of tuberculous disease in any commmunity.

In the vast majority of cases tuberculin positive individuals harbour tubercle bacilli in their bodies in the resting or inactive phase. In this phase the bacilli are non-pathogenic. Their presence in the body also exercises a somewhat protective function by maintaining a degree of hypersensitivity (and immunity) to further infection. On the other hand, in their presence within the body lie the seeds of future disease. When tubercular disease occurs the bacillary population goes into a state of flux changing to and fro between the active and non-active phases. It is only during the active phase of the bacilli, with increased metabolism, that they become responsive to chemotherapeutic agents. This changing responsiveness to chemotherapy requires that the duration of treatment be prolonged so that all the tubercle bacilli in the body can be eradicated.

The tuberculin non-reactors in the community are those individuals who have escaped primary infection by the bacillus. This sub-group also includes a very small proportion of people who were infected at one time in the past but in whom the bacilli have been eradicated by the body's defence mechanisms.

The prevalence of infection within a community is determined by the size of the reservoir of the disease. The number of active cases excreting bacilli in their sputa or, in the case of bovine tuberculosis, the number of infected cattle, constitute the reservoir of the disease. Amongst the infected individuals the development of the disease is very closely linked to the life stresses to which these individuals are subjected. At the individual level, the age of the host, nutritional status, intercurrent infections and biological stresses like those of pregnancy or puberty constitute some of the well documented stresses as described above. At the community level, the vital statistics of the community provide measures of such stresses. For example, there is a close parallel between mortality from tuberculosis and other vital statistics in many countries (table 14.3).

Table 14.3 Relationship between a community's stress situation and its tuberculosis situation

	East Africa (1961)	England & Wales (1901)	England & Wales (1961)
Vital statistics			
Infant mortality rate	180	150	21
Death rate 1–14 years (per million)	20 000	16 000	527
Crude death rate (per 1000 population)	25	18	12
Expectancy of life at birth (years)	40	50	72
Tuberculosis			
Incidence ⎱ per 100 000	250	270	35 *
Mortality ⎰ population yearly	170	180	6**
Proportionate mortality (per cent)	7	10	½**

* 1965   ** 1967

(*Source*: Kent P W. *E Afr med J* 1971; 48: 452)

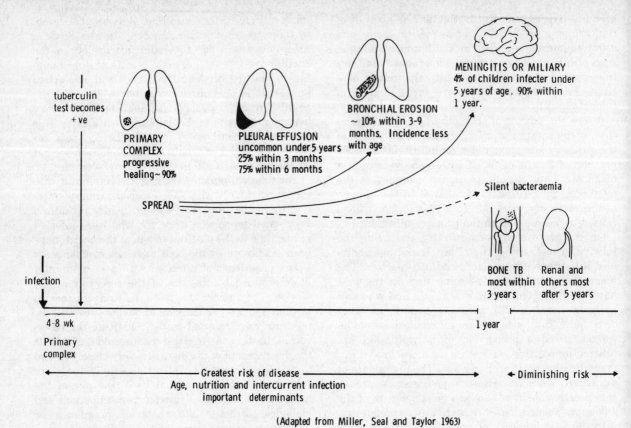

(Adapted from Miller, Seal and Taylor 1963)

Figure 14.3   Natural history of childhood tuberculosis

Complications of primary tuberculosis

Until such time as complete healing takes place the primary complex is a potential risk, mainly through its lymph node component (figure 14.3). Tuberculous lymph nodes have a tendency to enlarge and erode surrounding structures or to soften and discharge their contents of caseous material containing tubercle bacilli. Softening of nodes is most likely to occur within a year, but it can also happen soon after calcification has begun or, at times, even after several years of non-activity. The various events that may occur after the formation of the primary complex and the time sequence are summarised in figure 14.3.

Local complications in the lung (figures 14.4a, b and c)

These are mainly due to the enlarged hilar or para-tracheal lymph nodes pressing on the adjoining bronchi. The pressing lymph node can completely obstruct a bronchus and cause atelectasis. In some cases the occlusion may not be entirely due to extrinsic pressure; the caseous lymph node erodes through the wall of the bronchus and the lumen is filled with granulation tissue and caseous material. Usually the right middle lobe gets involved in this complication, which may later resolve with residual bronchiectasis.

The occlusion of the bronchus may be only partial, so that the lumen is patent in inspiration but is blocked during expiration, thereby producing a check-valve obstruction. This results in emphysema affecting a lobe, or an entire lung.

In rare instances a paratracheal lymph node erodes into the trachea, discharging caseous material into the lumen, or it may rupture into the pericardial sac, giving rise to pericarditis.

Bronchogenic spread

Caseous material from an enlarged hilar lymph

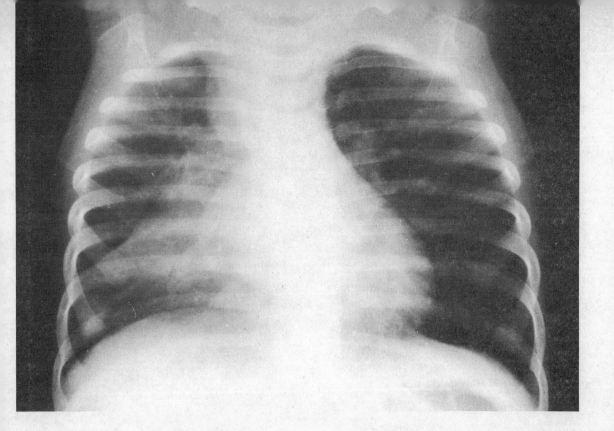

Figure 14.4a   Collapse of (R) middle lobe

Figure 14.4b   Emphysema (R) lung

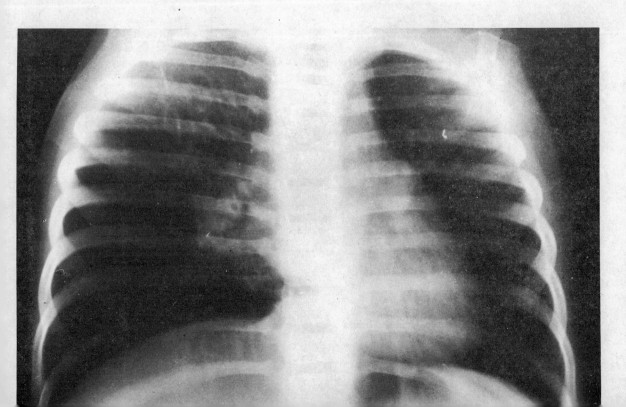

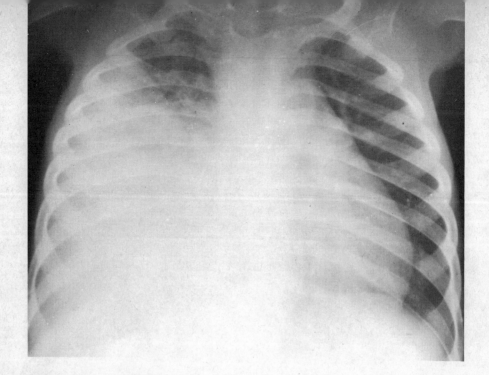

Figure 14.4c   Pleural effusion (R) side

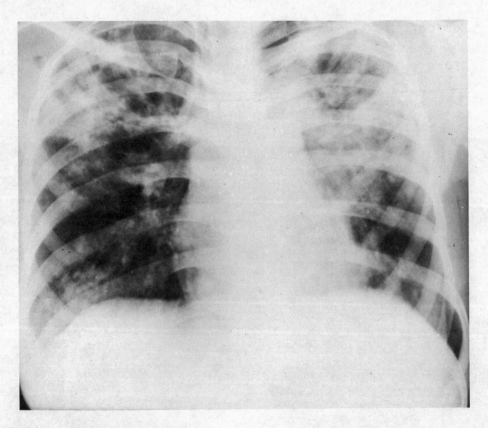

Figure 14.5   Advanced tuberculosis of the lungs

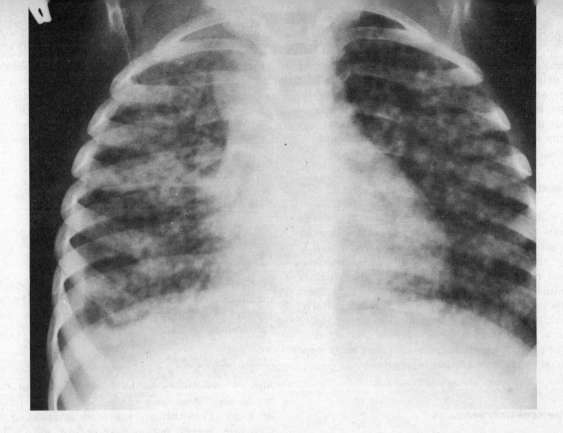

Figure 14.6   Miliary tuberculosis

node containing a large number of organisms is discharged into the lumen of a bronchus, from where it may be inhaled into different parts of the lobe or a segment of the lobe and cause tuberculous pneumonia or bronchopneumonia.

The adult type of fibrocaseous tuberculosis is occasionally seen in children, and is an indication of existing hypersensitivity due to earlier exposure to tuberculoproteins (figure 14.5). It is now known that in most cases the disease in the adult is the result of exacerbation of pre-existing tuberculous foci caused by a lowering of immunity as a result of malnutrition, intercurrent infection or stress like pregnancy.

Hematogenous dissemination (figure 14.6)

Acute miliary tuberculosis is due to erosion from the primary complex into a blood vessel, thereby discharging a large number of bacilli into the blood stream. Several organs of the body may be seeded with miliary tubercles.

From the primary complex bacilli continually escape in small numbers into the blood stream and reach distant organs where they may remain dormant for some time, only to cause a local form of disease at a later period, for example, in the bone, joints or the renal tract and genital organs. This is the chronic disseminated form of tuberculosis as distinct from the acute miliary tuberculosis.

Silent bacillaemia occurring from time to time may go unrecognised but cause serious disease later, for example, tuberculoma of the brain.

Clinical manifestations

Primary tuberculosis is recognised in one of several ways.

Non-symptomatic

In a majority of cases there may be no local or constitutional symptoms, the only sign being a recent conversion to tuberculin or a chance X-ray finding. Unless the child is below four years of age, this may need no more than a regular follow-up.

Occasionally a recent conversion to tuberculin may be detected in a child who comes from a household where one of the adults is a known case of tuberculosis. In such a case, even though the child may be more than four years of age, chemoprophylaxis may be more desirable than just regular supervision.

In association with other illnesses

In malnourished children tuberculosis is often an additional finding. Diagnosis can present difficulties because of diminished response to tuberculin and X-ray facilities are not always available. In malnourished children whose response to routine dietary treatment is slow, it is reasonable to suspect tuberculosis and take steps to confirm it. Similarly, in children recovering from measles or whooping cough, if the period of recovery is protracted or return to normal weight gain is delayed, early steps should be taken to exclude tuberculosis.

Hypersensitivity reactions

With the development of hypersensitivity to tuberculoprotein after an infection, constitutional symptoms occur in some children. These are seen about six to eight weeks after the infection, and may be in the form of *fever*, either irregular and low grade or sustained, and accompanied by other symptoms such as loss of appetite, lassitude, failure to gain weight, and so on. Other characteristic indications of hypersensitivity are *phlyctenular conjunctivitis* or *erythema nodosum*. The presence of either of these in association with a positive tuberculin test should lead to a thorough search for a primary focus.

Progressive primary infection

The child with a progressive primary infection may be just 'sickly' and suffer protracted ill-health, or can be very ill with symptoms and signs indicating a local lesion with constitutional symptoms. These local lesions are

(1) Absorptive collapse or obstructive emphysema. Pressure from an enlarged gland on the airway can cause cough which is often paroxysmal, not unlike that of pertussis. In some cases the airway is sufficiently narrowed to give rise to an asthma-like wheeze. These symptoms tend to be more common in the infant, and primary

tuberculosis should always be considered in the differential diagnosis of asthma or pertussis in the young infant. When obstructive emphysema occurs there is breathlessness with or without an asthma-like wheeze. X-rays provide an invaluable help in confirming collapse or emphysema.

(2) Pleural effusion may accompany the constitutional symptoms. Physical diagnosis is straightforward, and with adequate therapy complete recovery is the rule.

Post-primary spread

Post-primary spread can give rise to early or late manifestations of disease. The early lesions of post-primary spread are miliary tuberculosis and tuberculous meningitis.

Miliary tuberculosis

Miliary tuberculosis is so called because of the 'millet seed' appearance of the lesions in the lungs on X-ray. Even though respiratory symptoms predominate, several organs may be involved in the miliary spread, so that meningeal involvement or tuberculous lesions of the liver, the kidney or the bone may also be concomitantly present.

The child with miliary tuberculosis is ill and toxic. Fever and malaise of several days' duration can be the only presenting features. Anaemia and rapid loss of weight occur in the infant or the young child. If the lungs are extensively involved dyspnoea is also present. Clinical examination of the chest reveals widespread moist sounds on auscultation, often resulting in a mistaken diagnosis of bronchopneumonia. Presence of hepatosplenomegaly, anaemia and the appearance of the child, who looks more ill than the fever or clinical signs in the lungs suggest, should lead to X-rays and other tests. A positive tuberculin test in a child who had a recent contact with an 'open' case of tuberculosis and a suggestive X-ray, together with the clinical picture, add up to the correct diagnosis.

Tuberculous meningitis

Tuberculous meningitis is the most dreaded complication of primary tuberculosis. If not treated in the very early stages, it carries a high mortality and a risk of sequelae in those who recover. The onset is insidious with low grade fever, vomiting and apathy. Irritability alternating with drowsiness occurs in the early stage. The older child may complain of a headache if asked, but most of the time wishes to be left alone. In this early stage neck rigidity is absent and yet early diagnosis is essential for a satisfactory result of treatment. Diagnosis chiefly depends on the history of sudden alteration in behaviour in a normally happy child, the presence of irritability and the unusual lethargy and drowsiness.

Untreated, the disease will progress to the intermediate stage in a week or two and specific signs of involvement of the meninges and the nervous system now appear. There is neck stiffness or the presence of focal neurological signs such as cranial nerve palsy or hemiparesis. Ophthalmoscopy reveals papilloedema or the presence of choroid tubercles. The presence of the latter is diagnostic, and patient ophthalmoscopy is called for in a child showing progressive drowsiness and involvement of the central nervous system. The child in this stage typically lies curled up in bed turned away from light and resents examination. Even at this advanced stage there may yet be a good response to treatment, but neurological sequelae are common.

Progress of the disease to the final stage is rapid, with the child becoming comatose and signs of decerebrate rigidity appearing. Recovery from this advanced stage is difficult and when it does occur there is a high incidence of permanent brain damage such as mental deficiency, hydrocephalus, blindness, deafness, strabismus or paralysis.

Based on the state of consciousness three stages of progression in tuberculous meningitis are described as follows

(1) Stage I   Consciousness undisturbed. Focal neurological signs are absent or mild.
(2) Stage II   Consciousness is disturbed, but the patient is not comatose or delirious. Mild or moderate neurological signs may appear such as para paresis or hemiparesis, and cranial nerve palsies.
(3) Stage III Patient is comatose or delirious with recognisable neurological signs.

Tuberculous meningitis largely involves meninges at the base of the brain. The inflammation and exudate give rise to cranial nerve palsies affecting mostly the 3rd and the 6th, but also occasionally the 7th and 8th cranial nerves. An intense vasculitis accompanies the meningitis causing infarcts, and hence a variety of neurological deficits like motor paresis, decerebrate rigidity, cerebellar signs, hypothalamic disorders and spinal cord syndromes.

In the Transkei and surrounding regions *tubercular pericarditis* has been described as a common cause of congestive cardiac failure in children. The infection of the pericardium is either blood-borne or by direct extension from the mediastinal lymph nodes.

The *late lesions* of post primary spread occur in the bones, the joints, the kidneys or the genito-urinary tract and are often collectively referred to as 'surgical tuberculosis' because of the surgical intervention that may be needed for their management.

Diagnosis of childhood tuberculosis

Except for the well-advanced complication of tuberculous meningitis, there are no physical signs which may be described as characteristic of primary tuberculosis. A presumptive diagnosis is made on suspicion and confirmed by further tests and investigations. Suspicion is aroused in the case of the 'sickly' child who may not be thriving after an attack of measles or whooping cough or in the case of the child who has been in contact with an adult suffering from the disease. As a corollary to this it is important to remember that diagnosis of tuberculosis in an individual is never complete until all the contacts (at home, at work and in the school) have been examined.

Amongst the various diagnostic tools available the most effective tests are the ones which look for hypersensitivity to tuberculoproteins. Their basis is the cell-mediated response observed when tuberculin penetrates the skin of a sensitised person and is referred to as the tuberculin reaction. On penetration of the skin, tuberculin begins to be fixed in five to ten minutes after injection, and fixation is completed in one to two hours. Histologic study of the tuberculin reaction in the skin shows infiltration with granyloctyes a few hours after injection of tuberculin, followed later by small mononuclear cells. This increased cell content of the skin at the injection site is responsible for the induration seen. All non-specific reactions subside in 24 hours, so that the measurement of the induration at the end of 48–72 hours gives a measure of the degree of hypersensitivity. Since its introduction 50 years ago, various refinements in technique and in the preparation of tuberculin have helped to make the tuberculin reaction more meaningful. It has been shown that a linear relationship exists between the area of induration (expressed as the square of the diameter) and the logarithm of the intradermal dose in a constant volume. The tuberculin reaction depends upon the interaction of several factors such as the amount of tuberculoprotein injected, the total number of sensitised cells in the body, the local absorptive behaviour of the skin and the state of the immune responses of the host.

Old tuberculin and PPD

The original intradermal test utilised old tuberculin (OT), which is prepared from a six-week-old culture of tubercle bacilli in five per cent glycerine broth. The culture is evaporated to one-tenth of its volume, the bacilli are then killed by heat and filtered. The fluid obtained is stable, but dilutions tend to deteriorate. Tuberculin containing Tween 80 has better keeping quality and is commonly used.

More work on tuberculin to obtain a reliable standard product led to the development of the purified protein derivative (PPD) which has subsequently been refined to give a standard product (PPD-S).

Either OT or PPD-S can be used for diagnosis. The two products compare with each other as shown in table 14.4.

Table 14.4 A comparison of old tuberculin and purified protein derivative

Tuberculin Unit (TU)	OT dilution	PPD mg/dose
1	1:10 000	0.00002
5	1:2 000	0.0001
10	1:1 000	0.0002
250	1:40	0.005

In clinical work the test is usually carried out with 10 TU unless the patient is highly sensitive and shows reactions like erythema nodosum or phlyctenular conjunctivitis, in which case 1 TU is used as the starting dose. For all survey work a dose of 5 TU is used. PPD which is generally preferred is available made up in these dilutions so that 0.1 ml of the test solution may contain 1, 10 or 100 TU.

The test is read 48 hours after the intradermal injection, when induration and erythema may both be present. Only the induration is measured. If it is more than 10 mm in diameter, the tuberculin test is considered as positive.

A multiple puncture test was described by Heaf in 1951. It uses a multiple puncture apparatus to deliver six vertical needle punctures to a depth of 1–2mm. The puncture is made through a drop of full-strength OT or PPD and as the needles pene-

trate the skin the liquid on the surface is carried into the skin. The test is read after 48 hours and graded as follows:

Negative	-	only puncture marks or erythema
Grade I	-	induration around puncture marks
Grade II	-	induration around puncture marks running into each other to form a ring
Grade III	-	as in II and also the central hollow filled with induration
Grade IV	-	as in III plus surrounding induration

Grade IV and above should be treated with suspicion and further steps taken to confirm the diagnosis.

The Heaf test gives results intermediate betwen 5 TU and 100 TU Mantoux test, and for epidemiological use is preferable to Mantoux 5 TU test.

Variations in sensitivity

If a sufficiently strong dilution of tuberculin was used nearly everyone would show a positive reaction; the main problem was to find a strength which would help to pick out those individuals who were harbouring mycobacteria from the healthy ones. With trial and error it has been found that a dose of 10 TU is best suited to clinical diagnosis of tuberculosis and 2 TU of PPD RT23 is preferable for epidemiologic work. RT23 (which can be obtained from the State Serum Institute in Copenhagen or through the WHO and UNICEF) is a standardised tuberculin containing Tween 80 which improves its stability. More recently, the Heaf multiple puncture test has come to be used for initial screening and for surveys; those picked out by positive Heaf test can be further tested with serial dilutions of old tuberculin.

Mass surveys for tuberculin hypersensitivity have been carried out in many developing countries. An intriguing finding in these surveys has been the high preponderance of intermediate reactions to the standard dose amongst the healthy population. This has been ascribed to 'atypical' and avian mycobacteria which act as weak sensitising agents. In these countries, the usefulness of the tuberculin test as a diagnostic and epidemiologic tool may be reduced to a varying degree, depending upon the presence of low grade hypersensitivity in the population.

A further problem is created by lack of response

in malnourished children although they may be infected with miliary tuberculosis. The degree of impairment of response is related to the degree of growth impairment and may often be restored by a short period of good nutrition. Alternatively a higher strength of tuberculin may be used if a strong suspicion of tuberculosis exists and the response to the standard dose is negative. Besides malnutrition, negative tuberculin reaction may occur during virus illnesses like measles (including measles or yellow fever vaccination), with dehydration or during treatment with antihistamines or corticosteroids.

In the author's experience, for routine screening of hospital and out-patient attendances and for mass surveys, the multiple puncture method of Heaf is inexpensive, rapid and reliable. In the case of the individual child in whom there is a strong suspicion of tuberculosis, serial Mantoux tests with increasing strengths of tuberculin are the best.

Gastric lavage

In the young child it is very difficult to obtain sputum for staining. All coughed-up material tends to be swallowed, especially during sleep. Such material may be recovered by gastric lavage, especially in the early morning on a fasting stomach, and examined by microscopy for acid-fast bacilli. To carry out the test, the child needs to be admitted to hospital. Because of the possibilities of error it has to be done on at least three occasions before the test is declared negative.

Some authors have reported better results with laryngeal swabs. The technique is easy and quick and can be carried out even in out-patients. The difficulty is with the delay in obtaining the results, because culture may take as long as six to eight weeks.

X-rays

Radiography, though very useful in the diagnosis of the adult case, is of limited value in diagnosing the primary complex. The primary focus in the lung is too small to show on X-ray, and hilar enlargement, unless very marked, may be missed. However, if any of the pulmonary complications of the primary complex exist, like absorption collapse or emphysema, bronchopneumonia or pneumonia, or miliary mottling, they are easily seen on X-ray. The greatest usefulness of X-rays is in the long-term follow-up of a case which is receiving treatment.

It would thus appear that there is no short cut to the diagnosis of childhood tuberculosis. The process of diagnosis begins with suspicion, either from the history of vague symptomatology or of contact with an 'open' case of tuberculosis, and confirmed by the results of all the various investigations put together. In most cases, the diagnosis rests on a proper evaluation of the child and his environment.

Child	*Environment*
History and physical examination	Contact with an 'open' case
BCG – nutritional status	Frequency of exposure
Age – recent illnesses – results of investigation	The state of health of the immediate contacts

Management of childhood tuberculosis

Controlled therapeutic trials in several countries have helped to emphasise the importance of adequate chemotherapy and of patient co-operation for regular administration of drugs. Time honoured practices of complete bed rest, airy and spacious accommodation in a sanitorium, rich diet, or healthy climate have very little role in treatment. Hospital admissions should be restricted to only cases with complications, or with other associated illnesses such as anaemia and malnutrition or where there is a social problem in the family. There is also no reason for indiscriminate prescription of tonics and vitamins which the parents may consider more important than anti-tuberculous drugs and administer the former religiously while the real medicine is neglected.

In the typical pulmonary lesion of the adult patient three different types of bacillary populations may be identified. Inside the cavitary lesion a large (10^7–10^9) bacillary population is located in the liquid caseous layer covering the inner wall. Here the bacilli are extracellular and multiply actively because of favourable oxygen tension and presence of nutrients.

In addition to this main group two smaller bacillary populations (10^4–10^7) are also present. These are the bacilli (i) inside macrophages; and (ii) inside more solid caseous foci like lymph nodes. Here the bacilli multiply slowly or in intermittent bursts.

Drugs must be chosen for their specific activity against various types of bacterial populations in order to achieve quick and complete sterilisation of the lesion. For the large populations of bacilli actively multiplying on the walls of the cavities the most effective drugs are streptomycin, isoniazid and rifampicin. All of them are bactericidal. Ethambutol and PAS are bacteriostatic, whereas pyrazinamide is inactive. For the relatively smaller population of bacilli inside macrophages the most effective drugs are pyrazinamide, isoniazid and rifampicin. Streptomycin is inactive. In the solid lesions where the bacilli multiply intermittently rifampicin is bactericidal, and all other drugs are inactive.

In all the three bacterial populations, there also exist naturally occurring drug resistant mutants. Hence the need to deal with the sensitive bacilli urgently so as to give the body's defence mechanism a chance to deal with the resistant ones.

With this knowledge about the characteristics of the bacillary population, shorter and more effective courses of chemotherapy are possible compared to the previous standard regimens. The objective is to achieve complete sterilisation of the lesions as rapidly as possible.

A number of trials with short course chemotherapy in several countries have helped to establish the following principles

(1) The combination of rifampicin and isoniazid is essential in both the initial and continuation phases.
(2) Streptomycin and pyrazinamide are helpful as supplementary drugs in the initial phase, and if rifampicin is not available.
(3) The overall duration of the short course chemotherapy should be six to nine months.
(4) In the initial phase treatment must be intensive with daily administration of drugs.

The typical nine months regimen of short course chemotherapy is as follows:

An initial *intensive* phase of two months with daily administration of isoniazid 5mg/kg + rifampicin 10 mg/kg + ethambutol 20 mg/kg daily, followed by a *continuation* phase of daily isoniazid 5mg/kg + rifampicin 10 mg/kg until end of nine months.

Possible variations in the regimen are omission of ethambutol in the initial phase when sensitivity to isoniazid is certain, and isoniazid 15 mg/kg + rifampicin 10 mg/kg may be given twice weekly instead of daily in the continuation phase.

The typical six months regimen consists of:

An initial *intensive* phase of two months daily isoniazid 5 mg/kg + rifampicin 10 mg/kg + pyrazinamide 30 mg/kg with or without ethambutol 20 mg/kg, followed by a continuation phase of daily or twice weekly isoniazid 15 mg/kg + rifampicin 10 mg/kg until the end of six months.

Both regimens are given orally. Without pyrazinamide in the initial phase of the six months regimen relapse rates tend to be high.

The reported success rates for nine months' short course chemotherapy in ideal circumstances have been above 90 per cent. In well managed programmes in Tanzania, Mozambique, Malawi and Nicaragua success rates of 77–80 per cent have been reported compared to 58 per cent with the standard regimen.

On the basis of all reported studies the current recommendation for the treatment of pulmonary tuberculosis in the adult in the more developed countries is a six months regimen using isoniazid, rifampicin and pyrazinamide daily for two months followed by four months of daily or supervised twice weekly isoniazid and rifampicin. In cases of suspected drug resistance ethambutol or streptomycin may be added pending culture and sensitivity results.

Short course chemotherapy in children

Localised tuberculous lesions in children are typically caseous with relatively small number of mycobacteria. On the other hand the likelihood of dissemination like miliary or meningeal tuberculosis is greater in children. Hence adequate tissue penetration in a variety of organ systems is an important consideration in the choice of drugs. Isoniazid, rifampicin and pyrazinamide cross the blood-brain barrier adequately, whereas streptomycin does so only when the meninges are inflamed.

A number of studies in childhood tuberculosis indicate that a six months regimen is often adequate. The best studied regimen for pulmonary tuberculosis is an initial two months of daily isoniazid (10 mg/kg), rifampicin (10–15 mg/kg) and pyrazinamide (30 mg/kg) followed by four months of daily isoniazid (10 mg/kg) and rifampicin (10–15 mg/kg), or four months of supervised twice weekly isoniazid (20–25 mg/kg *per dose*) and rifampicin (10–15 mg/kg *per dose*). For suspected drug resistance, streptomycin (20 mg/kg) or ethambutol (15 mg/kg) should be added until culture results are available.

For the more serious forms of childhood tuberculosis like miliary, meningeal, pericardial and spinal disease, rifampicin should be included in the continuation phase, and the duration of treatment should be no less than nine months.

Treatment of tuberculous meningitis

In the early stage I of the disease a combination of isoniazid (10 mg/kg), rifampicin (15 mg/kg) and pyrazinamide (35 mg/kg) is effective. Treatment should last for at least one year, and longer if there is advanced disease or in the presence of a tuberculoma. Isoniazid is an important drug as it crosses the blood-brain barrier well. Rifampicin is also important and should be included in the continuation phase. Streptomycin crosses the blood-brain barrier when the meninges are inflamed, and is of value in the first few weeks. Thereafter it should be given intrathecally (1mg/kg to a maximum of 50 mg/day). Now with the more effective regimens intrathecal treatment is rarely required. Corticosteroids may be of benefit in stage II and III of the disease.

Treatment of extra-pulmonary tuberculosis

Chemotherapy is highly effective and surgery is rarely needed for spinal, bone or articular tuberculosis. All such lesions contain far fewer bacilli than pulmonary lesions, and ambulatory treatment with short course chemotherapy is adequate in the majority of cases.

Chemoprophylaxis

Protection may be required in the case of the very young child with a positive response to tuberculin. Since the likelihood of a post primary spread is greater the younger the child, chemoprophylaxis should be offered to all children under the age of four years.

In one study with 24 weeks on isoniazid alone there was a reduction in the incidence of disease by 65 per cent. When chemoprophylaxis was continued for one year there was a 75 per cent reduction. When four drugs were combined – isoniazid + streptomycin + rifampicin + pyrazinamide – the reduction in incidence was by 81.5 per cent on a two months' course, and 88 per cent on a three months' course. Since compliance is a problem in many developing countries, a two months' course with a four-drugs combination may be the best solution.

The older child, who is otherwise in good health, may be kept under observation with regular followups and, if possible, chest X-rays for a period of one year. The occasional child who, though older in age, is malnourished or is recovering from a severe illness, may need protection with chemoprophylaxis in the same way as in the case of the young child.

Chemoprophylaxis is also required for the young infant or toddler from a household with an 'open' case of tuberculosis. Such chemoprophylaxis should be continued until several sputum examinations on the adult patient have shown absence of bacilli, after which further protection can be provided by BCG.

Tuberculosis as a community problem

Three major indices indicate the extent of the tuberculosis problem in the community. These are

(1) The number of individuals with positive tuberculin reactions and their ages.
    The prevalence of a positive Mantoux test in children is the best indicator of the current transmission of infection in a community and if repeated surveys are done at regular intervals it may be possible to obtain an indication of the trend.
(2) The number of individuals excreting tubercle bacilli in their sputa.
    A positive sputum on microscopy is the best available information on the size of the reservoir of infection.
(3) The number of individuals with positive X-rays, but negative sputum.

Under natural conditions the reservoir of infection in the community is in equilibrium. A proportion may die and some patients improve temporarily so that they become sputum negative. On the other hand, new cases appear and a proportion of sputum negative cases deteriorate and begin to cough up the bacilli. Thus, the size of the pool remains virtually the same from year to year though changes occur over long periods (figure 14.7).

The existing reservoir of infection in the community causes fresh infections chiefly in the younger age groups. Some will ward off the infection and develop their own immunity whereas in others the infection will smoulder and break down later. Such occurrences add fresh cases to the pool.

A programme to deal with tuberculosis in the community must therefore have two major objectives as follows

(1) Elimination of the reservoir of infection by case-finding and adequate therapy.
(2) Protection of the younger age-groups by BCG vaccination.

In the rural areas of the developing countries there are few programmes of active case-finding. All new cases come to the notice of the health personnel on the initiative of the individual patient; this initiative often does not last beyond the first three to six months, so that drop-out rates are high.

EPIDEMIOLOGIC MODEL FOR TUBERCULOSIS IN THE AVERAGE DISTRICT IN INDIA

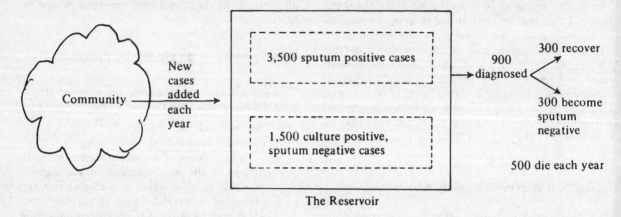

Figure 14.7   Tuberculosis in the community

When chemotherapy includes rifampicin, patients become non-infectious rapidly and long before the disappearance of acid fast bacilli from the sputum. For practical purposes patients are non-infectious after two weeks of chemotherapy which includes rifampicin. Thus risk of infection is much reduced compared to the previous standard regimen in which 50 per cent of patients remained sputum positive even after two months. The second advantage of the short course chemotherapy is the shorter duration of treatment thereby reducing the risk of resistance emerging.

If the risk of infection is reduced by four to five per cent annually, tuberculosis can cease to be a major health problem in developing countries within 20–30 years. If cure rates of 85 per cent can be maintained and case finding be improved to 60–65 per cent a 50 per cent reduction in the incidence of the disease can be expected in 10 to 12 years. With more efficient case finding rates the period to halving the incidence of tuberculosis can be shortened even more.

BCG coverage in developing countries is now about 80 per cent, although the average for sub-Saharan Africa is less than 60 per cent. It is generally agreed that BCG does not contribute significantly to reducing the transmission of infection, but it protects by limiting the spread of the bacilli after they gain entry into the body.

Further reading

Girling D J, Darbyshire J H, Humphries M J, O'Mahoney G. Extrapulmonary tuberculosis. *Br Med Bulletin* 1988; 44: 738–756.

Joint tuberculosis Committee of the British Thoracic Society. Control and prevention of tuberculosis; a code of practice. *Brit Med J* 1983; 287: 1118–1121.

Murray C J, Styblo K, Rouillon A. Tuberculosis in developing countries: burden, intervention and cost. *Bull Int Union Tuberc Lung Dis* 1990; 65: 6–24.

Snider (Jr.) D, Bridbord K, Hui F, (Eds). Research towards global control and prevention of tuberculosis with an emphasis on vaccine development. *Rev Inf Dis* 1989: Supplement 2.

Starke J R. Multidrug therapy for tuberculosis in children. *Ped Inf Dis J* 1990; 9: 785–793.

World Health Organisation. *Tuberculosis research and development*. Geneva: WHO 1991; document WHO/TB/91.160.

World Health Organisation. *Tuberculosis control and research strategy for the 1990s*. Geneva: WHO 1991; WHO/TB/91.157.Rev.1.

15 *Leprosy*

Leprosy is the most common communicable disease affecting the peripheral nervous system. Even though the obvious signs and symptoms are present in the skin, the peripheral nerves are the tissues largely affected resulting in disability, disfigurement and scarring. Without this progressive destruction of the peripheral nerve trunks and its consequences leprosy would largely remain a cutaneous condition of only cosmetic significance. The frequency and persistence of disabilities, the normal life span of the tuberculoid and indeterminate cases and the high cost of reconstructive surgery give leprosy a special place among communicable diseases.

Leprosy has been reported in almost all the countries of the world since the advent of history and was the dreaded scourge of ancient times. It has since receded from most of the countries of the western world and is today mainly confined to developing countries where poor socio-hygienic conditions, undernutrition and inadequate living standards contribute to its persistence. Of the estimated 10 million patients in the world, about a third are with significant deformities. About 62 per cent of all cases of leprosy are in Asia and 34 per cent in Africa (figure 15.1). Expressed in terms of mean prevalence, the disease is about three times as intense in Africa as it is in Asia. Countries with an estimated prevalence rate of more than 1 per 1000 population have a total population of 1.6 billion people. They constitute the population most at risk.

Several geographical differences in the prevalence rates of leprosy may be noted, even in the same country. For example, in India, a high prevalence rate of 10 per 1000 has been reported from the states of Tamil Nadu and Andhra Pradesh and a comparatively lower prevalence in the north. It has been observed that lepromatous leprosy is commoner among light-skinned people and the tuberculoid variety is seen in those who are darkly pigmented.

Leprosy is essentially a rural disease. Often the village communities are able to recognise the lepromatous case who is then forced by social pressure to leave home and seek the anonymity of the city where he constitutes a public health risk.

It has been universally appreciated that most infection with *Mycobacterium leprae* takes place in childhood. At the Ackworth leprosy clinic in Bombay, it has been observed that 12 per cent of all patients attending the clinic are in the paediatric age group, commonly between the ages of 8 and 14 years. Considering the very long incubation period of leprosy it is clear that infection must have occurred between the ages of 6 and 8 years. In a survey of school children in Bombay covering 50 697 students representing 10 per cent of the child population in the municipal schools, the prevalence rate of leprosy was found to be 3 per 1000. In a similar survey in a neighbourhood known to be endemic for leprosy, the prevalence rate was 11 per 1000. It was also shown that of 2000 cases in India, the lesion was first noted before the age of 20 years in 55.4 per cent of the cases. Similarly in East Africa, 27 per cent of all patients were found to be infected before the age of 15 and another 13 per cent between 15 and 20 years. Early infections are, of course, more common when there are infected parents living in the same house. Overcrowding and several families living together under one roof contribute to the transmission of the disease.

Mode of spread

Leprosy is known to spread by contact. Prolonged continuous contact is not always necessary and infection may be acquired even through one ideal contact, depending upon the resistance of the host. The intact skin acts as a barrier and provides no opportunity for the bacilli to emerge; on the other hand, ulcerative lesions may teem with bacilli. Secretions and discharges from ulcers may contain large numbers of bacilli and contaminated clothing or utensils are an important means of transmission

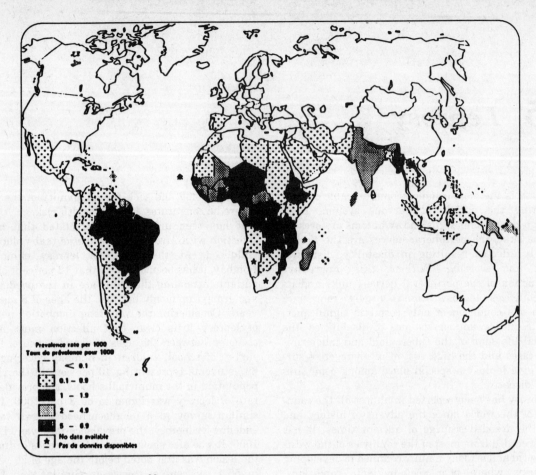

Figure 15.1 Prevalence rates of leprosy

of infection. The intact skin also offers resistance to entry but the scratched or abraded skin may allow entry to the organisms deposited on the surface. In this respect biting insects may have a role to play by causing scratching.

Recent work has shown that an important route of transmission is through nasal discharge and droplets. Endonasal examination in established cases of leprosy often shows specific lesions of the mucosa of an unsuspected extent. The organisms are viable for up to seven days outside the body. Thus the inhalation of infected droplets and swallowing of the bacilli entrapped in the nasal mucus is the commonest mode of entry for the organisms into the host.

Children in the family, household or compound run a special risk partly because of their age but mainly because of long periods of contact at night when they share a bed with an adult. Overcrowding in the home also favours transmission. In many peasant communities where families are close-knit and communal living is common, every individual must be regarded as a contact whenever leprosy is diagnosed.

In addition to the clinical cases of leprosy which act as the reservoir of the disease in the community, many of their contacts with no symptoms or lesions may harbour bacilli in the skin. Biopsies of skin taken from unselected sites in such individuals have shown the presence of acid fast bacilli. Whether they can also transmit disease and thus are acting as symptomless carriers in the community, needs further study.

The risk of acquiring the disease varies among individuals. In endemic areas leprosy is transmitted easily but 95 per cent of people who are infected never develop the disease. For each overt case of the disease as many as 200 individuals become infected without developing clinical manifestations. In early infection regression and spontaneous healing can also occur. The cell mediated immunity of the host is the main determinant as to whether infection will progress into disease, and also of the type of disease.

Pathology

The characteristic pathological lesion in leprosy is a granuloma. Depending upon the strength of the defence mounted by the body the characteristics of the granuloma vary, and this forms the basis of classification. At one end of the spectrum is *tuberculoid leprosy* where the lesions are few and circumscribed. They contain many lymphocytes and macrophages and hardly any bacteria. At the other *lepromatous* end of the spectrum the lesions are numerous, and are characterised by 'foamy' macrophages, few lymphocytes and a large number of bacteria. In between these two extremes are the borderline stages. A number of classifications have been proposed, but a simple and very practical classification is that proposed by the World Health Organisation viz. paucibacillary which includes tuberculoid (TT) and borderline tuberculoid (BT); and multibacillary – which includes borderline (BB), borderline lepromatous (BL) and lepromatous (LL).

Classification system				Spectrum of leprosy		
WHO	Paucibacillary			Multibacillary		
Madrid	Tuberculoid		Borderline		Lepromatous	
Ridley & Joplins	Polar Tuberculoid	Borderline Tuberculoid	Mid Borderline	Borderline Lepromatous	Polar Lepromatous	

In tuberculoid leprosy the inflammatory process begins in the peripheral nerve situated in the papillary layer of the dermis and extends to varying depths in the subcutaneous tissue along the nerve fibres. In lepromatous cases the skin shows signs of infiltrative processes. There is also early bacillary invasion of Schwann cells and swelling of nerve fibres. Later, there is cellular infiltration followed by fibrosis and strangulation of the nerve fibres. Many of the early pathological changes in nerve fibres suggest that the initial lesion is in the peripheral nerves from where the bacilli migrate to the skin.

The lepromin test is often used as a measure of the body's resistance and to differentiate lepromatous leprosy from the tuberculoid variety. Lepromin is a heat-killed suspension of *M. leprae*, and 0.1ml is injected intradermally into the patient's forearm. The immediate reaction is read between 24–48 hours and is usually allergic because of presence of various antigenic proteins in lepromin. The delayed reaction which is read after three weeks is more important and is said to indicate resistance.

In paucibacillary (tuberculoid) leprosy a positive test result is obtained indicating strong cell-mediated immunity.

Multibacillary (lepromatous) patients will have a negative test result indicating poor resistance. In borderline and intermediate varieties the results vary. The long waiting time between administration of lepromin and reading the test makes follow-up difficult especially in rural areas.

The lack of response to lepromin in multibacillary leprosy is evidence of deficient cell-mediated immunity. A number of studies have shown defective activation of T cells with markedly altered T4/T8 ratio, deficient secretion of interleukin–1 and utilisation of interleukin–2.

A number of serological tests are being developed. The currently available test is the fluorescent antibody absorption test to quantitate levels of antibody against *M. leprae*. The mean antibody titre is highest amongst lepromatous cases and lowest among those with tuberculoid diseases.

Clinical features

Leprosy always involves peripheral nerves, almost always involves the skin and frequently involves the mucus membrane. The cardinal signs are skin lesions, skin anaesthesia and enlarged peripheral nerves.

The clinical manifestations in the individual patient are due to three pathological mechanisms viz:

(1) bacterial proliferation;
(2) the immunologic response of the host; and
(3) peripheral neuritis caused by (1) and (2).

The onset is generally insidious, though general malaise may be noted in some children. The first presenting sign may be an area of hypopigmentation of the skin, in which, on further examination, sensations are found to be diminished or lost. In some cases, the first sign may be a burn or injury of the hands or feet of which the patient is usually unaware because of lack of pain. In the vast majority of cases, however, early leprosy is 'silent'. Patients enjoy good health and parents refuse to believe that the children show signs of a potentially serious disease. Early diagnosis is possible by regular examination of close contacts of the index case. Just as in the case of tuberculosis, so also in leprosy the diagnosis is incomplete unless a thorough search is made for the potential source from whom the patient received the infection and the possible contacts to whom he may have transmitted the disease.

Involvement of the peripheral nerve trunks produces local nerve tenderness, paraesthesia or neuralgia. The affected nerves become palpable as cords, and the ones easily felt are the ulnar, the median, the external popliteal, the posterior tibial and the great auricular. Involvement of the motor fibres in these nerves causes paralysis of muscles and deformities, usually in the hands and feet. The common deformities are claw hands or toes, dropped feet, or inversion of the feet. Because of the deformities and anaesthesia in the hands and feet, minor injuries are difficult to avoid and are not felt. Sepsis can result in trophic ulcers. In the late stages the vicious circle of sepsis, trophic ulcers, extension of the disease to bones, deformities and the anaesthesia of the hands and feet can cause disorganisation of joints and there may be disappearance of parts of fingers and toes.

Depending upon the interaction between the resistance of the host and the invading microorganisms, various clinical forms of the disease may be recognised. *Lepromatous leprosy* is characterised by infiltration in the skin and in later stages by the occurrence of nodules. Clinical signs of nerve involvement occur at a later stage in the lepromatous form as compared to the other forms. All lesions of lepromatous leprosy are full of bacilli which may be found even in the unaffected skin. There is invasion of the other organs in addition to the skin and the bacilli may be obtained from liver, spleen, kidneys or the bone marrow. Invasion of the mucous membrane of the upper respiratory passages occurs early and *M. leprae* may be found in large numbers in the nasal mucus and the secretions. Patients with lepromatous leprosy will have episodes of increased activity of the disease called lepra reactions. These episodes are brought about by intercurrent infections, use of certain drugs or at times with no obvious cause. They are characterised by pyrexia, enlargement and swelling of the old lesions and appearance of new ones, tenderness and swelling of peripheral nerves and inflammation of respiratory

mucosae. Each episode leaves the patient weak and debilitated.

Tuberculoid leprosy is not as virulent as the lepromatous type. There are hypopigmented patches in the skin, some of which heal spontaneously. The main brunt of the attack is on the peripheral nerves which are enlarged and tender. Sensory impairment occurs early in the course of the illness and various degrees of motor paralysis occur as the disease advances. The skin does not show many bacilli by the ordinary methods of testing.

Diagnosis

Diagnosis of the lepromatous form is established by the demonstration of *M. leprae* in the skin. A superficial incision 3–4 mm deep is taken in the skin at the involved site. The point of the scalpel is then rotated through 90° in the incision, so that the edge scrapes the sides of the incision. The drop of tissue fluid and scraping so obtained is spread on a glass slide and stained by the Ziehl-Neelsen method for acid fast bacilli. *M. leprae* is less acid fast than *M. tuberculosis* and the decolorisation during staining should be less.

In lepromatous and near lepromatous leprosy the mucosa lying over the septum and the anterior aspects of the middle and lower turbinates harbours leprosy bacilli which are discharged in large numbers in the nasal mucus. In early cases *M. leprae* bacilli are not seen in the nasal mucus until the infection is widespread and the apparently healthy skin harbours the bacilli in large numbers.

Thus, examination of the nasal mucus for *M. leprae* is not a useful early screening test. On the other hand, the nasal mucus often reveals bacilli when they are no longer found in the skin by standard techniques and during a relapse bacilli appear in the nasal discharge long before they can be found routinely in the skin. If the nasal discharge contains viable bacilli, the patient is to be considered contagious since large numbers of bacilli will be shed during sneezing and coughing.

In the absence of bacilli, the diagnosis of leprosy will rest on the clinical demonstration of nerve damage, in the form of loss of temperature, touch and pain sensations or as motor paralysis. Anhidrosis is also another form of nerve damage. In doubtful cases skin biopsy and the characteristic histologic changes as well as demonstration of acid-fast organisms help to confirm the diagnosis.

Treatment

In the typical multibacillary patient there are essentially three populations of M. leprae viz:

(1) fully drug susceptible organisms;
(2) a small population of drug resistant mutants; and
(3) a small population of non-multiplying bacilli (persisters) that are not eliminated by treatment with presently available drugs.

Similarly three populations of M. leprae can be expected in the paucibacillary case except that the total bacterial load is smaller.

The currently recommended treatment is a multidrug regimen as follows

Multidrug Therapy (MDT)

	Paucibacillary Leprosy	Multibacillary Leprosy
Regimen	Rifampicin 20mg/kg to max. of 600mg, once monthly – supervised + Dapsone 1–2mg/kg daily (max.100mg) self-administered	Rifampicin 20mg/kg (max.600mg) once monthly – supervised + Dapsone 1–2mg/kg (max.100mg) daily self-administered + * Clofazimine 300mg once monthly supervised and 50mg daily self-administered
Duration of treatment	6 months	At least 2 years or until skin smears -ve
Follow up	Annually for at least 2 years	Annually for at least 5 years

* If clofazimine unacceptable, substitute ethionamide or prothionamide daily self-administered 5–10mg/kg

With MDT relapse rates have been low after stopping therapy unlike in the case of previous monotherapy with dapsone. In field trials relapse rates have been of the magnitude of 4.17 per 1000 person-years in paucibacillary leprosy in the first year after completion of MDT. No relapse rates were reported in more than 8000 person-years of follow up in multibacillary leprosy. In well-managed programmes relapse rates have been less than 0.1 per cent per year among 85 000 cases of paucibacillary and less than 0.06 per cent per year among 22 000 cases of multibacillary leprosy.

Depending on the results of field trials currently in progress, minocycline may be added to the list of drugs for the treatment of leprosy.

Disabilities

About 30 per cent of known leprosy patients suffer from deformities and disabilities caused by damage to the peripheral nerves. Loss of skin sensation leading to recurrent damage and paralysis of muscle movements are the main cause of disabilities. The feet and hands are the most susceptible. Early diagnosis and a high degree of suspicion are the best measures for preventing disabilities. Protective devices to prevent injury to hands and feet, appropriate footwear, physiotherapy and surgical intervention may be required as indicated.

Patient compliance has always been a major obstacle in the management of leprosy. Studies in Asia and Africa have shown that patient compliance may be as low as a third to a half with self-administered dapsone. A number of approaches like patient education, community mobilisation and home visiting have been tried to improve compliance. Recently calendar packs with bubble presentation of individual tablets have been introduced to improve compliance, and to avoid wastage of drugs.

Prevention

Man is the only known source of M. leprae and hence the total number of persons with the illness comprise the reservoir of infection in the community. If the individual cases can be found early and treated so as to render them non-contagious, the cycle of transmission can be broken. Case-finding, contact tracing and adequate treatment of those who are affected will hold out the best chances for the control of leprosy in the community.

(1) Case-finding by means of house to house visits or whole population surveys may be considered for communities where leprosy is highly endemic. Such surveys are expensive and not very practicable and may be undertaken only for those areas where the prevalence of leprosy exceeds one per cent.

Rifampicin is rapidly bactericidal, achieving a 99 per cent kill rate of M. leprae in three to four days. With dapsone and clofazimine such a magnitude of kill rate is obtained in about four months. Thus, with MDT it is possible to render a patient non-infectious in a short time. In communities where the annual incidence rate of leprosy has been regularly monitored, a 40 per cent reduction in incidence was noted three years after the introduction of MDT.

(2) *Contact tracing.* Epidemiologic investigation in the pre-sulphone era has shown that in an endemic area the risk of acquiring leprosy for a household contact of lepromatous patients was eight times that of a member of a household not infected with leprosy. It was four times in the case of a household contact of tuberculoid leprosy. Recent work shows that leprosy is more highly infectious than prevalence studies indicate, and that a sub-clinical infection commonly follows exposure to *M. leprae.* The development of disease is related to the intensity of exposure and the resistance of the host. Thus, regular examination of household, occupational and family contacts of patients is necessary for early detection of the disease.

(3) In many developing countries a high proportion of beggars in the cities may have leprosy. Regular supervision and treatment of this group is essential because of their mobility in the city.

BCG vaccination

In addition to measures directed against the reservoir of the infection in the community, a control programme should also aim at the protection of the vulnerable groups. No vaccine against *M. leprae* is available but BCG is holding out some promise. In laboratory experiments it has been shown that BCG can almost completely suppress the multiplication of *M. leprae* in mice. In a large scale trial in Uganda,

it was found that BCG can cause 80 per cent reduction in the incidence of leprosy at the end of 26 months and 87 per cent reduction at the end of 44 months. In a similar trial in New Guinea it was found that BCG vaccination led to a reduction in the incidence of tuberculoid leprosy by 50 per cent.

More recent approaches to vaccine production have involved two strategies: use of *M. leprae* itself, or of immunologically related non-pathogenic organisms other than BCG. Vaccine prepared from both these approaches are currently undergoing field trials.

Molecular genetics have also opened up new opportunities. The major protein antigens of *M. leprae* and *M. tuberculosis* have been cloned in vectors like *E. coli*, and the most effective epitopes for vaccines may be determined by this approach.

It would appear that with a well co-ordinated programme of reducing the reservoir of infection in the community by case-finding and treatment, and by vaccination with BCG, this ancient scourge can be brought under control. New drugs like rifampicin may further contribute by making complete cure possible and reducing the duration of treatment.

Further reading

Ellard G A. The Chemotherapy of Leprosy. Part 1. *Int J Lep* 1990; 58: 704–716. Part 2. *Int J Lep* 1991; 59: 82–94.
Hastings R C, Gillis T P, Krahenbuhl J L, Franzblau S G. Leprosy. *Clinical Microbiology Reviews* 1988; 1: 330–348.
Kaufmann S A E. Immunology of leprosy: new findings. *Microbial Pathogenesis* 1986; 1: 107–114.
Noordeen S K. The epidemiology of leprosy. *In* Hastings R C (Ed). *Leprosy.* London: Churchill-Livingstone. 1985.
Sutherland I. Research into the control of tuberculosis and leprosy in the community. *Brit Medical Bulletin* 1988; 44: 665–678.

Section IV

Epidemic Illnesses

16 *Cholera*

Cholera is endemic in many countries of South-east Asia. Before 1961 it was restricted to a few centres around the Bay of Bengal in the region of the delta of the great rivers – the Ganges, and Brahmaputra and the Irawaddy. Here the relatively stagnant waters of the sluggishly flowing rivers, the concentration of large populations combined with poor hygienic conditions maintained the causative organisms. From time to time in the past cholera spread out from the endemic foci and gave rise to epidemics. In all eight pandemics have occurred. Six of them were in the nineteenth century and two in the present one. The last pandemic occurred in the sixties. In the year 1961 confirmed cases of clinical cholera began to appear in South-east Asia caused by a new biotype of the vibrio, namely, the vibrio El-Tor. Soon

afterwards the vibrio spread to Indonesia and north and east to Hong Kong, the Philippines, Korea and possibly the Chinese mainland. It swept back through South-east Asia including India and the Middle East (figure 16.1). It then invaded new territories in the USSR, north, east and west African countries and even a few European countries. In all the outbreaks recorded, the infecting strain was El-Tor and not the cholera vibrio. El-Tor is more resistant to adverse environmental conditions and hence can survive longer in food and fomites. Also, the ratio of mild and symptomless infections to the typical disease is much higher in the cases of El-Tor compared to classical infection. Thus the number of symptomless carriers tends to be higher, favouring spread of the disease.

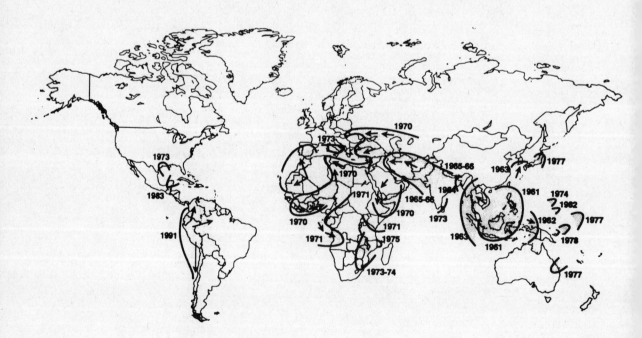

Figure 16.1 The cholera epidemic 1961–1991

As a result of the last pandemic, cholera has become endemic in some countries such as the Philippines, whereas in others, for example, Korea and Taiwan, the disease seems to have disappeared after the initial outbreak. In India, a country highly infected with cholera for several centuries, a number of centres of endemicity exist. For example, seven states (out of a total of 21) containing a third of the population of the country, contributed over 75 per cent of the reported cholera cases and 80 per cent of cholera deaths during the epidemic.

Over half a million cases of cholera were notified in 1991. Seventy per cent of the cases were reported from 13 Latin American countries with Peru reporting the maximum number. Africa was the most heavily afflicted continent with 19 countries reporting outbreaks of the disease. Control measures in Latin America helped to contain the epidemic and kept the fatality rate low at about one per cent. In Africa case fatality ranged from eight to ten per cent.

In endemic areas, cholera predominates amongst children, but in newly invaded areas, where the population has no basic immunity, there is no age difference. In rural areas where facilities for adequate treatment are not available, the greatest mortality occurs at the two extremes of age, again demonstrating the importance of the disease in the young.

Transmission

Vibrio cholerae occurs in more than 60 serogroups, but only serogroup 01 can cause cholera. *V.cholerae 01* occurs as two biotypes – classical and El-Tor. The latter has been responsible for nearly all the recent outbreaks of cholera, although the classical biotype is still present on the Indian subcontinent.

The El-Tor biotype has a higher infection-to-case ratio and survives longer than the classical biotypes in the environment for example, in water, nightsoil used as fertiliser, and sewage. It may survive as a free-living organism in association with aquatic plants and animals without cholera cases occurring in the area. By contrast the classical biotype has not been isolated from water or from aquatic plants and animals in the absence of human infection.

Man is the only known host. The transmission of the disease requires the transfer of the vibrios from a patient to the new host and their multiplication in the gut of the host. In most instances such a transfer is via the oro-faecal route.

In the acute stage of the disease a typical patient excretes 10 to 20 litres of stool per day containing 10^8 to 10^9 vibrios/ml and is able to contaminate a large area in his neighbourhood. The milder case passes a smaller number of organisms in the stool, between 10^2 and 10^5 vibrios/ml but in fact poses a greater hazard by being ambulant. In any given community, symptomless infections are more common. Only about one per cent of those infected develop clinical cholera and about 10 per cent develop mild diarrhoea or loose motions. It is known that 70 per cent of patients stop excreting vibrios by the end of the first week, 90 per cent by the end of the second and 98 per cent by the end of the third. Similar figures probably apply to asymptomatic cases.

Various figures varying from 5–20 per cent are given for inter-family spread. These figures are low compared to the large number of vibrios passed and indicate that cholera does not spread readily by direct contact. For spread in the community the vibrios must contaminate the water supply.

The survival time of vibrios in water depends on a number of factors, such as, temperature, pH of the water and its bacterial, salt and organic content. In clean water taken from a well or a tank and stored in the laboratory, vibrios generally do not survive for more than 7 – 13 days. In water containing a large number of other bacteria (for example, river water) the survival time of vibrios is very short, about one to two days, but in sterile filtered or autoclaved water the survival time varies from 17 days at room temperature to 42 days at 5 – 10°C. These observations show that contamination of water can play a role in the spread of cholera, though only for a limited period of time unless there is repeated contamination by a human source.

The vibrios do not tolerate drying, exposure to sunlight or competition with other organisms. Water is found to be contaminated only in association with infected individuals. In endemic areas in India, it has hardly ever been possible to isolate the organisms from natural surface water sources such as rivers and tanks, in the absence of cholera in the neighbourhood. Furthermore, it has been observed that contaminated water will become free of vibrios in a few days if such individuals are removed.

The vibrios remain viable for several days in food that is alkaline and moist provided competing organisms do not overgrow it. The commonest source of food-borne cholera is contaminated water used for cleaning vegetables or cooking, or the contaminated hands of a carrier. Milk and milk products and some kinds of boiled rice are good media of transmission; the addition of salt to fresh fish, meat, water-melon, and boiled rice makes them support the growth and multiplication of the vibrios. On the other hand, vibrios die after a few days when placed on a wide variety of other foods. Flies may physically transport vibrios from excreta to food, although they have not been shown to play a significant role in the spread of cholera. Vibrios may remain viable for long periods of time in clothing or bedding contaminated with cholera stools and these items have been implicated in the transmission of the disease when they were washed in river water that was also used for drinking.

Man the host

In endemic areas cholera attacks more children than adults. This may be due to acquired immunity in the adult. During an epidemic, however, no such difference is noted because the entire population may lack immunity.

Mass movement of population resulting in people living in overcrowded refugee camps create special hazards. Such movements are also responsible for the establishment of new foci of endemicity along the routes of migration.

In malnourished individuals, diarrhoea may persist longer than usual and the shedding of vibrios goes on for a longer period. This may be due to decreased local immunity of the mucosal cells as well as their slow turn-over because of malnutrition.

After an infection some individuals recover and become chronic carriers, because of a persistent infection in the biliary tract. Such carriers have been noted to shed organisms intermittently for an indefinite period. Such a person becomes a reservoir of the disease in the community and is responsible for the persistence of the disease and recurrent epidemics in the community. The detection of such carriers is difficult because the vibrios are shed intermittently and although they are noted to have persistent high levels of antibodies, serological screening of large populations is not yet practical.

Pathophysiology

The acidity of gastric juice acts as the host's first line of defence since the ingested vibrios are acid-sensitive. How this defence mechanism is overcome in established infections is not known. On reaching the small intestine the vibrio must multiply and adhere to the mucosa to cause symptoms. It secretes an enterotoxin which has two sub units. The light (L) sub unit binds with a ganglioside in the mucosal cell membrane. The heavy (H) sub unit releases various polypeptides which activate the enzyme adenyl cyclase. The activity of this enzyme results in the production of cyclic AMP (3,5 adenosine monophosphate) from adenosine triphosphate. Cyclic AMP paralyses the sodium pump of the enterocyte and leads to the outpouring of a large amount of fluid into the gut. The pathologic state in cholera is due to the massive intestinal loss of a fluid with the following electrolyte content: sodium 126 ± 9 m eq/l, potassium 19 ± 9 m eq/l, bicarbonate 47 ± 10 m eq/l and chloride 95 ± 9 m eq/l. The rate of loss of fluid in the adult can be as high as 1 l/hour. In addition to the acute and severe dehydration, acidosis and hypoglycaemia may be important complications in children.

Clinical picture

The clinical spectrum varies from asymptomatic states and mild cases to severe dehydration. In the classical infection the proportion of asymptomatic infection is estimated to be 10 to 1 clinical case. In the case of the El-Tor infection, it can be as high as 100 to 1. The mild cases have no distinguishing features and can be recognised only by stool culture. Such cases may not be brought to the notice of the health authorities and will remain untreated. They are, however, of epidemiologic importance because they maintain the microbe in the community.

Both the classical vibrio and El-Tor produce an identical clinical syndrome of abrupt onset of effortless vomiting and watery diarrhoea which quickly takes on the appearance of 'rice water'.

In the untreated cases, the mortality can be as high as 60 per cent, but with adequate treatment the water and electrolyte loss and acidosis can be corrected within two to three hours of admission in adults and about eight hours in children. Diarrhoea may persist for another two to six days with total stool production of several litres.

In the case of children, certain additional features are seen, for example: (1) the sensorium is altered to a greater degree; (2) siezures occur frequently. (In some children they are associated with hypoglycaemia or severe electrolyte disturbances, but the cause is not always known.); (3) high fever is frequently seen in children, but not in adults. A cholera-like syndrome has been seen in infections with non-agglutinable vibrios and certain strains of E.coli. The single distinguishing feature of this syndrome is its short duration.

Diagnosis

During an epidemic diagnosis is made on the basis of the clinical picture in most cases. Special diagnostic facilities do not exist at most rural health centres and dispensaries and yet cholera is predominantly a rural disease. The speed with which the diagnosis is made in the index case will help in preventing a large out-break. A high degree of suspicion and awareness of the existing diagnostic facilities in the district can often help the health team to stem a major epidemic in its early stages.

In the first day or two of diarrhoea, vibrios can be easily seen under the microscope. Later they are not so plentiful and culture may be necessary. In recent years dark field microscopy has been used for early diagnosis. By this method up to 80 per cent cases can be diagnosed within a few minutes if stools are examined early in the course of the disease. Contacts should be tested as soon as possible after detection of the index case. Where facilities exist and in endemic areas, stool culture should be carried out if there is a suspicion of cholera. Three grammes of stool are placed in a sterile tube containing 50 – 100 ml of alkaline peptone water. On arrival in the laboratory the specimen is incubated for eight hours and then plated on both selective and non-selective media.

Treatment

The immediate need is to replace the losses of water and electrolytes and to correct acidosis and hypoglycaemia if present. The degree of dehydration is graded by clinical assessment and the weight loss. The quantity of replacement fluid is judged as follows

		Replacement fluid required
Mild dehydration	– 5% weight loss	150 ml/kg
Moderate dehydration	– 8% weight loss	200 ml/kg
Severe dehydration	– 10% weight loss	300 ml/kg

Unless the patient is severely dehydrated approaching ten per cent and in shock, he can be treated by the oral route. Up to a third to a quarter of the calculated losses are replaced rapidly in the first two to four hours and the remainder in the next four to six hours more slowly. If the patient is in shock, the early replacement of losses is done intravenously by administration of Ringer lactate followed by oral rehydration.

Current research on the patho-physiology of diarrhoea and correction of dehydration by the oral route using a glucose-electrolyte solution (as discussed in chapter 11) began with cholera. Oral rehydration is now a firmly established method of treatment both in cholera as well as in all diarrhoeas. Eighty to 90 per cent of cases can be adequately treated by the oral route. Moreover this form of treatment helps to extend the care of the patient to remote rural areas where prompt action can be life saving. Because of prompt rehydration fewer than one per cent of over 200 000 reported cholera cases have died in recent outbreaks. Packets of glucose and salt containing sodium chloride 3.5 g, potassium chloride 1.5 g, sodium citrate 2.9 g (or sodium bicarbonate 2.5 g) and glucose 20 g are now widely available. The contents are dissolved in 1 litre of water and administered as an oral drink or by nasogastric tube at the rate of 50 to 100 ml/kg in four to six hours. The aim is to get as much fluid into the patient as is passed in the stool. Where pre-packed salts are not available the ingredients can be weighed separately and dissolved in water for administration. Cane sugar (40g) or rice powder (50g) may be used instead of glucose.

Vomiting can cause difficulty with administration of oral fluids. Experience has shown that 70 per cent of patients have copious vomiting in the acute stage. Of these 60 per cent vomit a total of less than 1.5 litres, another 25 per cent vomit more than 1.5 litres, but less than 3.5 litres, and only two per cent of patients vomit more than 5 litres in 24 hours. In spite of vomiting it has been possible to achieve positive gut balance with oral therapy in mild-moderate cases.

The vibrios are susceptible to several antibiotics. The most commonly used is tetracycline because of its low cost. It is given in a dose of 12.5 mg/kg every six hours for children until all diarrhoea has stopped. Doxycycline, a long acting form of tetracycline may be preferred in large epidemics since it needs to be administered only once daily. If purging continues after 48 hours of antibiotic treatment resistance is likely. Other antimicrobial agents which may be used in such a situation are furazolidine (1.25 mg/kg four times /day for three days) trimethoprim – sulfamethoxazole (TMP 5 mg/kg; SMX 25 mg/kg twice daily for three days), erythromycin (125 – 250 mg/kg six hourly), and chloramphenicol (50 – 100 mg/kg daily in four doses).

Preventative measures
Vaccine

The conventional vaccine consists of killed *V.cho-lerae 01* and requiring two injections provides a variable degree of short lived protection, and is no longer recommended.

Two new oral vaccines are presently undergoing field trials. These are:

Killed whole-cell/B subunit (WC/B)

The vaccine consists of killed *V.cholerae 01* of both sero-types (Inaba, Ogawa), and both biotypes (Classical, El-Tor). To this WC component is added a purified component of cholera toxin (B sub unit) which is immunogenic but harmless.

The vaccine stimulates both local and serum antibody responses. In field trials the WC/B vaccine has been shown to provide 85 per cent protection in the first six months, and 50 to 52 per cent protection for three years. After this the protection wanes. The protection in children is much less (24 to 47 per cent) compared to older persons, and lasts for a shorter duration.

Live oral vaccine (CVD–103 HgR)

The vaccine consists of live *V.cholerae* which have been genetically manipulated to delete the genes encoding for the cholera toxin. There is a small risk of mild diarrhoea of short duration in susceptible individuals. One single dose of the vaccine is more immunogenic than three doses of WC/B. The vaccine still needs to undergo extensive field trials before it can be released for general use.

Protection of water supply

In most areas where cholera is endemic, villages depend upon surface water and wells for individual water supply. Most of these are grossly contaminated, and during outbreaks of cholera need protection. This can be achieved by regular chlorination of all points of water supply carried out on the same day, together with regular supervision of their use by the public.

For chlorination of water a fresh *stock solution* may be prepared daily by adding 4 teaspoons (16g) of swimming pool hypochlorite or 10 teaspoons (40g) of bleaching powder to 1 litre of water. For making water safe the stock solution is added in the following proportions:

Quantity of water	Volume of stock solution needed
1 litre	3 drops
30 litres	1 teaspoonful
4550 litres	1 litre

After adding the stock solution the water should be allowed to stand for 20 to 30 minutes.

Early detection and removal to hospital of the index case and supervision of contact carriers may help to reduce the transmission.

During outbreaks hygienic disposal of human waste, clean water supply and food hygiene should be rigorously ensured. The principles of controlling outbreaks comprise isolation of cases for treatment to render them non-infectious; monitoring of contacts; ensuring of environmental sanitation; and the protection of drinking water as well as food.

Further reading

Holmgren J, Svennerholm A M. Mechanism of disease and immunity in cholera. *J infect Dis* 1977; 136 (suppl.): 105

Sandle G L. Oral therapy in cholera. *New Engl J Med* 1978; 298: 797–8.

World Health Organisation. Guidelines for cholera control. *WHO/CDD/SER/80.4 Rev.2 1991*. Geneva: World Health Organisation. 1991.

Clemens J D, Sack D A, Harris J R *et al*. Field trial of oral cholera vaccines in Bangladesh: results from 3 year follow-up. *Lancet* 1990; 335:270–73.

Holmgren J, Clemens J, Sack D A *et al*. Oral immunisation against cholera. *Current topics in microbiology and Immunology*. 1989; 146:197–204.

Levine M M. Modern vaccines: enteric infection. *Lancet* 1990; 335:958–61

Glass R I, Claeson M, Black P A, Waldman R J, Pierce N F. Cholera in Africa: lessons on transmission and control for Latin America. *Lancet* 1991; 338:791–795.

17 Dengue haemorrhagic fever*

Dengue haemorrhagic fever (DHF) is an acute febrile illness caused by any one of the four serotypes of the dengue virus. DHF is characterised clinically by high continuous fever, a haemorrhagic diathesis and a tendency to develop shock (dengue shock syndrome – DSS) which may be fatal. Thrombocytopenia and haemo-concentration are constant laboratory findings. Dengue haemorrhagic fever differs from classical dengue fever (DF) which is a mild febrile illness accompanied by skin rash, and muscle and joint pains.

History

The disease was first recognised in Manila, Philippines, in 1954 as a new disease outbreak in children associated with haemorrhagic manifestations and shock with high mortality. The clinical and epidemiological characteristics of this new disease were sufficiently novel for the disease to be named Philippine haemorrhagic fever. Subsequent epidemics in Thailand in 1958 and Singapore in 1960 thus prompted the names Thai and Singapore haemorrhagic fevers. The disease has spread further thereafter to several other countries in the South-east Asia and the western Pacific regions. It has now become an increasing public health problem in most tropical and sub-tropical Asian countries as it is among the ten leading causes of hospitalisation and death in children.

During 1977–1980 dengue infection spread to Cuba with 45 per cent of the population becoming infected by dengue virus type 1. The outbreak was characterised by mild symptoms. In 1981 dengue virus type 2 caused a major outbreak in Cuba with more than 10 000 cases of shock syndrome being recorded. The Cuban epidemic is the first reported outbreak outside South-east Asia in recent times.

DHF is a new clinical entity or a new variant of dengue infection because of its unusual haemorrhages and/or shock syndrome. The so-called dengue shock syndrome (DSS) marks the difference between DHF and the benign dengue or classical dengue fever (DF). The manifestations of ordinary dengue illness, which have been known for more than a century, are largely age-dependent. This disease is mild in children and almost unrecognised in infants, but more severe in adults. Infants and children with normal dengue infection have syndromes ranging from undifferentiated fever to mild febrile illness, sometimes with rash. Older children and, more frequently, adults suffer a more severe form of classical dengue syndrome with the triad of high fever, pain in various parts of the body, and maculopapular rash. The disease is known as non-fatal, death is rather exceptional. DHF, on the contrary, attacks mostly children under the age of 15 years and causes significant mortality among pre-school age children of the tropical and sub-tropical Asian countries where classical dengue syndrome is a rare incidence among indigenous people.

Etiology

The dengue virus belongs to the group of flaviviruses. It is a small RNA virus. There are four serotypes (DEN 1, DEN 2, DEN 3 and DEN 4) which are antigenically similar yet different enough to elicit only partial cross-protection after infection by one of them. In a first infection viraemia occurs following an incubation period of four to six days. Antibody titres rise slowly to a modest level, and the antibody is relatively monospecific. Immunity develops to the specific type of the infecting virus, but there is only partial protection against the other types. Following a second infection antibody titres rise rapidly, and this time the antibody can react against a wide variety of flavivirus antigens.

Any of the four dengue serotypes can cause DHF

* By S. Nimmanitya, Children's Hospital. Rajarithee Road, Ryathai, Bangkok, Thailand, and G. J. Ebrahim.

or a mild illness depending on the immune status of the host. Generally DHF occurs in children who have had previous dengue infection and in infants with waning levels of maternally derived dengue antibody. Studies in Thailand and evidence in Cuba indicate that the sequence of infecting serotypes, especially a DEN 1 infection followed by DEN 2 infection, may influence the occurrence of DHF/DSS.

Epidemiology

Dengue viruses can be transmitted by several species of *Aedes* mosquitoes of the Stegomyia family. *Aedes aegypti*, which is abundant everywhere in tropical and sub-tropical Asia, is, however, a principal vector responsible for DHF epidemics in most places. *Aedes aegypti* which breeds largely indoors, takes many blood meals, is closely associated with man and is an extremely efficient vector. *Aedes aegypti* bite only during the day. After feeding on a patient whose blood contains the virus, the female *Aedes aegypti* can transmit dengue either after an incubation period (three to ten days) during which the virus multiplies in its salivary glands, or immediately by change of host when its blood meal is interrupted. *Aedes aegypti* mosquitoes are usually found in and around houses and because of their limited flying range of 200 metres, a distant spread of an epidemic is mainly through movement of man rather than mosquitoes. It is apparent that the spread of epidemics usually follows main lines of communications. The advanced transportation systems and the rapid growing urbanisations with inadequate piped water supply are important factors contributing to the wide spread of DHF. The greater the density of human and vector populations, the greater the potential for virus transmission and the establishment of endemicity.

In most places there seems to be a distinct seasonal pattern in disease outbreak with the peak incidence of cases coinciding with the mid-rainy season. The seasonal variation is presumably caused by fluctuations in the vector population biting activity or a decrease in longevity of female mosquitoes. Increased exposure to the vector during the rainy season, when children stay indoors more during the day time, may also be a factor contributing to seasonal fluctuation.

DHF is mainly a disease of children. The majority of cases are under the age of 15, with the peak incidence between ages two to eight years. In endemic areas with crowded populations of both man and vectors, infections with dengue viruses of all types are frequent and second infections with heterologous types are common. All the older and much of the younger segment (early months of life) of the population are immune. However cases in children as young as two months and young adults in their twenties have been reported.

Children over the age of one year comprise approximately 90 per cent or more of patients with DHF/DSS. As many as 99 per cent of the children with DHF/DSS have had a previous infection. It has also been observed that infants less than one year old who develop DHF/DSS during primary infections are born to dengue immune mothers.

Epidemiological studies in various places revealed the association of DHF with second dengue infection and it is observed that DHF occurs where two or more dengue types are simultaneously endemic or sequentially epidemic. These observations implicate 'the two infections hypothesis' in the pathogenesis of DHF. It has been postulated that during a second infection with a dengue virus, different from the one that caused the primary infection, an enhanced immune response occurs with formation of large amounts of virus antibody complexes. These complexes cause the immunopathology which plays a central role in disease picture.

Dengue viruses replicate in mononuclear phagocytes. The greater the number of phagocytes infected the more severe the illness. Subneutralising concentration of antibody enhances dengue virus infection in these cells. This phenomenon has been described for a number of other flaviviruses besides dengue type 1 to 4.

Occasionally, shock and severe haemorrhage are observed in patients with primary dengue infection, more frequently in infants under the age of one year.

Clinical pictures

The clinical spectrum of dengue illness ranges from mild dengue fever to a life threatening disease, DHF or DSS. Generally dengue fever is age dependent. In infants and young children there may be an undifferentiated febrile illness occasionally associated with a maculopapular rash.

Classical DF with abrupt onset of high fever accompanied by severe headache, muscle and joint pain, and a skin rash is more common in older children and adults. Occasionally dengue fever may be associated with petechiae and other haemorrhagic diatheses. Rarely severe haemorrhage (DF with unusual haemorrhage) has caused death in some outbreaks.

DHF is more common in children and is characterised by four major clinical manifestations viz. high continuous fever, haemorrhagic diathesis, hepatomegaly, and a tendency to develop shock. Moderate to marked thrombocytopenia with concurrent haemoconcentration is a distinctive laboratory finding. The major pathophysiologic change which determines the severity of disease in DHF and differentiates it from DF is the leakage of plasma as manifested by a rising haematocrit. In typical cases of DHF the illness commonly begins with a sudden rise of temperature. This is accompanied by other constitutional symptoms resembling DF. Fever persists high for two to seven days in most cases, then falls by lysis. During the first two to three days of the illness a positive tourniquet test and the presence of petechiae are suggestive evidence for the clinical diagnosis of dengue.

In mild or moderate cases all signs and symptoms abate after lysis of fever.

The more severe forms of dengue fever like DHF and DSS are now common elements of dengue outbreaks in some countries. These illnesses begin with symptoms indistinguishable from those of simple dengue fever followed by rapid deterioration two to five days later (figure 17.1).

In a severe case, following fever of a few days duration, the patient's condition suddenly deteriorates. Accompanying or shortly after the fall in temperature there are signs of circulatory failure; the skin becomes cool, blotchy and congested and circumoral cyanosis is frequently observed. The pulse becomes rapid and feeble. Although the patient may appear lethargic, he becomes restless and then rapidly goes into a critical stage of shock. Abdominal pain is a frequent complaint shortly before the onset of shock.

Shock, as a result of insufficient tissue perfusion, is characterised by a rapid and weak pulse with narrowing of the pulse pressure or hypotension with cold, clammy skin and restlessness. The course of shock is short and stormy: the patient may pass into a stage of profound shock, the pulse and the blood pressure become imperceptible and the patient may die within 24 hours after the onset of shock. Prolonged shock may give rise to a more complicated

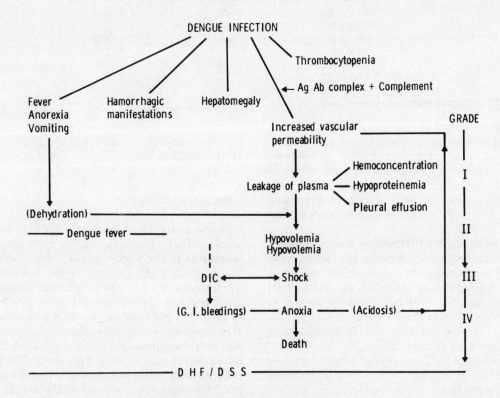

THE SPECTRUM OF DENGUE DISEASES

Figure 17.1   Major manifestation of DHF

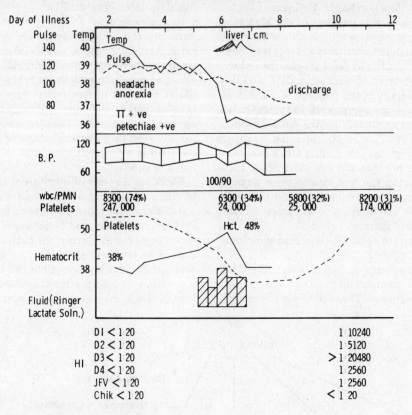

Figure 17.2   Clinical manifestation of DHF

course with metabolic acidosis, severe gastro-intestinal bleeding and a poor prognosis. If, however, the patient is given appropriate supportive therapy before irreversible shock takes place, rapid, uneventful recovery is the rule, even with profound shock. Transient diuresis often occurs as the patient recovers.

Convalescence after DHF with or without shock is short and uncomplicated. Bradycardia, occasionally absolute bradycardia or sinus arrhythmia is a common finding during convalescence but without clinical significance. Patients rapidly return to normal within two to three days after termination of shock. The course of illness in DHF ranges from seven to ten days in most cases.

The severity of DHF is classified into four grades: Grades I and II are non-shock illnesses; Grade II presents with spontaneous haemorrhage while a positive tourniquet test is the only haemorrhagic sign in Grade I; Grades III and IV are those with shock, regardless of the haemorrhagic manifestations. The moribund patients with profound shock,

no blood pressure or pulse, are classified as Grade IV (figure 17.3).

Laboratory findings

Changes in the blood leucocytes are not characteristic for DHF. Leucocyte counts may range from leucopenia to slight leucocytosis, with relative lymphocytosis towards the end of the febrile period. Thrombocytopenia and haemoconcentration are constant findings. A platelet count below 100 000/mm^3 is usually found between the third and eighth day. Haemoconcentration, an evidence of plasma leakage, is always present even in mild cases but to a lesser degree than in those with shock. The platelet count drops and the haematocrit rises concurrently, preceding subsidence of fever and/or shock. Abnormal coagulation may be found in severe cases.

Other physiopathologic changes include hypoproteinaemia, hyponatraemia, mildly elevated serum transaminase and blood urea nitrogen levels.

Metabolic acidosis may be found in cases with pro-longed shock.

A transient mild albuminuria is sometimes present and infrequently associated with microscopic haematuria. Occult blood is often found in stools.

Electrocardiographic changes are commonly found as a low voltage with non-specific ST and T wave changes in the standard and left precordial leads.

Diagnosis

The most alarming aspect of DHF contributing to mortality is the shock syndrome. The diagnosis is not difficult once the identity of an epidemic has been established and even becomes relatively easy when the patient is ushered in with shock. As the prognosis depends upon an early recognition of the disease and the monitoring of pre-shock conditions, clinical criteria for guidance in the diagnosis of DHF are most desirable. The following criteria based on major clinical manifestations frequently observed have been selected for use with good results at the Children's Hospital, Bangkok. Their use could provide the basis for accurate and rapid diagnosis

before shock or irreversible shock occurs and yet avoid over-diagnosis of the disease.

Criteria for guidance in the diagnosis of DHF

Clinical

(1) Fever, acute onset, high continuous for two to seven days;
(2) Haemorrhagic manifestations including a positive tourniquet test and any of the following: petechiae, purpura, ecchymosis, epistaxis, gum bleeding, haematemesis/malaena;
(3) Enlargement of liver;
(4) Shock.

Laboratory

(1) Thrombocytopenia (100 000/mm³ or less);
(2) Haemoconcentration (20 per cent or more increased haematocrit). The sequence of clinical course is illustrated in figure 17.2.).

The presence of the first two clinical criteria, fever and haemorrhagic manifestation is essential for suspicion of DHF in a patient with an acute febrile illness. An enlarged liver and thrombocytopenia associated with the above are sufficient to establish a clinical diagnosis of DHF, before the onset of shock. When shock occurs with a high haematocrit

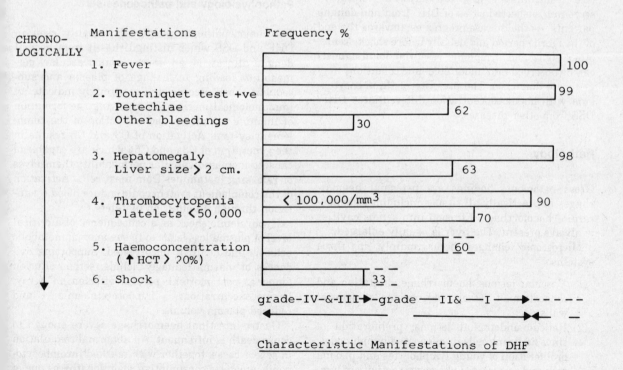

Figure 17.3 Classification of DHF according to major manifestations

reading (except in patients with severe bleeding) and marked thrombocytopenia, the diagnosis of DHF is quite clear.

Virological diagnosis

The etiologic diagnosis can be confirmed by serological tests or isolation of the virus from blood. Antibody to dengue antigens rises very rapidly in DHF patients with secondary infection. A diagnostic (four-fold) rise in dengue haemagglutination inhibition antibody can usually be demonstrated if sera are obtained early in the febrile phase or on admission, and three to five days later. A third specimen two weeks after onset is still required to assure laboratory diagnosis of primary infection.

Differential diagnosis

Early in the febrile phase, the differential diagnosis includes a wide spectrum of viral and bacterial infections. In endemic areas DHF should be considered as one possibility in any child with acute pyrexia of unknown origin, and the essential criteria for DHF diagnosis should be looked for carefully. The tourniquet test which often gives a positive result in the first few days, is helpful in screening suspected cases of DHF from non-dengue patients. As the disease progresses, towards the end of the febrile period and usually before shock occurs, other signs and symptoms essential for diagnosis can be observed and under epidemic conditions may facilitate diagnosis. The presence of thrombocytopenia with haemoconcentration differentiates DHF/DSS from other diseases.

Pathology

Gross pathologic findings are petechial haemorrhages in practically all tissues including subendocardial haemorrhage. Effusion into serous cavities is always present. The liver is usually enlarged.

Microscopic changes occur mainly in three systems.

(1) Vascular lesions: haemorrhage, dilatation and congestion of vessels and oedema of arterial walls.
(2) Reticulo-endothelial lesions: proliferation of sinusoid lining cells in spleen and lymph nodes; proliferation of young lymphocytes and plasma cells and accelerated phagocytic activity of lymphocytes.

(3) Hepatic lesions: necrosis of liver and Kupffer's cells; cellular infiltration in portal area; formation of councilman-like bodies.

Bone marrow biopsy shows maturation arrest of megakaryocytes in early stages of the disease resembling bone marrow changes in idiopathic thrombocytopenic purpura. There are also slight depressions in other cellular elements, mainly erythroids and myeloids. Relative hypercellular marrow is observed during the next four to six days and megakaryocytes are the first to proliferate. The bone marrow usually returns to normal cellular architecture by day eight or ten. It has been observed at autopsy that an increased number of megakaryocytes were seen in the capillaries of the lungs.

Recent immuno-fluorescent studies of kidney biopsy in patients recovering from DHF have been able to demonstrate immune complexes, IgG, dengue antigen and the third component of complement localised in the glomeruli. Electron microscopy showed focal thickening of glomerular basement membrane with some degree of hypertrophy of mesangial cells at the sites where immune complex was shown.

Pathophysiology and pathogenesis

The major pathophysiologic abnormality seen in DHF and DSS which distinguishes it from normal dengue illness is an increase in vascular permeability leading to leakage of plasma and subsequent shock. Recent studies strongly indicate an immunological mechanism involving the formation of immune complexes and activation of the complement system. Activation of C3 and C5 results in the generation of C3a and C5a which are capable of causing increased vascular permeability themselves or releasing histamines from mast cells. Activation of the complement system could induce blood coagulation through an effect on platelets.

Hypovolemic shock as a consequence of a critical level of plasma loss leads to tissue anoxia, metabolic acidosis and death if uncorrected. Supporting evidences of plasma leakage include: serous effusion found at post mortem; pleural effusion on X-ray; haemoconcentration; hypoproteinaemia and reduced plasma volume.

Gastro-intestinal haemorrhage severe enough to cause death is infrequent. An abnormal coagulation in severe cases, together with marked thrombocytopenia, suggests consumptive coagulopathy as one of the causes of severe bleeding in DHF. The evidence that in most cases of DHF, early and effective replacement of plasma volume results in favourable outcome and that with early treatment of shock the incidence of severe bleeding, despite the presence of marked thrombocytopenia, is further reduced strongly indicates the major role of increased vascular permeability and extravasation of plasma in the pathogenesis of DHF/DSS. Consumptive coagulopathy, with subsequent haemorrhage, may however play a significant role as shock progresses and result in an irreversible stage.

Treatment

As in other viral infections, there is no specific treatment. No antiviral agent or antibiotics available at present are of any benefit in the treatment of DHF. Symptomatic and supportive measures are, however, effective provided all are taken before irreversible shock occurs. General symptomatic and supportive measures are as follows

(1) In patients with high temperature, particularly in children with a history of febrile convulsions or in patients with severe headache, muscle or joint pain, antipyretic and/or analgesic drugs may be indicated. Salicylates should be avoided since they are known to cause bleeding and acid-base imbalance.

(2) High fever, anorexia and vomiting in most patients usually result in fluid loss and thirst. Fluid intake by mouth should be ample as tolerated. Fruit juice is preferable to plain water because there is a deficit of some electrolytes. Cold drinks seem to be fairly well tolerated. Electrolyte and dextrose solution as used in diarrhoeal disease is recommended.

(3) Patients require careful observation for early signs and symptoms of shock. The critical period is the transition from the febrile to afebrile phase which is usually about the third day on. The presence of any signs of circulatory disturbances should prompt hospitalisation and be immediately treated.

(4) Serial platelet counts and haematocrit determinations. A drop in the platelet count usually precedes the haematocrit rise and the onset of shock. Haematocrit determination is an essential guide to therapy since it reflects the degree of plasma leakage and the need for intravenous fluid. Qualitative estimation of platelet function and haematocrit determinations are simple and reliable tools, which can be done in the out-patient clinic and used as a guide for when to admit the patients to the hospital.

In large outbreaks hospital facilities are likely to get swamped. There is no need to hospitalise every case. Shock develops in about a third of the patients. A drop in the platelet count, indicating a tendency for spontaneous bleeding, precedes the rise in the haematocrit, which in turn is a sign of capillary fragility with leakage of plasma. Daily platelet count and haematocrit from the third day of illness until the temperature remains normal for one to two days are essential for monitoring progress.

Management of severe cases

The major abnormality in DSS is increase in vascular permeability, causing leakage of plasma. In severe cases up to 20 per cent reduction in the circulating plasma volume can occur. Hypovolaemic shock in such cases leads to tissue anoxia, metabolic acidosis and death. In DHF there are additional problems of haemostasis due to capillary fragility (as evidenced by a positive tourniquet test), thrombocytopenia and disorder of coagulation. Up to 80 per cent of patients with DSS and 17 per cent without shock show signs of disseminated intravascular coagulation (DIC).

Blood transfusion is needed for those patients with signs of bleeding. About a third of cases with DSS tend to suffer internal bleeding, mainly in the gastrointestinal tract.

DSS is rapidly reversible. Prompt action will in most cases prevent DIC. Thus in the management of the severe case early recognition of shock with good monitoring is essential, especially in the critical phase of transition from the febrile to the afebrile phase on the third day of illness. Repeated haematocrit measurements provide an indication of the degree of plasma leakage, and are a guide to treatment. Haemoconcentration normally precedes changes in blood pressure and pulse rate. Clinical signs like restlessness or lethargy, acute abdominal pain, cold extremities and oliguria are together with frequent charting of the pulse rate and blood pressure also helpful in early diagnosis of shock.

As in all hypovolemic shock, an immediate volume replacement is vital. The following steps are recommended

(1) Immediate rapid replacement of an existing plasma loss with plasma or plasma expander and/or Ringer's Lactate until there is definite improvement in vital signs.

(2) Continue replacement of further plasma leakage to maintain sufficient circulatory blood volume for another 12–24 hours, usually not longer than 48 hours. It is very important to stop intravenous fluid therapy as soon as there is no further leakage as manifested by stable haematocrit and vital signs. A good volume of urine and increased frequency indicate sufficient tissue perfusion. As soon as the leakage stops, the extra-vasated plasma is reabsorbed so there is a danger of over-hydration which will result in heart failure and/or pulmonary oedema if fluid therapy is continued.

(3) Specific correction of electrolyte and acid-base disturbances. Commonly hyponatraemia and occasionally metabolic acidosis occur. The latter, in particular, if uncorrected may lead to disseminated intravascular clotting resulting in a more complicated course.

(4) Blood transfusion is indicated only in cases with massive bleedings. Fresh blood is preferable.

(5) Close observation around the clock is imperative. Frequent recording of vital signs and haematocrit determinations are important in evaluating results of treatment.

At the Children's Hospital in Bangkok steady improvements in mortality have been reported since the early 1960s when the epidemic first struck. These improvements are largely ascribed to early recognition of the illness as well as early and appropriate treatment of shock with good nursing care to monitor the patients' condition.

Further reading

Halstead S B. Pathogenesis of dengue: challenges to molecular biology. *Science* 1988: 23: 476–481.

Henchal E A., Putnak J R. The dengue viruses. *Clinical Microbiology Rev* 1990: 3: 376–96.

Kouri G P, Guzman M G, Bravo J R, Triana C. Dengue haemorrhagic fever/dengue shock syndrome: lessons from the Cuban epidemic, 1981. *Bull Wld Hlth Org* 1989; 67: 375–380.

World Health Organisation. *Dengue Haemorrhagic Fever: diagnosis, treatment and control.* Geneva: W.H.O. 1986.

18 *Epidemic meningitis (cerebro-spinal meningitis)*

In several countries of Africa lying between the Sahara and the equator, major epidemics of meningitis occur from time to time due to meningococcus (figure 18.1). In temperate countries outbreaks have been described in institutions and army barracks. More recently Brazil experienced a major epidemic with over 13 000 reported cases and since then seasonal cycles of infection have been observed in several European countries.

Saudi Arabia experienced an epidemic during the Haj of 1987, and this spread into a number of neighbouring countries including sub-Saharan Africa. In late 1989 epidemics occurred in Kenya, Tanzania, Uganda, Malawi and Mozambique.

The seasonal epidemics of the Cerebro-Spinal Meningitis Belt in Africa occur mainly during the winter months when environmental conditions favour spread of infection. Because of the cold nights

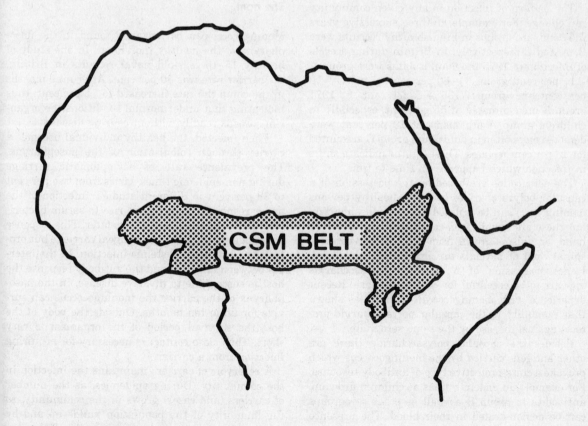

Figure 18.1 CSM belt in Africa

and a strong seasonal wind in the winter, people tend to huddle together in huts, thereby favouring droplet infection.

Like all epidemics, those of meningococcal infection occur when the relationship between parasite host and environment favour spread of infection. These three ingredients of an epidemic require detailed study in order to create effective programmes of prevention.

The organism

Nisseria meningitidis is classified into several serogroups according to antigenic characteristics. Serogroup A has been responsible for most epidemics in Africa although other serogroups have been identified in the community between epidemics. Serogroups A and C were mainly responsible for the epidemic in Brazil in the early seventies. In America, serogroup B used to prevail but in more recent years has been replaced by group C. Besides these three major groups, other serogroups, namely, X, Y, Z and W135 have also been identified.

The pattern of infection in any given community can change. For example, in three successive years the dominant groups in Finnish army recruits were B, A and C respectively. In Britain during a cycle of infection in 1975 the main isolates were group A – 11 per cent, group B – 60 per cent, group C – 19 per cent and group W135 – 8 per cent. In 1977 group B predominated at 55 per cent, especially in children; group A organisms at 19 per cent were detected more often in adults and group C accounted for 18 per cent isolates. These figures indicate shifts in infection which happen from time to time.

The serogroups are based on the possession of a capsular polysaccharide. In many healthy persons meningococci can be isolated from the nasopharynx but these are usually non-capsulated. On the other hand, organisms grown from the blood or cerebrospinal fluid of patients are invariably capsulated. Hence possession of a capsular polysaccharide appears to be essential for causing disease. Recent experience with meningococcal vaccine has shown that immunity to the capsular polysaccharide protects against disease by the same serogroup.

Besides the capsular polysaccharide there are other antigens carried by the meningococcus which provoke a cross-protective type of antibody response. For example, in endemic areas as children grow up, antibodies to group B as well as other serogroups can be demonstrated in their blood. The presence of such antibodies correlates well with decreasing prevalence of infection. It would thus appear that

as children come into repeated contact with the meningococcus in their environment, they develop immunity which is not only to the strain they carry but also to a wide range of serogroups. The antigens responsible for such a cross-protective immune response are protein in nature.

In order to cause disease an invading organism must penetrate the mucus secretions overlying the epithelial surface and adhere to the underlying cell. *N. meningitidis* is able to achieve this by means of small projections, the pili, on the surface of the organism.

In established infections, meningococci produce an endotoxin which is responsible for their pathogenicity. In fatal infections a constant feature is vascular lesions in the form of widely spread thrombi, intravascular coagulation and vasculitis. Haemorrhagic infarction of the adrenal gland is the classical lesion of meningococcal septicaemia. Immune complexes are also common and are responsible for such symptoms as arthritis, episcleritis and cutaneous lesions.

The host

Meningococci can be normally found in the nasopharynx of the healthy individual. In one study of healthy 15–16-year-old naval recruits in Britain, the carrier rate was 30 per cent. After nine months in the camp the rate increased to 71 per cent, thus indicating that under normal conditions the organism spreads readily without causing disease.

When infected, the healthy individual becomes a carrier through colonisation of the nasopharynx. The prevalence rate of asymptomatic carriage during non-epidemic times varies from two per cent to 38 per cent in different studies. Infection of the upper respiratory tract gives rise to serum bactericidal antibody seven to ten days later. This response does not eliminate nasopharyngeal carriage but protects the host from systemic infection. In the interval between infection and the antibody response the host is susceptible to invasive disease. In the nasopharynx of the carrier the meningococcus can survive for up to ten months. Outside the body of the host the survival period of the organism is very short. Thus close contact is necessary for acquiring infection from a carrier.

A reservoir of carriers maintains the infection in the community. During epidemics, as the number of carriers (and cases) grows in the community, so the immunity of the population builds up and by the time the season changes practically all the susceptible population has become immune.

In a small number of individuals the meningococci overwhelm the defences and enter the blood stream. This may be due to a heavy dose of infection, weak defences because of age or undernutrition, local trauma or possibly a familial immune defect resulting in a decreased ability to respond to polysaccharide antigens. When the blood stream is invaded, the meninges are secondarily infected. The septicaemia also results in the dissemination of meningococci into capillaries causing local lesions as well as release of endotoxin. A series of immune reactions are triggered by the endotoxin including formation of immune complexes and disseminated intravascular coagulation.

The environment

In the CSM belt of Africa the dry winter months with their cold nights and the desert wind result in people huddling together inside their poorly ventilated homes. Similar overcrowding is usual in army barracks and institutions. Even worse overcrowding is now building up in the shanty towns and slums of the cities of the Third World. In all such situations a great increase occurs in the number of airborne bacteria. For example, a ten-fold increase in bacterial counts has been demonstrated in the huts of the CSM belt during the epidemic season. A close correlation has been observed in the number of airborne bacteria, crowding and the incidence of meningitis. In these circumstances the carriers among the group are responsible for a widespread dissemination of meningococci. The evolution of the epidemic is abrupt with the sudden occurrence of many clinical cases after a wide spread of infection amongst the susceptibles.

Clinical picture

The various clinical syndromes in meningococcal infections such as acute septicaemia with its purpuric rash and joint as well as muscle pains, the Waterhouse-Friderichsen syndrome of acute adrenal failure, fulminating meningococcal encephalitis and meningitis are described in standard text books and will not be considered further. However, it is important to emphasise the rapid progression of illness, especially in children under the age of two years. The interval between the first onset of symptoms and death in young children can be as short as 14–40 hours. A high degree of suspicion is necessary in the endemic areas especially during the

season, and in non-endemic areas if a large number of cases are being reported in the community. Hence an efficient system of notification is essential for timely intervention.

In areas where meningococcal infections are not of common occurrence early diagnosis presents several difficulties. The cerebrospinal fluid (CSF) often has the normal number of cells in the early stages even though it may eventually yield a positive culture. A simple rule to observe is that in young children all CSF should be cultured regardless of cellularity. A second type of difficulty arises when the initial CSF is normal on microscopy and sterile on culture but a repeat lumbar puncture shows unequivocal meningitis. A septicaemic child with a normal CSF should have further lumbar puncture if his condition warrants it.

The haemorrhagic or purpuric rash, a sign of intra-vascular coagulation, is an important clinical sign and is usually seen within three to 24 hours of the onset of symptoms. On the pigmented skin the rash may not be easily noticeable and a careful examination is necessary. The onset of shock is a grave prognostic sign and treatment needs to be started before its onset to be effective.

Meningococcal septicaemia ranges from a fulminating lethal illness to a low grade infection. The course is determined more by host resistance than by the strain of the organism.

Fulminating septicaemia comes with startling suddenness. After a brief period of unexplained change in behaviour there is rapid deterioration of consciousness, fever, shock, cardiac and renal failure, and disseminated intravascular coagulopathy. Death can occur within 48 hours.

Unfavourable clinical signs in meningococcal septicaemia are: hyperpyrexia, absence of marked leucocytosis, thrombocytopaenia, prompt appearance of petechiae, and low blood pressure.

Chronic low grade septicaemia can also occur, and lasts for weeks with a rash, joint pains and malaise.

Treatment and chemoprophylaxis

In the established case the drug of choice is benzylpenicillin 300 000 u/kg/day administered six hourly by the intravenous route. Ampicillin (300mg/kg/day) is also effective and can be used with chloramphenicol (100mg/kg/day). It is recommended to add rifampicin for two days before discharge from the hospital. Antibiotic treatment should be continued for two or three days more after the fever has settled, and depending on the general condition of the patient.

Treatment for shock with intravenous fluids and cortisone may be necessary in the severely ill cases. If there is clinical or laboratory evidence of disseminated intravascular coagulation treatment with heparin is recommended by some experts.

Chemoprophylaxis

Chemoprophylaxis must be considered whenever a clinical case occurs. Epidemiologic data indicate that more than half the secondary cases occur less than five days after the index case. In the close family, especially when the living conditions are crowded, the risk of infection can be as much as 1000 fold compared to the general population. In one community survey in Florida, 35 per cent close contacts yielded *N. meningitidis* from the initial pharyngeal culture compared with only one per cent in controls.

From clinical and epidemiological observations, two high risk groups can be identified for chemoprophylaxis. Firstly, the child under the age of five in a household where meningococcal disease has been diagnosed as well as the very young contact in a day nursery. Secondly, the close household contact, particularly the ones sharing sleeping accommodation with the patient. Similar reasoning also applies where there are many susceptibles as, for example, in a boarding school or a recruit camp. The secondary attack rate amongst close household contacts has been calculated to be six per cent but is twice that in children aged one to four years.

If the organism is sensitive to sulphonamides, sulphadiazine has been found to be highly effective for chemoprophylaxis. The dose for children 1–12 years old is 500 mg twice daily for two days. Older children and adults need 1 g twice daily for two days. In the case of resistance to sulphonamides, rifampicin and minocycline (related to tetracyclines) have been found effective. With rifampicin a clearance rate of 88 per cent has been reported after two days of treatment, and with minocycline after a similar duration of therapy the clearance rate was 67.6 per cent. During the epidemic in Brazil caused by group C meningococci, the carriage rates two weeks after treatment were 49 per cent with sulphadiazine, 17 per cent with minocycline and 9 per cent with rifampicin. With a combination of rifampicin and minocycline the carriage rates were reduced to nil but a third of the subjects suffered side effects.

Vaccines

The capsular polysaccharides of group A and C meningococci are potent antigens and give rise to protective group-specific antibodies.

Quadrivalent polysaccharide vaccine (Group A, C, Y and W135) is currently available, but the protection is short lived. It is largely used for the control of epidemics. Another drawback is that the vaccine is not effective against group A infections in infants less than three months old. Improved group A and C vaccines consisting of polysaccharide protein conjugates are likely to become available in the future. Unfortunately a vaccine against group B meningococcal disease does not seem amenable to such a strategy at present.

Further reading

Peltola H. Meningococcal disease still with us. *Rev Inf Dis* 1983; 5: 71–87.

Schwartz B, Moore P S, Broome C V. Global epidemiology of meningococcal disease. *Clin Micro Rev* 1989; 2: supplement s118-s124.

Frasch C E. Vaccines for prevention of meningococcal disease. *Clin Micro Rev* 1989; 2: Supplement s135-s137.

Feldman H A. The meningococcus: a twenty year perspective. *Rev Inf Dis* 1986; 8: 288–94.

Jones D M. Control of meningococcal disease. *Brit Med J* 1989; 298: 542–543.

19 *Human immunodeficiency virus (HIV) infection*

It is estimated that some 6 to 8 million people are infected with HIV infection. This number is expected to rise to 15–20 million by the year 2000 according to most conservative estimates. The end-stage of the infection, the acquired immunodeficiency syndrome (AIDS) is estimated to have affected 1 million adults and 500 000 children by 1991. The cumulative total of AIDS in adults projected by the World Health Organisation for the year 2000 is close to 10 million, of whom almost 90 per cent are expected to be in developing countries. In addition to infections occurring in the paediatric age group it is expected that more than 10 million children will be orphaned in the coming decade as their mothers, or both parents, die of AIDS.

Characteristics of the human immunodeficiency virus (figure 19.1)

HIV is a retrovirus which belongs to the sub-family of lentiviruses. The lentiviruses cause slowly progressive infections involving the nervous system, the immune system and other body organs. Characteristically there are periods of clinical latency, weak immune response, and persistent viraemia. Examples of lentivirus infections causing immunodeficiency in the hosts are the simian immunodeficiency virus, and the feline immunodeficiency virus.

Most retroviruses are simple structures containing only three genes – a gene coding for the core polypeptides (the *gag* gene), one coding for the surface envelope protein (the *env* gene) and a gene which codes for the reverse transcriptase and other enzymes (the *pol* gene). HIV contains not only these three genes, but also six additional ones which probably explains its enhanced pathogenicity.

The enzyme reverse transcriptase lends its name to the retroviruses. It allows these viruses to set up permanent infections in the host by incorporating the viral genes into the DNA of the infected host cells. Under appropriate conditions the viral gene is expressed by the host cell nucleus and new viral particles get synthesised harnessing the cellular machinery of the host.

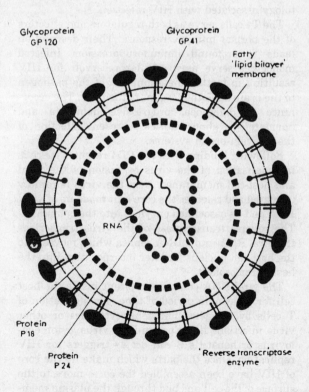

Figure 19.1 Structure of the human immunodeficiency virus

195

Transmission

HIV is a fragile virus and survives poorly outside the body. Its mode of transmission closely resembles that of hepatitis B – viz. sexual, blood to blood transmission (including through blood products and contaminated syringes, needles or other equipment), and maternofetal.

Natural history of infection with HIV (figure 19.2)

Infection with HIV begins with the binding of the envelope protein of the virus (gp120) to the surface receptor molecule CD4 on the target cells. CD4 is most commonly found on a subset of T lymphocytes known as the helper/inducer or T4 lymphocytes. CD4 receptor molecule is also found on the surface of monocytes, macrophages and glial cells. The CD4 receptor is the principal though not the sole high-affinity cellular receptor for HIV. The virus can also infect the gut epithelium, and bone marrow cells. This pattern of infection explains the symptomatology associated with HIV infection.

The T4 cells serve as both regulators and effectors of the normal immune response. Their destruction leads to profound immunosuppression. Infected monocytes serve as a cellular reservoir for HIV resulting in further dissemination of the pathogen to the brain and other organs of the body. The occurrence of diarrhoea, progressive dementia and haematologic abnormalities represent infection of the relevant organ systems.

Following binding with the CD4 receptor there is internalisation of the virus by fusion of the viral and host-cell membranes. Next the virus is rapidly uncoated and releases the core unit made up of viral RNA and its associated enzymes into the cytoplasm. The reverse transcriptase of the virus transcribes the viral RNA into a DNA replica which moves into the host cell nucleus for later incorporation into the host chromosomes.

The viral DNA can remain latent inside the host cell for a variable period of time. The activation of T cells by antigens, mitogens, cytokines or other virus infections like Epstein-Barr virus, cytomegalovirus or hepatitis B can act as triggers for HIV replication. Once the parts which make up the core of HIV have been assembled the cores move to the surface of the cell and bud through the plasma membrane, acquiring their envelope coating as they do so.

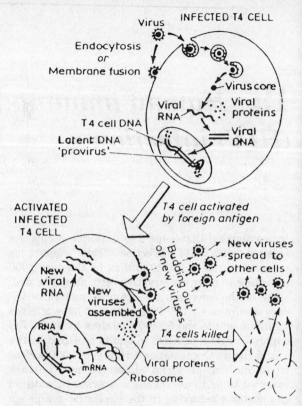

Figure 19.2   Multiplication of the human immunodeficiency virus

Infection with HIV leads to the production of antibodies within about three months of infection. They do not neutralise the virus, but serve as a marker of infection. The most widely used marker is the serum P24 (core protein) antigen. In general it reflects the level of HIV replication activity. A more accurate measure for assessing progress of infection is the number of T4 cells infected and the level of plasma viraemia.

Clinical signs and symptoms

The pattern of symptoms characteristic of HIV infection has been described through observations in adults. A similar pattern may be observed also in older children who are infected by contaminated blood, blood products or syringes and needles.

At the time of infection there may occur transient non-specific illness with swelling of lymph nodes, aching joints and muscles, sore throat and skin rash, which is easily mistaken for glandular fever. In most cases, however, infection is sub-clinical.

Amongst those who sero convert some enter a latent phase. In those who progress to chronic infection the infection may remain asymptomatic, or develop into illness of varying degrees of severity ranging from persistent generalised lymphadenopathy (PGL), aids related complex (ARC), acquired immune deficiency syndrome (AIDS), or neurologic manifestations.

Persistent generalised lymphadenopathy (PGL) is characterised by enlargement of lymph nodes at least 1 cm in diameter in two or more non-contagious extra-inguinal sites persisting for at least three months in the absence of any current illness or medication. A large proportion of those affected remain well. About 10 to 30 per cent progress to AIDS.

The aids related complex (ARC) is diagnosed when any two of the following signs or symptoms have been present for three months or longer, and any two or more of the abnormal laboratory values are obtained.

Aids related complex

(Presence of any two or more symptoms/signs for $\leq$ three months,
and
two or more abnormal laboratory findings)

Symptoms/signs
Fever $\leq$ 38°C intermittent or continuous
Weight loss > 10 per cent
Enlarged lymph nodes, for example PGL
Diarrhoea intermittent or continuous
Easy fatigability
Night sweats

Abnormal laboratory findings
Anaemia
Thrombocytopenia
Leucopenia especially lymphopenia
Reduced T helper cells
Reduced ratio of T4:T8
Raised gamma globulin

Those with ARC stand the highest risk of progression to full AIDS syndrome compared to those who are seropositive and well, or those who have PGL.

AIDS is diagnosed at the onset of opportunistic infections or tumours. The infections most frequently involve the lungs, gut and the nervous system with *pneumocystis carinii* pneumonia being very common. Another common infection is reactivation of latent foci of tuberculosis with unusual forms of presentation. The most common tumour is Kaposi's sarcoma.

HIV infection in children

The most common form of transmission of HIV infection in the paediatric age group is perinatal transmission and, less commonly, through blood transfusion or blood products. Infection by the transplacental route in foetal life has also been reported. Accidental transmission through contaminated equipment including needles and syringes is an ever-present risk.

Studies of infants born to HIV positive mothers suggests a transmission rate of 25 to 35 per cent. In those who are infected the majority (>80 per cent) show clinical or laboratory features of infection by the age of six months. By the age of one year 17 per cent die of HIV related disease and about a quarter have symptoms of AIDS. Subsequently in the second year the progress of the disease is slower. The duration of survival is particularly short in those presenting with *pneumocystis carinii* pneumonia and encephalopathy.

In young children, besides the usual opportunistic infections other 'indicator' illnesses are lymphocytic interstitial pneumonitis; recurrent candida infection especially of the oesophagus; wasting with or without cryptosporidiosis; encephalopathy, and recurrent bacterial infections.

Diagnosis

Clinical suspicion of immunodeficiency can be confirmed by the following laboratory tests

(1) White cell count and differential
(2) Total and differential count for lymphocytes (and T lymphocyte subsets if facilities allow)
(3) Immunoglobulins
(4) Complement (if facilities are available)
(5) Intradermal test of hypersensitivity

In the differential diagnosis the classical syndromes of immunodeficiency, malnutrition and viral infections may need to be ruled out.

A number of screening tests using the ELISA technique have been developed to screen for HIV infection. These tests detect antibodies against either the core protein (gp24), or the envelope

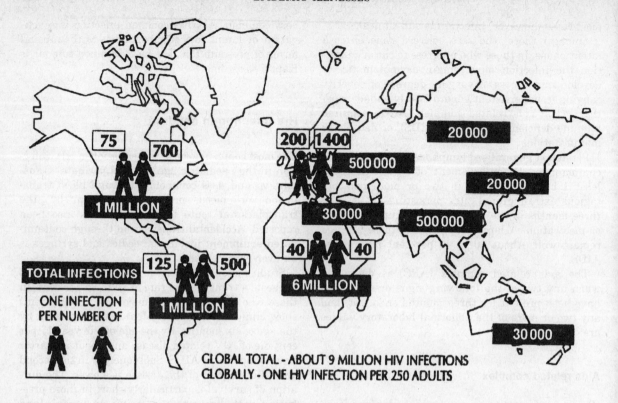

Figure 19.3   Global distribution of adult HIV infections – 1991 (Source – WHO)

protein (gp120). False positive or negative results are common with these tests. At present western blot analysis is the most common confirmatory test in clinical use, but may not be widely available in developing countries. Other screening tests which utilise latex particle or a dipstick are being developed.

Management

There is no specific cure. A great deal of research is in progress to develop drugs which would block specific stages of the infection. For example, zidovudine (ZDV, previously AZT) acts by inhibiting the reverse transcriptase of the retroviruses including HIV. It improves survival time but does not bring about cure. Several other dideoxynucleosides, the family of compounds to which ZDV belongs, like dideoxyinosine (ddI) and dideoxycytidine (ddc) are currently undergoing trials.

Like any other chronic and fatal illness HIV infec-

tion carries major upsets for the family. As many as 90 per cent of HIV infected children suffer neurological and developmental complications. In addition there are problems of stigma and altered social experiences. Very often the mother or other members of the family are also affected, and some may have died so that the care provider is either a foster parent, a member of the extended family, or an institution. Because the incubation period in the vertically infected infant is three to ten months compared to ten years in the adult, the mother often learns about her own infection *after* the diagnosis has been made in the infant. This may lead to rejection. For all these reasons the focus of care must be the family, even though it is centred on the child. At the same time care must be interdisciplinary involving social and psychiatric services as much as health services.

As the pandemic of HIV infection gathers momentum in the 1990s, not only can a large number of paediatric AIDS cases be expected, but also hundreds of thousands of uninfected children will be orphaned because of deaths in their HIV infected parents due to AIDS.

Programmes of prevention

Prevention in a given locality must be based on patterns of transmission. Globally, three broad patterns have been identified (figure 19.3).

In pattern 1 areas, for example Western Europe and North America, the primary population groups affected are homosexual men and intravenous drug users. Heterosexual spread, though on the increase, is on a small scale. Paediatric AIDS is seen on a small scale.

In pattern 2 areas, characterised by sub-Saharan Africa and parts of the Caribbean, heterosexual spread is the predominant form of transmission. Since many women of childbearing age have become infected, perinatal transmission is a major problem. Poorly developed laboratory and screening services mean that blood transfusions and other forms of intravenous therapy are an ever present risk. Similarly inadequately sterilised needles and syringes present a risk.

In pattern 3 areas, characterised by Asia and most Pacific countries, HIV was introduced much later but now is spreading amongst intravenous drug users and those working in the sex industry.

Patterns of transmission can change as the pandemic gathers momentum. For example many countries of Latin America are moving from pattern 1 to 2, and a similar change is forecast for Asia. In the 1990s many countries are likely to experience worsening of mortality rates among women and children because of AIDS.

Vaccines

A number of initiatives for the development of a vaccine have been taken, but no suitable product is expected in the near future.

Further reading

Chin J. Current and future dimensions of the HIV/AIDS pandemic in women and children *Lancet* 1990; 336: 221–224.

European Collaborative Study. Children born to women with HIV–1 infection: natural history and risk of transmission. *Lancet* 1991; 337: 253–260.

Greene W C. The molecular biology of human immunodeficiency virus Type 1 infection. *New Eng J Med* 1991; 324: 308–315.

Baltimore D, Feinberg M B. HIV revealed. Towards a natural history of the infection. *New Eng J Med* 1989; 321: 1673–1675.

UNICEF *Children and AIDS: an impending calamity.* New York: UNICEF, 1990.

Jones P, Watson J G. Aids. *In*: David (Ed). *Recent Advances in Paediatrics.* London: Churchill – Livingstone, 1990.

Section V

Parasitic Diseases

20 *Malaria*

Malaria is the leading communicable disease for a large segment of the population in many developing countries. Almost one third of the world's population is exposed to the risk of infection (figure 20.1). It has been estimated that in some parts of tropical Africa about ten per cent of all deaths occurring in infants and children below the age of three years are due to malaria. The total mortality in Africa in both infants and adults is in excess of one million deaths annually and 15 per cent of all clinical illness in tropical Africa can be attributed to malaria. In those countries where successful malaria eradication programmes have been carried out the infant mortality has fallen by a half to a third, as for

example in the case of Sri Lanka. It may be argued that some of the improvement in infant mortality may be due to the development of the health infrastructure necessary for operating a malaria eradication campaign, and this may well be so. On the other hand, there is no disputing the fact that the community pays a heavy price in terms of infant and pre-school mortality in all malarious regions.

In Africa alone on conservative estimates 200 million episodes of clinical malaria occur each year among children under the age of five. The average child in rural areas suffers one to five attacks a year, and a slightly lower number of attacks in the cities. One to two per cent of children with malaria

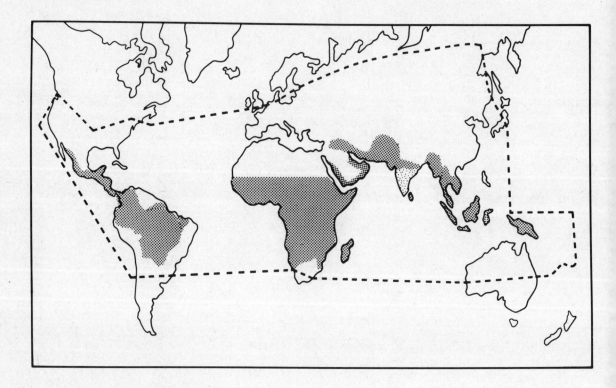

Figure 20.1 The prevalence of malaria

develop a severe disease, with a mortality risk of 10–30 per cent. Each clinical attack carries a mortality risk of 0.5 to 1 per cent.

The rapid spread of chloroquine resistance in Africa where there is a high prevalence of *P. falciparum* is particularly worrying. Similarly there have been setbacks in the strategies for the control of malaria. National programme goals have had to be changed from eradication (in 1955) to control (in 1976) to the more recent one of attempts to reduce morbidity and mortality through development of primary health care services.

The incidence of malaria in the community is measured by means of two indices, namely, the parasite rate and the splenic rate. The *parasite rate* is measured by examining blood smears of a random selection of the population and finding the percent-

age with malaria parasites in the blood. The *splenic rate* is measured by examining a sample of children and determining the percentage with enlarged spleens.

According to the number of clinical cases seen each year, malaria may be described as sporadic, epidemic or endemic. It is *sporadic* when the cases are few and scattered, *epidemic* when there is a seasonal or other periodic sharp rise of the number of cases, and *endemic* when there is a fairly constant incidence of cases. In the latter situation, if there is a perennial high degree of transmission malaria is said to be hyper or holo endemic in that area.

In the transmission of malaria, three factors are involved, namely, the parasite, the vector and the host (figure 20.2). The parasite, a protozoon, is known by the generic name *Plasmodium*. There are

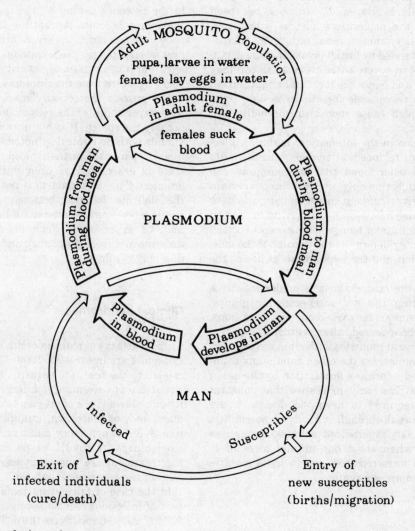

Figure 20.2 The malaria cycle

several types, some affecting man and some with a predilection for other animals. Those affecting man are of four different kinds distributed in various regions of the tropical world. They can be identified in the peripheral blood because of specific morphologic characteristics, and are named *P. vivax, P. ovale, P. malariae* and *P. falciparum*. Vivax and falciparum malaria together represent 95 per cent of all infections. Each variety has two life cycles, one in the host where the invasion of body organs and red blood cells takes place and the other in the vector where the sexual forms of the parasite combine to form a fertilised egg. *P. vivax* and *P. ovale* are characterised by persistent tissue forms chiefly in the liver, from whence fresh attacks of clinical malaria can arise even in the absence of reinfection. Thus, clinical malaria has been reported after periods as long as seven to ten years after leaving a malarious area. *P. malariae* has been implicated in the nephrotic syndrome with a progressive illness ending in renal failure. *P. falciparum* is characterised by heavy invasion of the erythrocytes so that in severe cases every tenth cell may be parasitised and hence the term malignant tertian malaria. It is responsible for all the severe forms of malaria which cause such high morbidity and mortality.

The difference in the intensity of malarial infection in different regions is often due to the mosquito *vector*. It has been found that the mosquito can transmit the infection only after reaching a certain stage of maturity. Different species of mosquito have different feeding habits, some preferring to feed on cattle than on human beings. The general ecology of the region may determine the density of the mosquito population and the expectation of life of the mosquito.

As regards the *host*, malaria is predominantly a disease affecting the low socio-economic groups. With improvement in socio-economic conditions, malaria has disappeared, after centuries of prevalence, from several countries without massive eradication programmes. On the other hand many countries had hoped to achieve eradication by the use of modern insecticides only to realise that constant vigilance is required to keep the disease under check, and a break-through is always a possibility. Thus, Sri Lanka experienced a break-through in recent years when about one million cases of *P. vivax* malaria were reported, and in India malaria is beginning to appear again.

Host immunity

Infection by the malaria parasite causes an immune response in the host and an antibody against *Plasmodium* has been demonstrated in the gamma globulin fraction of the blood proteins. The very high levels of IgG in adult Africans are perhaps due to the almost continuous exposure to malaria. The extent to which this immunity provides protection is not known. In the case of an infective agent like *Plasmodium* which undergoes several changes in form during its life cycle in the host, several surface antigens are exposed to the body's immune mechanisms at various times and the antibody may not be very specific. It is known that malarial antibody in the mother can cross the placenta and is one of the factors responsible for the low incidence of malaria in the newborn period. As the antibody level falls, the infant becomes susceptible to malaria and at about the age of four to six months he develops the first febrile episode. Such episodes recur at intervals with varying degrees of severity until the school years by which time the child has sufficient immunity to provide protection. This is often associated with hypertrophy of the reticulo-endothelial organs, notably the spleen. It is not uncommon to find individuals with no clinical symptoms and yet carrying malaria parasites in their blood (figure 20.3). This state is designated as premunition. The state of 'immunity' against malaria is not specific and often the delicate balance between premunition and invasiveness may be altered and clinical symptoms may be experienced. Such an occurrence is not uncommon during pregnancy and haemolytic anaemia may result.

Clinical syndromes

Clinical attacks of malaria occur when levels of parasitaemia are in excess of 1000- 110 000 /ul. Factors related to the host, the parasite, the vector and the environment determine to a large extent the severity of malaria. Lack of previous exposure and consequent lack of protective immunity, genetic factors like G–6-P-D deficiency and a carrier gene for haemoglobinopathy, the HLA type, and a delay in seeking treatment are important host factors in determining the severity of malaria.

In the case of falciparum malaria about one per cent of infections lead to severe illness with a case fatality rate of about one third. In clinical practice severe disease presents as cerebral malaria or

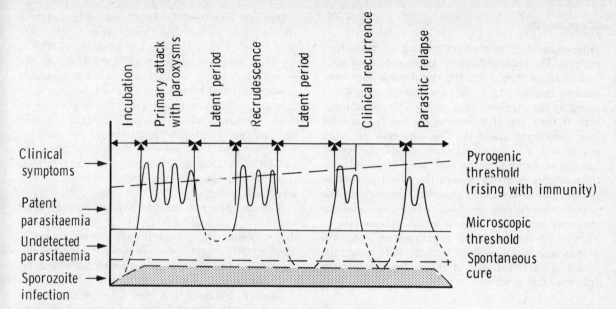

Figure 20.3 Parasitaemia and clinical malaria

severe anaemia. The degree of parasitaemia and the host response including the production of Tumour Necrosis Factor $\propto$ (TNF$\propto$) and other inflammatory responses are significant risk factors for cerebral malaria. In the case of cerebral malaria there is excess release of TNF$\propto$ from monocytes following T cell mediated release of interleukin 3 and other cytokines. TNF$\propto$ has widespread physiological effects including cytoadherence and endothelial damage. Excess TNF$\propto$ levels increase the risks of fatal outcome. In survivors of cerebral malaria mean plasma levels of TNF$\propto$ are twice those in healthy controls, and in fatal cases they are ten times as high.

Placental infection

It has been observed that even with heavy malarial parasitaemia in the mother, transmission of infection to the foetus is rare. However, the placenta invariably shows heavy infection. As expected, placental function deteriorates so that the baby suffers intrauterine growth retardation and is born small-for-dates. Thus, malaria is an important cause of low birth weight in many tropical countries. In several island communities birth weights have shown an upward swing within months of commencing an antimalarial campaign.

Heavy malarial infection in the last month of pregnancy is an important cause of premature labour. It is likely that in endemic areas malaria is an important cause of abortion, late foetal and neonatal deaths.

During pregnancy immunity to malaria is reduced and there is increased parasitaemia. The resulting haemolysis can give rise to severe anaemia which is preventable by chemoprophylaxis. Malaria tends to be particularly severe in pregnancy and especially in primeparae. Serious consideration should be given to the use of chemoprophylaxis in pregnant women.

Anaemia of infancy

Heavy malarial infection in the infant is known to precipitate severe anaemia. This is especially so when the iron stores of the baby at birth are poor either due to maternal anaemia in pregnancy, low birth weight or multiple pregnancy. The blood picture is one of severe iron deficiency anaemia and the bone marrow shows poor iron stores.

Anaemia and cerebral malaria have come to be recognised as the common presenting features of severe malaria. Parasitaemia is often low but abundant malarial pigment is to be found in monocytes and other phagocytic cells indicating recent or resolving infection. It is important to bear in mind that secondary bacterial infection may often be associated with severe anaemia.

Splenomegaly

Splenomegaly is a common finding in malarious regions. The enlarged spleen traps red blood cells and removes them from the circulation. The bone marrow responds by stepping up haemopoiesis and using up the available iron stores. The clinical picture is thus one of splenomegaly associated with iron deficiency anaemia. The anaemia is often severe and it is not uncommon to find the lowest haemoglobins in patients with very large spleens. Splenectomy helps to restore the blood picture to normal but carries long term risks in making the patient susceptible to fulminating bacterial or malarial infections. Alternatively, spleen size is known to revert to normal in patients on long-term prophylaxis with proguanil, or other anti-malarials, which is the treatment of choice for the tropical splenomegaly syndrome.

Cerebral malaria

Cerebral malaria, is the most severe and dreaded complication of malaria. It occurs with *P. falciparum* infections and is characterised by heavy parasitaemia, high fever and neurological symptoms.

The history is usually of a short illness, often less than two days. The onset is dramatic with a generalised convulsion followed by persisting unconsciousness. Coma should persist for at least 30 minutes after a generalised convulsion to distinguish it from post-ictal coma. The modified Glasgow Coma Scale may be used to assess the degree of unconsciousness on a scale of 0–5 as follows

Eye movements	Directed (e.g. to the face of the speaker or mother)	1
	Not directed	0
Verbal response	Appropriate	2
	Inappropriate or just a moan	1
	None	0
Best motor response	Localises painful stimulus	2
	Withdraws limb from pain	1
	Non-specific or absent response	0
	Total	0–5

Neck rigidity and photophobia are absent, but mild neck stiffness and opisthotonus may occur. Various forms of decerebrate rigidity may occur and raise suspicion of meningitis or encephalitis. Papilloedema does not commonly occur. Retinal haemorrhages, when present, are a bad prognostic sign.

Lumbar puncture is often not indicated and should not be undertaken lightly. It is important to bear in mind that the opening pressure of CSF is elevated, and sometimes very high. Many of the neurological signs of cerebral malaria resemble those of cerebral herniation. On the other hand differentiation from meningitis may not be possible on clinical grounds alone. In such a situation it may be necessary to treat empirically for cerebral malaria as well as possible meningitis until the patient's condition improves, before doing a lumbar puncture. In the CSF the protein and lactic acid levels are raised.

It is important to exclude hypoglycaemia (blood sugar < 2.2mmol/l;<40mg/dl) impending shock (b.p.< 50mm Hg), renal failure (urine output < 12ml/kg/24h) and disseminated intravascular coagulation, as well as superadded infection, for example aspiration pneumonia.

Cerebral malaria is a medical emergency. The essential pathological feature of severe *P. falciparum* is sequestration of erythrocytes containing mature forms of the parasite in the vascular beds of internal organs. The sequestration is greatest in the brain. Besides mechanical obstruction to the blood supply, such sequestration causes metabolic derangement, release of inflammatory agents and possibly also the release of unidentified toxic factors. One such agent is the cytokine tissue necrosis factor (TNF).

In *chloroquine-sensitive* infection, chloroquine is given by continuous slow intravenous infusion in a dose of 10mg base/kg body weight over eight hours, followed by three 8-hour infusions of 5mg/kg each (that is 15mg/kg in all administered over the next 24 hours).

Oral therapy should be commenced as soon as possible to complete the course of a total dose of 25 mg of base/kg body weight. *Or* chloroquine 5mg base/kg body weight given IV over six hours, to be repeated every six hours until five such administrations have been given (that is a total of 25 mg base/kg body weight). If intravenous administration is not possible chloroquine may be administered by injection (intramuscular or subcutaneous) in a dose of 3.5mg base/kg every six hours until a total of 25mg base/kg has been administered. (The medication may be changed to oral administration when the patient can swallow to complete the treatment.)

In areas of *chloroquine resistance* (figure 20.4) quinine is the drug of choice, to be administered with a loading dose of 20mg salt/kg body weight intravenously over four hours. This is followed by a maintenance dose given eight to ten hours later of 10mg salt/kg body weight over four hours. This maintenance dose is repeated every eight to ten hours on the second day of treatment until the patient can take oral medication. The oral treatment comprises quinine 10mg/kg body weight, eight hourly for seven days. If intravenous therapy is to continue into the third or subsequent day of treatment the dose of quinine is halved to 5mg salt/kg body weight over four hours. If resistance to quinine is suspected, an oral course of halofantrine 8mg base/kg body weight every six hours for three doses may be added. Mefloquine 15mg/kg in two doses 12 hours apart is also useful, but should not be commenced until 12 hours after completion of parenteral administration of quinine.

In addition to anti-malarial therapy, a single intramuscular injection of phenobarbital sodium 10–15 mg/kg body weight helps to prevent convulsions. If convulsions do occur they can be controlled by intramuscular injection of paraldehyde (0.1 ml/kg body weight using a glass syringe), or

diazepam (0.5–1.0 mg/kg body weight) administered rectally.

The mortality of cerebral malaria is 10–40 per cent in different studies. In those who survive up to 10 per cent may show neurological sequelae like haemiplegia; cortical blindness; cranial nerve palsies; behaviour disturbances and other focal neurological deficits. Gradual improvement occurs with the passage of time.

Febrile convulsions

The sudden onset of high fever with rigors in infants can give rise to a febrile convulsion and often it is necessary to differentiate such episodes from cerebral malaria. The child is well in between fits, is conscious and shows no neurological deficits. Antipyretics and the routine treatment of malaria suffice in most cases. To prevent recurrence of fits, phenobarbitone may be necessary.

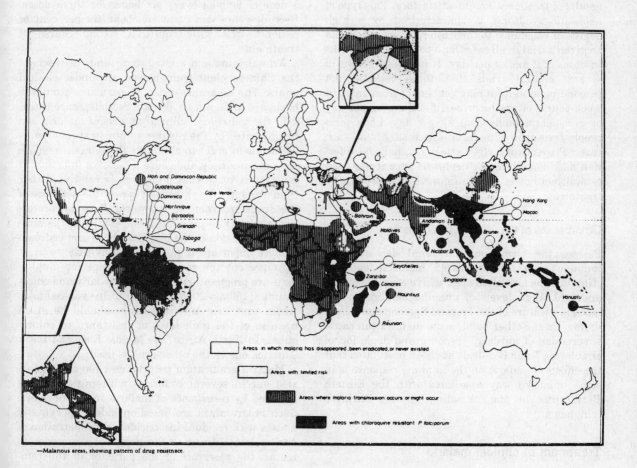

—Malarious areas, showing pattern of drug resistance.

Figure 20.4 Malarious areas with patterns of drug resistance

Renal disease

Three main types of renal lesions are known to occur in malaria. Acute renal failure may complicate falciparum malaria and is due to interference with microcirculation in the kidneys. It is usually reversible with prompt treatment. Glomerulonephritis and the nephrotic syndrome have also been described in falciparum infections. There is proteinuria occurring within a week or two of infection. Renal biopsies show deposits of 1gM and complement together with antigen in the glomerular basement membrane, and accompanied by proliferation of mesangial and endothelial cells. Like the acute renal failure, both these conditions in falciparum malaria are reversible.

Nephrotic syndrome with progressive deterioration in renal function and a relentless progress to renal failure is associated with *P. malariae* infections. It is caused by the deposition of soluble antigen-antibody complexes in the glomerulus. The results of treatment are unsatisfactory. This type of nephrotic syndrome is characterised by a high degree of resistance to corticosteroids which should be given a trial in all cases for a period of four weeks in doses of 2 mg/kg per day. It has been shown in several clinical trials that those children not responding to steroids may yet benefit from an eight week course of azathioprine 1.5–2.5 mg/kg per day or cyclophosphamide 3 mg/kg per day. Long term prophylaxis against malaria is necessary in all such cases. Preventing further attacks of malarial infection may do nothing for nephrosis once it has been established but is said to improve the response to treatment.

Disturbances of the immune mechanisms

Besides the formation and renal deposition of immune complexes, repeated malarial episodes stimulate the formation of excessive amounts of IgG and IgM. High levels of immunoglobulins in the blood is a feature of the Tropical Splenomegaly Syndrome. On the other hand, acute malaria can cause suppression of antibody response and depletion of circulating T and B cells. It has been postulated that the effects of malaria on the immune response is in some unknown way associated with the Ebstein Barr virus in the causation of the Burkitt's lymphoma.

Treatment of clinical malaria

Resistance to chloroquine is now widespread in the case of *P. falciparum* in Asia, sub-Saharan Africa and in tropical South America. Hence treatment is commenced with quinine or mefloquine in such areas.

Quinine is administered in a dose of 10mg/kg every eight hours for seven days followed by Fansidar (pyrimethamine 25 mg + sulfadoxine 500mg) half to one tablet according to age as a single dose.

Alternatively mefloquine (20mg/kg) may be given instead of quinine in two divided doses six to eight hours apart. It is not necessary to follow up with Fansidar.

In the case of chloroquine sensitive strains of *P. falciparum* and in all benign malaria (*P. vivax, P. ovale* and *P. malariae*) chloroquine is the drug of choice. It is given as an initial dose of 10mg/kg of the base, then six to eight hours later 5mg/kg as a single dose followed by 5mg/kg daily as a single dose for two days.

Halofantrine is a new antimalarial which is effective against all varieties of malaria. It is given in a dose of 8mg/kg every six hours for three doses. Recrudescence can occur in about six per cent of patients who will require a second course of treatment.

Artemisinine and related compounds (extracts of the Chinese plant Quinghaosu) are under clinical trials. The clearance rates of parasites from the blood are high, but so also are recrudescence rates.

In the individual, clinical attacks of malaria can be prevented by the regular administration of anti-malarials in order to eliminate the parasites before they can multiply and cause a massive infection. It must be stressed that protection is relative rather than absolute. Breakthrough is possible with any of the drugs anywhere in the world. Personal protection against mosquito bites, and control of the mosquito population in the neighbourhood and bedroom is more important than chemoprophylaxis.

At present the recommended drugs for prophylaxis are proguanil (100mg–150mg) daily and chloroquine (150mg–200mg) weekly. In sub-Saharan Africa and Asia both the drugs should be given because of the high level of resistance to chloroquine. In North Africa, the Middle East and Latin America one or the other drug is used.

Malaria eradication programmes have been carried out in several countries with initial success followed by resurgence of malaria in recent years. Such programmes are based on indoor spraying of houses with residual insecticides, administration of anti-malarial drugs to the population in order to reduce the reservoir of the parasite in the community and regular surveillance of the community for early detection and treatment of any cases that

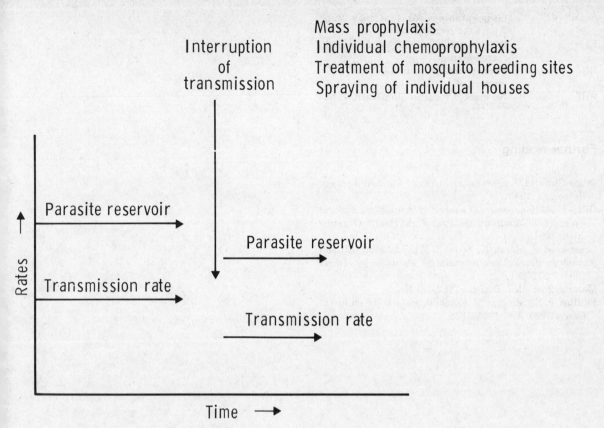

Figure 20.5   Reducing malaria transmission

may occur sporadically. Such a programme requires a well developed health infrastructure and adequately trained personnel to work efficiently. The experience in many countries has helped to identify several difficulties. The mosquito eventually develops resistance to residual insecticides such as DDT and dieldrin. The population in rural areas tends to be mobile, moving from one area to another or from one plot of land to another, and the dwellings may not be permanent structures but mud and wattle huts as in most of Africa. All these difficulties stand in the way of successful eradication.

In countries where malaria eradication programmes cannot be instituted, it is still possible to carry out community measures aimed at reducing transmission rates (figure 20.5).

In recent years bednets impregnated with synthetic pyrethroids are being recommended as a means of personal protection especially for pregnant women and young children. Similarly, premethlin-impregnated bed curtains have been shown to

reduce the incidence of malaria episodes in some studies.

Breeding grounds of the mosquito in the neighbourhood should be controlled by filling, draining and trimming of canals. Surface water should be covered with larvicides such as Paris green during the mosquito-breeding season and the residents should be encouraged to use preventive measures including mosquito nets, insecticide sprays, etc. to protect against mosquito bites. Antimalarials should be used regularly for suppressive therapy in the under-fives' and ante-natal clinics and they should be freely available to the community. A combination of these measures will help to reduce the parasite reservoir in the community and also the transmission rate, thereby reducing the prevalence of malaria.

In hospitals and health centres it is necessary to document the emerging resistance of malaria to the commonly used antimalarials. Resistance (or otherwise) is defined along the following criteria

Sensitive 'S'   -   disappearance of parasitaemia within
                      7 days (no recrudescence)
RI   -   the same as 'S' but early or late
                      recrudescence
RII   -   Parasitaemia is reduced but not
                      eliminated
RIII   -   No marked reduction in parasitaemia

Further reading

Bruce-Chwatt L J. *Essential malariology* – 2nd ed. London:
    Heineman, 1985.
Gilles H M. *Management of severe and complicated malaria
    – a practical handbook*. Geneva: World Health Organis-
    ation, 1991.
Greenwood B, Marsh K, Snow R. Why do some African
    children develop severe malaria? *Parasitology Today*
    1991; 7:277–281.
Malaria. *Brit. Med. Bulletin* 1982: 38: No. 2.
Phillips R E, Solomon T. Cerebral malaria in children.
    Lancet 1990; 336: 1355–1359.

21 Parasites invading the gastro-intestinal system

Many of the parasites affecting man have complex life cycles dependent upon the close proximity of one or more intermediate hosts. Hence geographic and ecologic conditions are important in the prevalence of the parasitic infestations. Activities which may affect the ecologic balance may produce an effect on the prevalence of parasites. Thus, the construction of dams and irrigation canals in many parts of Africa has led to the spread of schistosomiasis. Dietary and personal habits as well as customs may also contribute to the spread of parasitic disease. For example, the eating of under-cooked meat, common in many countries of the Middle East and in the Mediterranean regions is responsible for taeniasis; on the other hand strong attachment to household pets such as cats and dogs is held responsible for *Toxocara* infestation.

Many of the common parasites of man inhabit the gastro-intestinal tract, where pathological changes occur in any of the following ways

(1) Loss of body constituents, for example, blood loss in ankylostomiasis
(2) Interference with the absorption of nutrients, for example, in taeniasis and giardiasis
(3) Disruption of the morphologic structure of the intestine, for example, in strongyloides
(4) Tissue injury because of the invasive nature of the parasite, for example amoebiasis and fascioliasis
(5) Mechanical block, for example intestinal obstruction due to heavy infestation with *Ascaris*.

In the affluent societies of Western Europe, socio-economic improvement has resulted in a reduced prevalence of parasitic illnesses. In recent years, however, with increased travel and arrival of immigrant workers from the tropical and sub-tropical countries, the risk of reintroduction of parasitic illness is considerably increased.

The clinical and pathological findings of the common parasites affecting the gastro-intestinal tract are discussed below.

Amoebiasis

Entamoeba histolytica infects about ten per cent of the world's population. After malaria and schistosomiasis it is the third leading cause of death from parasitic diseases. Infection is acquired through faecal contamination of food and water, and manifests as asymptomatic intestinal carriage, acute or chronic invasive colitis or liver abscess. Asymptomatic carriage is the most common outcome. Most infected individuals eliminate the parasite in about 12 months.

Entamoeba histolytica lives primarily as a commensal in the large intestine feeding mainly on bacteria and on superficial cells of the mucosa. In laboratory experiments it has been demonstrated that amoebae would not colonise the bacteria-free guinea-pig caecum. Some colonisation was produced after the caecal mucosa had been damaged but the lesions were small. Normal lesions occurred only when the germ-free guinea-pigs were contaminated with *Clostridium perfringens* or *Bacterium subtilis*. Severe amoebiasis may complicate infection with *Strongyloides stercoralis* with fatal outcome. In Malaysian aborigines amoebic dysentery is often found with *Trichuris trichuria*. The nutritional status of the host also appears to be a factor in invasiveness. Thus, in the healthy individual, amoebae are avirulent and under some stimulus, which so far remains undefined, they change to a virulent form giving rise to ulceration in the large intestine.

Life cycle

Infection is acquired by ingestion of the cyst, either through drinking contaminated water or eating vegetables and foods handled by a carrier or washed in water containing cysts.

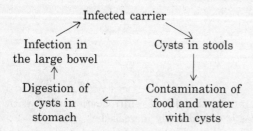

E. histolytica is primarily a parasite of the large bowel where it mostly affects the caecum and the ascending colon. In severe infection extension into the small intestine or the appendix may also occur. Dissemination to other tissues of the body from the initial gut lesion is common. Though extensive intestinal involvement appears to favour dissemination, it can also occur with relatively few intestinal lesions. Most frequent dissemination is to the liver where a colony of trophozoites may be established. Colliquative necrosis of the liver cells gives rise to an amoebic abscess. In fatal cases of amoebiasis the frequency of liver abscess varies from 36.5 to 94.5 per cent in different series described in the literature. A large majority of such descriptions are in adults but in one study 41 cases were reported from the children's hospital in Mexico and the youngest in the series was an infant seven days old. The natural history of an amoebic abscess is to continue growing until it ruptures into the peritoneal cavity, into an abdominal organ or through the diaphragm into the lung. Other common complications which may arise from intestinal amoebiasis are: direct extension to the skin resulting in a painful and growing ulcer in the perianal area; and peritonitis with or without perforation. In different series the incidence of peritonitis has varied from 1.5–21 per cent.

Diagnosis

Diagnosis may present a problem, especially in areas where amoebic infection is not commonly seen. All stool specimens must be examined fresh within one hour of passage.

The mild attack presents with some looseness of bowels and passage of mucus and blood. In the absence of specific treatment there are recurrent relapses with intervening periods of quiescence, often leading to a mistaken diagnosis of ulcerative colitis. Treatment with corticosteroids can cause acute exacerbation in such cases. In the same way, hepatic or pleuropulmonary amoebiasis can be mistaken for other conditions.

In recent years the development of indirect fluorescent antibody technique and other serologic tests holds promise of improving the diagnostic capability. Serological tests have their limitations. The tests can remain positive for a varying period of time after cure, even as long as five years. Thus, a positive test indicates amoebic infection at some time but does not necessarily mean active disease. Serological tests have their greatest use in screening for amoebic infection in a critically ill patient and where examination of stool is not possible.

The test for salivary IgA antibodies to *E. histolytica* membrane extract has a high predictive value for infection at different levels of prevalence in the community. The test, however, cannot differentiate between asymptomatic carriers and those with invasive disease. Its main use is for immunoepidemiologic surveys.

Treatment

The mainstay of treatment for chronic intestinal amoebiasis or asymptomatic carriage of pathogenic strains is *diloxanide furoate* (20mg/kg for 10 days). *Metronidazole* (200mg – 400mg every eight hours for five days) is effective in amoebic dysentery, and reaches good tissue concentration. A subsequent cycle of diloxanide may be used to remove luminal forms. For amoebic abscesses metronidazole is effective in the above dose, and may be repeated after a fortnight if necessary. Aspiration of the abscess is indicated if there is no improvement after three days of metronidazole. Aspiration improves tissue penetration of the drug. Chloroquine may be added to metronidazole.

Giardiasis

Giardia lamblia is a flagellate protozoan which has both a trophozoic and a cystic stage. It inhabits the duodenum and jejunum and is amongst one of the most common parasites of man. Incidence rates vary – a rate of 47 per cent was reported from hospital patients in Columbia; surveys in primary school children in Rangoon, Burma have shown prevalence rates of 21 per cent for *Giardia* and 5.7 per cent for *E. histolytica*; a similar survey in Mexico City revealed rates of 13.7 per cent and 14.3 per cent respectively. In endemic areas, children are in the main reported to be symptomatic and to suffer malabsorption.

Transmission occurs from person to person through ingestion of food and water contaminated with cysts. Flies may also play an important role in the transmission. Many of the cases of so-called 'travellers' diarrhoea' may be due to infection with this parasite. Though an acute attack of diarrhoea as seen in 'travellers' diarrhoea' can also occur in giardial infection, there is usually an incubation period of one to four weeks.

Results of exposure to *G. lamblia* are variable depending upon variation in the parasite or in host factors like age, nutrition and immune status. In an experimental study, 40 volunteers were fed a single strain of the parasite at different dose levels and only 21 became infected. As few as 10 cysts were sufficient to cause infection in some individuals, though an average of 100 or more cysts were required to guarantee infection. It is likely that many individuals harbour the parasite in an essentially commensal relationship.

Clinical symptoms vary from no symptoms to severe diarrhoea. The latter may be acute and of a short duration or may become prolonged and chronic. With chronicity signs and symptoms of malabsorption may occur in some individuals. Alteration in the morphology of the jejunal mucosa has been demonstrated in cases of giardiasis presenting with malabsorption. Shortening and thickening of the villi and increased cellularity of the lamina propria have been constant findings. In addition, acute inflammation in the mucosa may be seen in the more severely ill patients. There is an increased epithelial cell turnover, as evidenced by increased epithelial mitotic activity, in response to epithelial injury. These morphological changes in the jejunal mucosa lead to decreased absorptive capacity resulting in malabsorption and a sprue-like syndrome. The histologic changes have been shown to revert to normal after successful treatment.

Giardia infection is an associated finding in patients with gastro-intestinal immunodeficiency syndromes like hypo-γ-globulinaemic sprue with a flat mucosa and nodular lymphoid hyperplasia. Successful therapy leads to amelioration of steatorrhoea with improved absorption and histological improvement. It is likely that in such cases the defective immune mechanism leads to an opportunistic infection by *Giardia*. Similarly, giardiasis with diarrhoea is common in marasmic children and the infection may be an important factor in the etiology of malnutrition.

Diagnosis

In the acute case, examination of freshly voided stool may show the presence of the trophozoite with its characteristic features and flagellar movements. The cysts are more commonly found and can be seen even in well-formed stools. However, in many infected individuals several stool examinations may be negative. A definite periodicity of presence or absence of cysts in stools has been demonstrated in experimental infections. In such cases microscopic examination of duodenal juice and small intestinal biopsy may reveal presence of the trophozoites. Such investigations are justified only in long-standing diarrhoea and malabsorption states.

Treatment

Metronidazole in a dose of 0.25 g two or three times a day for a period of five to ten days is now considered the drug of choice and has superseded mepacrine in the treatment of giardiasis. With the above regimen, a cure of 80 per cent or more can be expected from a single course of treatment.

Cryptosporidiasis

Cryptosporidium is a unicellular coccidian parasite which infects the epithelial cells lining the gut and the respiratory tract. Other coccidian parasites which are closely related to cryptosporidium are *Isospora belli* (definitive host is the pig and other farm animals; also infects humans), and *Toxoplasma gondii* (definitive host is the cat; also infects humans). Various species of cryptosporidium have been isolated from fishes, reptiles, birds and mammals. Severe bovine diarrhoea in calves and lambs, and respiratory illness in poultry due to this parasite are well known in veterinary medicine.

The immune status of the host is a major determinant of the outcome of infection. In immunocompetent individuals the infection may be subclinical and go unrecognised, or present as profuse watery diarrhoea which is self-limiting. Occasionally non-specific symptoms like myalgia, malaise and headache may be present. However, in immunocompromised individuals the illness is severe, prolonged and life threatening with marked weight loss. Cryptosporidium as a major cause of the wasting syndrome 'Slim disease' came to light with the spread of HIV infection in Central and Eastern Africa. In cases of AIDS, infection with cryptosporidium causes diarrhoea which becomes progressively worse. Infection begins with the organism colonising the jejunum or ileum, and becomes life threatening when a large portion of the gastro-intestinal tract is covered. The diarrhoea is profuse and cholera like with average losses of three to six litres of watery stools per day. It is estimated that in 15 per cent of AIDS patients who have diarrhoea the cause is infection by cryptosporidium. The rate may be much higher in developing countries, and figures of 41 per cent have been reported from Haiti, and of 85 per cent from Kinshasa. A severe form of illness may also occur when the immune response of the host is dampened for any other reason, for example, in malnutrition, or following virus infections like measles and CMV.

Cryptosporidium is an ubiquitous parasite. More than 40 mammals including a variety of farm animals serve as hosts. The parasite readily crosses the host barrier, and so most infections are some form of zoonotic transmission. Runoffs from dairy or grazing land contaminating surface or drinking water is a frequent cause of outbreaks. Person to person transmission is also a possibility since there are several reports of outbreaks in day care centres, and of hospital acquired infections. Waterborne outbreaks have been described in several countries. The mechanisms and pathways of waterborne transmission are similar to those in the case of giardiasis, except that the oocysts of cryptosporidium are 10 to 15 times more resistant to levels of chlorine routinely employed in water treatment plants.

The life cycle of cryptosporidium is similar to other coccidia. Six major milestones in the life cycle have been described viz. excystation following the ingestion of the oocyst which releases the infective sporozoites; asexual multiplication inside the host cells; gamete formation; fertilisation; oocyst wall formation; development of infective sporozoites within the oocysts. The thick wall of the oocysts provides protection against most common disinfectants, for example ammonia at 50 per cent concentration, or formalin at 10 per cent concentration for half an hour. Routine treatment of drinking water (1 p.p.m. of chlorine or 0.4 p.p.m. of ozone) has little or no effect. Heat at 60°C or more for 30 minutes kills the oocysts. During outbreaks, boiling of all drinking water is the most effective preventive measure. Up to 20 per cent of oocysts do not form a thick outer membrane. Soon after release from the host cell they infect other enterocytes and reinitiate the life cycle. They are the auto infective forms which are responsible for chronicity and severity of the infection.

The most common clinical presentation is with profuse and watery diarrhoea (92 per cent of cases), which is often 'cholera-like'. Abdominal pain (45 per cent), vomiting (51 per cent) low grade fever (36 per cent) are other associated symptoms. In well nourished subjects the diarrhoea lasts from three to 12 days, and is self limited. In poorly nourished hosts the diarrhoea can be persistent (more than two weeks) and associated with excessive fluid loss. The cholera-like diarrhoea indicates toxin-mediated hypersecretion into the gut. There is also parasite induced villous damage causing impaired digestion and malabsorption. Failure to thrive as a result of persistent diarrhoea may also be responsible for maintaining the chronicity of the infection in infants and young children in communities where sanitation and hygiene are poor. In immunodeficient subjects respiratory problems like coughing, wheezing and shortness of breath may predominate. Rarely cholecystitis, hepatitis or pancreatitis may be the presenting features. Future research will help to define the role of cryptosporidium in respiratory illness which so commonly accompanies diarrhoea in malnourished children in developing countries.

In the acute stage diagnosis is usually made by identifying oocysts by microscopy in freshly passed stools, in sputum, or in body fluids like tracheal aspirates, bronchoalveolar lavage fluid, and alveolar exudates. Specimens must be examined fresh or transported in 10 per cent formalin. Stool concentration methods using either the flotation or sedimentation technique may be employed in the same manner as in the case of ova or other gut parasites. Serodiagnosis is indicative of past exposure, or subclinical infection. In some difficult cases jejunal biopsy may help to establish the diagnosis.

There is no effective treatment. The immune response of the host is the important determinant of the outcome of infection. In endemic areas breast feeding provides a degree of protection. Reports from Costa Rica, Guatemala, Haiti and Liberia indicate that cryptosporidium infection is less prevalent in breast fed compared to artificially fed infants. Attempts to produce hyper-immune cow's milk or colostrum by immunising pregnant cows with oocyst/sporozoite antigens has not been shown to have any protection for calves or humans. At present the most important preventive measures are sanitation and food as well as personal hygiene. In developing countries these measures are usually absent in communities which are at greatest risk.

Ascariasis

Ascariasis infestation is widespread. In the United States, ascariasis is more prevalent in southern than in northern states and also more common in rural than in urban areas. In Europe, the incidence is low in large cities (for example, Prague 4 per cent, Warsaw 4.9 per cent, Rome 1.23 per cent) and is greater in rural areas. In Kenya, 58.1 per cent of children in rural families are infected.

In a study conducted in Taiwan it was estimated that the average infected individual harboured 12 parasites. On the other hand in a similar study in Sri Lanka, 500 to 700 worms per person were seen amongst those living in poor socio-economic conditions. The soil can determine the rates of prevalence and transmission. Eggs deposited in soil became infective when the soil temperature reached 20°C in summer months. When placed one centimetre deep in the soil, they were killed when soil humidity fell below four per cent.

Life cycle

The life span of the adult worm is six months to one year. The fertile female deposits an average of 200 000 ova daily. For optimal development the eggs need moist shady soil with an environmental temperature of between 23 and 33°C.

When the eggs are swallowed, the outer coat dissolves in the stomach and hatched larvae pass into the small intestine. They penetrate the surface epithelium of the intestinal mucosa and enter the venules of the portal system along which they travel to the liver, where they move freely in the sinusoids causing minimal inflammatory reaction.

The larvae travel to the right side of the heart and thence, through the pulmonary circulation, to the lungs where they break through the capillary wall and enter the respiratory spaces. In experimental animals larvae may be seen in the lungs within 24 hours although the majority reach the pulmonary vessels between the fifth and sixth day after swallowing eggs. In the pulmonary space the larvae grow considerably in size. At this stage inflammatory reaction can be seen in the alveoli and the bronchial walls.

The grown larvae travel up the tracheobronchial tree, to reach the hypopharynx where they are swallowed. In the small intestine they continue to grow and about two or three months after ingestion of the ova, the parasite attains sexual maturity.

Symptoms

In some cases, pulmonary symptoms such as cough, dyspnoea and asthmatic attacks occur with or without fever, about one week after ingestion of eggs. Clinical signs such as rhonchi and rales may be present – rarely signs of consolidation occur. X-ray of chest shows increased bronchial markings, diffuse mottling or areas of consolidation depending upon the degree of parenchymal involvement. Spontaneous improvement occurs in about a week's time.

Abdominal symptoms depend upon the parasitic load, and vary from no symptoms or vague abdominal pains and bowel upsets to serious complications. The latter are due to large numbers of parasites in the intestinal lumen and to their tendency to wrap themselves round one another into tight bundles. This may cause acute abdomen due to obstruction (figure 21.1). Of all acute abdominal emergencies in children in Capetown 12.8 per cent are caused by ascaris.

Adult ascaris in the host intestine have been shown to concentrate a great deal of cellular material in their gut, which is lined with microvilli. When the host is on marginal nutrition, a heavy infestation may precipitate deficiency disorders. It has been shown that in children infected with 13 to 40 worms (average 26) approximately 4 g of protein per day can be lost out of a daily intake of 35 to 50 g.

Digestive disturbances, fevers or other irritations in their environment can cause adult worms to migrate giving rise to surgical complications. Thus, bile duct obstruction, liver abscess and haemorrhagic pancreatitis have been reported as complications of ascariasis. Appendicitis is a recognised complication of ascaris infection and intestinal perforation with peritonitis has also been reported. After abdominal surgery, any existing ascaris infection is a potential hazard since the worms may penetrate suture lines and cause peritonitis.

Treatment

The presently available chemotherapeutic agents act only on adult worms in the intestinal lumen; no drug is known to be able to deal with the larval stages in the body. Piperazine has been used widely during the past 25 years and is the drug of choice. It acts by causing a neuromuscular block in the ascaris so that the worm loses its ability to maintain its position against peristalsis. A single dose of 3–4 gm of piperazine gives an 85 to 90 per cent cure rate

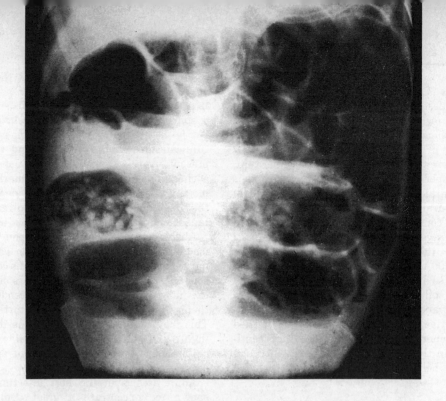

Figure 21.1 Intestinal obstruction with multiple fluid levels in ascariasis

and a considerable reduction of the worm load in the remainder.

Levamisole is now being preferred because of freedom from any side effects. The single dose for children is 2.5 mg/kg. The efficacy of treatment with levamisole has been recorded as 77 per cent (in heavy infections) to 96 per cent. However, levamisole is effective against ascariasis only and in mixed infections, which are common in many countries, its use will be limited, besides being more expensive than piperazine.

Mebendazole is a broad spectrum drug effective against *Ascaris*, hookworm and *Trichuris* infections. In a daily dose of 50–150 mg for children given for four consecutive days its efficacy has been between 84 to 100 per cent.

Pyrantel embonate also has broad spectrum activity. In a single dose of 2.5 to 10 mg/kg it is effective against *Ascaris* as well as hookworm. The lower dose given over two days and repeated every other month has been used in the mass treatment of *Ascaris* and hookworm.

The availability of effective and safe drugs makes the control of ascariasis in small village communities possible through mass treatment. The aim is to achieve eradication of worms in a large number of persons in the community, thereby reducing the reservoir of infection and interrupting transmission. In many places transmission is continuous all the year round. Here mass treatment at intervals of two or three months may help to reduce the reservoir of infection. In some areas there are large seasonal variations in transmission rates. In such cases mass treatment in children's clinics, schools and by home visits should commence four to six weeks after transmission begins and continue at two monthly intervals while transmission lasts.

In island communities mass treatment with a single dose of albendazole in school children in four cycles at intervals of four months has shown a fall in prevalence rates in the target population as well as in adults.

Other roundworm infections

Ascaris of other animals can infect man. There are several reports in the literature of human infection by *Ascaris sum*, the porcine *Ascaris*, which is probably due to ingestion of eggs through pig manure.

A newly discovered species of roundworm – *Capillaria philippinensis* – was the causal parasite in an epidemic of severe and often fatal diarrhoea in the Philippines. In the epidemic 1000 cases were reported with more than ten per cent confirmed case fatalities. In the affected areas, a survey in one village with a population of 700 showed that 32 per cent were affected, and all those passing eggs of *C. philippinensis* in their stools eventually became symptomatic. In untreated cases mortality rates of 19–35 per cent were reported. The main clinical symptoms were of abdominal pain, diarrhoea, muscle wasting and oedema leading to debility and death in two to four months without treatment. Clinical studies have shown the presence of a severe protein-losing enteropathy with malabsorption of fats and sugars in those with heavy infestations. Treatment with thiabendazole caused dramatic improvement. Presently mebendazole is the treatment of choice in a dose of 100–400 mg per day for 10–30 days.

Of the known 250 species of *Capillaria*, three have been found in man. The life cycle of *C. philippinensis* has not been fully elucidated. It is thought that it has a direct cycle with no intermediate hosts but may utilise certain fish and crustaceans as transport hosts. Eggs passed in stools become embryonated in ten days and are infective to certain fresh water fish. After three weeks of development in the intestine of the fish the larvae are infective to primates.

Most of the cases in the literature have been described from the northern Philippines where several outbreaks with high mortality have been confirmed. More recently there have been reports from Thailand of several outbreaks.

Toxocara canis and catis, the common roundworms of dogs and cats, can occasionally give rise to serious illness in man. Typically, symptoms occur in children one to four years old with a history of pica or close association with domestic animals. The characteristic symptoms are persistent eosinophilia, hepatomegaly, fever, asthmatic attacks, bronchitis and other signs of pulmonary involvement associated with anaemia, leucocytosis and raised immunoglobulins in the blood. Usually the condition improves spontaneously over a period of months, though fatalities have also been described. The occurrence of symptoms is related to the number of eggs ingested, and unless larvae invade vital organs such as the brain or the eye, ingestion of a small number of eggs may go unnoticed.

Toxocaral invasion of the eye occurs as an isolated lesion usually in older children who may show no other signs of visceral toxocariasis. It is nearly always unilateral. Pathologically, the lesion is a chronic endophthalmitis with or without retinal detachment. The presenting complaint is strabismus or contraction of the visual field. The natural history of ocular toxocariasis is one of resolution of the inflammatory mass leaving a residual scar and a degree of blindness which depends on the size of the scar and its nearness to macula. Encephalopathy is another manifestation of toxocaral infection and a wide spectrum of neurologic signs including convulsions may result. In several cases *T. canis* larvae have been demonstrated in brain tissue at necropsy. In a group of 349 patients with epilepsy, 7.5 per cent gave a positive reaction to toxocara skin test – a proportion three and a half times as great as among the healthy population. This has raised the possibility of a relationship between epilepsy and toxocariasis.

The natural habitat of *Toxocara* is the small intestine of cats and dogs. The eggs are passed in the faeces and are swallowed by mice, rats and a wide variety of animals in whom they develop into larvae. When dogs or cats eat infected rats and mice these larvae develop into adults in their guts. The most usual method of infection in dogs is during intrauterine life. When the dogs swallow *T. cani* eggs the resulting larvae migrate into tissues and persist for long periods. From these tissues, particularly the retroperitoneal tissue in the pregnant bitch, they enter the foetus by a route the details of which are unknown.

When infective *T. canis* or *T. catis* eggs are swallowed by man, larvae emerge from the eggs in the human intestine, penetrate the bowel wall and travel in portal blood to the liver and thence to the lungs and beyond to other tissues of the body. The size and shape of the larvae determines the extent to which it can travel in the blood vessel because it appears to leave the vessel at a point at which its diameter approaches that of the blood vessel. This fact may explain why *Ascaris* larvae are filtered out of the circulation in man in the liver and lungs and do not pass beyond these organs to other tissues, since they are about twice the size of the *Toxocara* larvae.

Since toxocaral infection can present in several different ways, the diagnosis may be difficult. It should be suspected in choroidoretinitis, hepatomegaly, asthma or pneumonitis especially when these conditions are associated with eosinophilia of undetermined origin. A presumptive diagnosis is made if the skin test is positive. In this test the toxocara antigen is injected into the skin of the patient in a 1/1000 dilution. In sensitised individuals it produces a wheal. The test is sensitive; in experimental animals a small infective dose of twenty eggs was sufficient to cause conversion. It does not give cross-reaction with *Enterobius*, *Trichuris* and hookworm infection but false positive results may be obtained in *Ascaris* infection since *Toxocara* seems to share many antigenic components with these species. The skin test does not distinguish between infections which are recent and active and those which are long-standing and inactive. Active infection may be detected by a fluorescent antibody test or by haemagglutination techniques.

Treatment

Thiabendazole (50 mg/kg daily for five days) and diethylcarbamazine (3 mg/kg thrice daily for 21 days) cause death of the larvae in the tissues and amelioration of symptoms in some cases. Corticosteroids are advisable in the presence of ocular involvement.

Enterobiasis

The threadworm is a small intestinal roundworm. Man is the only known natural host. There is no period of development outside the human body and no intermediate host. Hence transmission occurs from man to man.

The normal habitat of the worm is the caecum and the appendix. In heavy infections the ileum may also be affected. The male worm dies soon after copulation and is unimportant in the pathogenesis. The gravid females descend to the rectum, pass through the anal sphincter at night and lay eggs in the perianal and the perineal region. The female threadworm is known to lay up to 10 000 eggs on emerging from the anal canal. It usually dies after oviposition. The life cycle of the worm is completed when the infective eggs are ingested. On reaching the duodenum, rhabditiform larvae are hatched which undergo several moults before becoming adult worms.

Threadworm ova are resistant to adverse environmental conditions. Unlike those of ascaris, they are rarely found in the soil, but they occur in dust especially after bedmaking, in the bedclothes, pyjamas, on toys and furniture. In one study it was found that there were 199 eggs on each square foot of the walls in the school dining hall, 305 on the classroom walls and 5000 on the lavatory walls. Thus, they can be easily transferred to the same or other human hosts in close contacts.

Pathological lesions due to the worm are commonly seen in the area of the caecum, the appendix and the lower ileum. Depending upon the degree of infection, the lesions vary from mild catarrhal inflammation to areas of erosions in the mucosa and in some cases, large ulcers. Pyogenic infection can give rise to single or multiple mucosal or submucosal abscesses. In a histological study of 691 appendices removed from children, enterobius was found in 52. Of these, 8 showed abscess formation, 14 had early evidence of appendicitis and 30 showed morphological picture of acute appendicitis. The most common presenting symptom is anal pruritis which can be intense and may lead to skin changes secondary to itching. Symptoms relating to the gastrointestinal tract are less common and are usually non-specific, for example, anorexia, vague abdominal discomfort, weight loss etc. Examination of stools does not show presence of eggs and the diagnosis is made by swabbing the perineal region with sticky cellophane (Sellotape) and examining it under the microscope.

Treatment

Mebendazole (100mg as a single dose) is the drug of choice. Pyrantel (a single dose of 5mg/kg) is equally effective. Ideally, the whole family including the parents should receive treatment.

Trichuriasis

In the tropics and the sub-tropics the prevalence rates are similar to those of ascariasis. In a study of 9256 Puerto Rican children, prevalence rates of 87 per cent were reported as compared to 40 per cent for ascariasis and 26 per cent for hookworm. In Singapore, prevalence rates of 62–57 per cent were reported amongst male patients attending the General Hospital. In Europe, similar high rates have been reported in Yugoslavia, Albania, rural France and Italy.

The adult worms are flesh-coloured, thin and hair-like at the anterior three-fifths, and thicker and fleshy in the posterior two-fifths. The usual habitat is the caecum but they may also be found in the appendix, any portion of the colon and in some cases may even extend to the ileum. The anterior hair-like part of the body of the worm is deeply attached to the mucosa.

Freshly-passed eggs must gain access to warm, moist and shaded soil where they become infective after about three weeks. Man is infected by ingestion of embryonated eggs. The larvae are set free in the small intestine and enter nearby crypts for temporary nourishment. Later the mature larvae move to the large bowel where they develop further into adult worms.

The bowel may show no lesions in mild infections. In massive infections the mucosal cells show degenerative changes with necrosis, inflammation and small subepithelial haemorrhages. There may be lymphocytic or eosiniphilic infiltration in the area adjacent to the worm.

Vague abdominal discomfort may be the only symptom in mild infection. In massive infections there is diarrhoea with mucus and blood, tenesmus, loss of weight, and, occasionally, rectal prolapse. Studies with radioisotopes suggest that the adult worm draws a small amount of blood from the host of the order of 0.005 ml per day, and that in children with poor nutrition, iron deficiency anaemia may be precipitated.

Mebendazole (100mg as a single dose) is effective. Similarly, newer preparations like albendazole and ivermectin have shown good results in clinical trials.

Ankylostomiasis

Ankylostomiasis is a disease of hot humid regions; in temperate climates the prevalence of the disease depends upon the degree of atmospheric humidity and the temperature. In tropical countries, where the rainy season is clear-cut, the most favourable transmission periods for the parasite are at the beginning and towards the end of the rains. In areas with extensive irrigation systems or in the delta regions, the ground may be moist even in the absence of rain, and hookworm transmission can occur all the year round. Agricultural practices like the use of night soils as the main source of fertilisers help to facilitate transmission.

There are two distinct human hookworms, namely, *Ankylostoma duodenale* and *Necator americanus*. Both these parasites are widespread throughout the tropics and the sub-tropics and rigid demarcations are no longer possible.

The adult worm lives in the upper small intestine, firmly attached to the mucosa where it sucks the host's blood to obtain oxygen and glucose. It has been estimated that the amount of blood lost per day is 0.03 ml per worm in the case of *Necator americanus* and 0.015–0.02 ml per worm in the case of *Ankylostoma duodenale*. Eggs are passed in the faeces where they continue to develop, and under optimal conditions at 23–30°C, they are hatched within a day.

When the eggs are hatched the emerging larvae feed on the faecal microflora and other organic material and pass through several stages of develop-

ment before reaching the infective stage. The infective larvae are capable of active vertical movement in the soil but they do not disperse horizontally. Thus, in the soil they are found in aggregates at sites where stools have been deposited. In the infective stage the larvae depend upon their own food reserves which are diminishing rapidly. Hence only a few are able to survive for prolonged periods, especially if the soil surface becomes dry in the summer heat.

Environmental conditions are important for the transmission of infection, which is highest about six weeks after the rainy season. Physical properties of the soil affect the development and maturation of the larvae. A soil rich in organic matter is preferred and larvae will remain alive in such soil for up to six weeks.

Man is infected through the penetration of the exposed skin by the larvae. On gaining entry through the skin, the larvae enter the lymphatics and find their way to the pulmonary circulation. In the lungs, they burrow their way into the alveolar sacs, and travel along the bronchial passages to the trachea and the hypopharynx where they are swallowed and thus reach the gastro-intestinal tract.

In experimental infections with several hundred larvae it was noticed that initially there were discrete skin lesions, catarrh, dysphagia and nasal irritation. A month after the infection there is abdominal pain which is at times acute and can simulate peptic dyspepsia.

In heavy infections, worm loads of up to 6000 have been recorded. Such a large number of worms can cause considerable blood loss every day, resulting in an iron deficiency state. Hookworm infection is the commonest cause of iron deficiency anaemia in many tropical countries.

Hookworm infection can lead to considerable mucosal damage. Direct observation in infected dogs has shown that the worms change their site of attachment every four to six hours to seek out new feeding areas and for purposes of mating. At each site the buccal capsule of the worm is attached to one of the villi and a plug of host tissue is pulled free from the lamina propria causing rupture of capillaries and bleeding. The bolus of mucosa in the worm's gut undergoes progressive digestion followed by successive plugs of tissue being ingested. A maximally developed mucosal lesion involves about nine villi and an individual worm causes up to six such lesions per day. After detachment of the worm reparative changes are rapid because of the constant turnover of epithelial cells in the gut mucosa.

Besides iron, albumin is also lost into the gut in quantities proportional to the blood loss and the mucosal tissue ingested by the worm. Most adults, on an adequate diet, are able to compensate for the albumin loss by an increased turnover of albumin, but in children and in poorly nourished adults such compensation is not possible and hypo-proteinaemia with oedema may result. There are contradictory reports on the association of hookworm disease with malabsorption. Several authors have described villous atrophy in the intestinal mucosa and it is possible that some degree of malabsorption may occur in heavy infestations.

Treatment

Bephenium is still widely used and has minimal side effects. A single dose of 1.25g–2.5g is administered and repeated a couple of days later. Pyrantel (a single dose of 5mg/kg) is also effective. Mebendazole, a broad spectrum anthelmintic which is effective against enterobius, ascaris, trichuris and ankylostoma may be used in a dose of 100 mg twice daily for three days.

The availability of highly effective and non-toxic preparations with a broad spectrum of action has increased the possibility of regular mass treatments of defined rural communities in order to reduce the reservoir of the parasite in the community and thereby reduce transmission. The most favourable time for mass campaigns is immediately after the period in which maximum transmission occurs. In most cases this is generally two months after the end of the rainy season.

Strongyloides

The prevalence of Strongyloides varies according to geography and climate. In warm semi-arid areas the prevalence is seldom above three per cent. In the tropics the rates vary from 35 to 40 per cent, whereas in the sub-tropics, with well distributed yearly rainfall, as in some areas of Brazil, the prevalence rates can be as high as 85 per cent. The adult female inhabits the crypts of the duodenum and the first part of the jejunum, where eggs are deposited in the intestinal mucosa within serpentine channels burrowed by the female. The larvae hatch in the mucosa and gain access to the intestinal lumen by piercing the epithelium. Occasionally, some larvae may burrow in the opposite direction – through the muscularis and the serosa into the peritoneal cavity.

Most of the larvae, however, are passed in the faeces of the host. In favourable circumstances the larvae grow rapidly in the soil to become adult worms; copulation takes place and eggs develop which, on hatching, produce rhabditiform larvae. These metamorphose into infective larvae. Under unfavourable circumstances, the larvae passed in the stools do not develop into adult worms but change into infective larvae. In some instances, the larvae within the gut lumen may metamorphose into infective larvae and reinfect the host by penetrating the colonic mucosa, thereby causing the hyperinfection syndrome.

Free-living infective larvae in the soil gain entry into the body of the host by penetrating the skin and travel through the blood stream to the pulmonary circulation. They remain in the lungs for several days growing into adults. Fertilisation of the female possibly occurs in the lungs. The adult worm travels along the respiratory passages to the hypopharynx where it is swallowed and enters the gastro-intestinal tract.

Heavy infection with Strongyloides, gives rise to a duodenitis and jejunitis with malabsorption and steatorrhoea. The mucosa is damaged by the gravid female making burrows to lay eggs and by the larvae penetrating the epithelium to reach the lumen (figure 21.2). Intestinal lesions vary from mild catarrhal enteritis with congestion, haemorrhage and micro-ulceration to oedema of the mucosa, flattening and atrophy of the villi. In severe infections or in cases with disturbed immune mechanism as occurs in treatment with corticosteroids or immunosuppressive drugs there may be ulcerative enteritis with mucosal atrophy, macroscopic ulceration and a severe inflammatory response due to secondary bacterial invasion. The lesion can lead to a form of stenosis with vomiting and consequent malnutrition. In some instances the malnutrition may come to dominate the clinical picture. Duodenal lesions are seen on a barium meal as mucosal oedema, duodenal dilation and delay in the emptying of the third part of the duodenum. When large ulcers occur, healing takes place with fibrosis and permanent stricture results. The common presenting symptoms are abdominal pain, nausea and vomiting, anorexia and loose stools. The diarrhoea is blood-tinged in about 25 per cent of heavy infections and can be severe enough to give rise to electrolyte imbalance. Pulmonary symptoms with pneumonitis and bronchopneumonia may dominate the clinical pictures. In areas where Strongyloides infection is prevalent it should be considered in the differential diagnosis in any patient presenting with gastro-intestinal symptoms with cough, dyspnoea and hemoptysis.

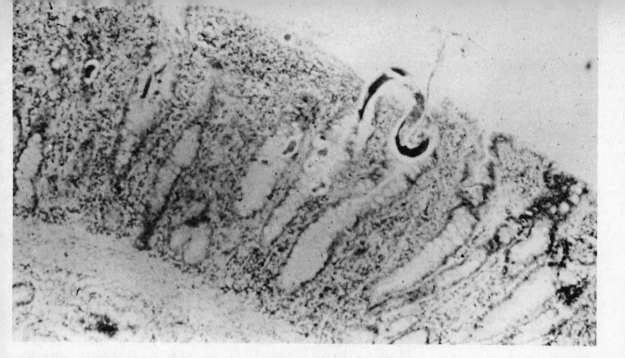

Figure 21.2   Strongyloides – the gravid female penetrating the gut mucosa

Treatment

Thiabendazole, a broad-spectrum anthelmintic, has gained acceptance as the drug of choice in the treatment of *Strongyloides*. A mean cure rate of 96 per cent has been reported with this drug. Side effects of dizziness, nausea, vomiting and abdominal pain occur in a few cases. Mebendazole, a recently introduced broad spectrum anthelmintic, is also effective against *Strongyloides* and has virtually no side effects.

Intestinal taeniasis

The distribution and prevalence of *Taenia* infection depends on the dietary habit of eating under-cooked or raw meat and fish. High incidence rates occur in many countries of tropical Africa, the Middle East and southern Mediterranean countries. The fish tape-worm, *Diphyllobotrium latum*, occurs among the Eskimo in Quebec, in Finland, in parts of Romania and Turkey.

Life cycle

When the eggs are swallowed the shell is dissolved by the action of pancreatin and bile salts and embryos emerge in the duodenum and the upper small intestine. The embryos then penetrate the wall of the intestine and travel in the blood stream or lymphatics to reach body tissues (skeletal muscle, myocardium, diaphragm and tongue) where they encyst and produce a bladder-like structure containing fluid. The cells of the wall of this cyst give rise to scolex and neck, and become the cysticercus. (In the case of *Echinococcus granulosus*, the dog tapeworm, the cyst contains a germinal layer that gives rise to many scolices and is called a hydatid.) When the cyst is ingested by the definitive host, the scolex evaginates and attaches itself to the intestinal wall of the host by means of suction cups, grooves or hooks, and grows into an adult parasite. Below the scolex is the neck region from which proglottids (segments) develop. In the beef tapeworm (*Taenia saginata*) the fully grown parasite is known to achieve a length of five metres. Each proglottid has male and female reproductive organs. The surface has a pattern of microvilli for absorption of nutrients. There is also a network of excretory canals. Eggs appear in the faeces of the human host. When ingested by cattle they develop into cysticerci in their tissues.

No definitive intestinal lesions or symptoms have been reported. Loose stools, excessive appetite and hunger pains can occur in infected individuals. Presence of the fish tapeworm in the gut has been associated with vitamin B_{12} deficiency and macrocytic anaemia in the host.

Treatment

The treatment has been much simplified since the availability of niclosamide. It is given as a single dose of 500mg – 1g depending on age, followed by a purgative two hours later. Praziquantel is equally effective in a single dose of 10–20 mg/kg after a light breakfast.

Tapeworms of other animals causing human disease

Hymenolepis nana

The usual host is the mouse. When eggs are swallowed by man, they hatch in the stomach or the small intestine, penetrate the villi and become cystericercoids. In about a fortnight, the villus disintegrates and the larva attaches itself to the wall where it grows into an adult.

Echinococcus (hydatic disease)

The common hydatid-producing tapeworm is *E. granulosus*. The mature tapeworm lives in the small intestine of the dog; almost all mammals can be the intermediate hosts but the optimal one appears to be the sheep. A cycle of transmission between livestock and dogs maintains the persistence of the worm. Other less important worms causing hydatid disease are:

(1) *E. multilocularis* where domestic cats and foxes carry the mature adult worm and various rodents constitute the intermediate hosts.
(2) *E. oligarthus* – the definitive hosts are cats and members of the cat family and intermediate hosts are small rodents.

The eggs of *Echinococcus* are remarkably resistant to environmental conditions. They can survive temperatures of –16°C and viable eggs can be recovered after 35 days of exposure to sun. Human disease occurs when the eggs are swallowed by man, for example, in communities where there is intimate contact with dogs. The eggs are digested releasing a free embryo in the duodenum. It penetrates the mucosa until it enters a venule and travels along it until held up in a narrow capillary. Embryos develop into small bladder-like cysts which grow to reach a diameter of 40–50 mm after three months. The fluid in the cyst contains granules called 'hydatid sand' which are actually brood capsules with

developing scolices. (When a hydatid cyst is ingested by the definitive host, for example, dogs eating the flesh of dead livestock, the embryos are freed from the cyst, become attached to the intestinal mucosa and grow into adult worms. Thus, the parasite reproduces itself in the final host by producing a large number of eggs, and in the intermediate host by formation of numerous scolices.)

In the intermediate host a large majority (60 per cent) of the embryos get trapped in the sinusoids of the liver which is the organ most commonly affected (93 per cent) in hydatid disease. Some embryos (20 per cent) escape the hepatic vascular bed and get arrested in the pulmonary circulation and the rest reach the systemic circulation. Hydatid cysts grow at the rate of 1 cm per year, and symptoms of a space-occupying lesion usually develop when they reach a size of 10 cm in diameter.

The Cassoni's test has been used for many years to make a diagnosis of hydatid disease. In recent years, serological tests like indirect haemagglutination and the latex agglutination which demonstrate the presence of complement-fixing antibody have been developed. High titres occur in patients with active infection. Low levels of the antibody may persist for some years after the removal of cysts; low levels have also been found in people working in some cattle and sheep farming areas.

Albendazole is effective if adequate concentration can be achieved inside the cyst. It is also effective for inoperable cases, and for prophylaxis prior to surgery. The recommended dose is 10–15 mg/kg daily in three divided doses as four courses of one month's duration each, with an interval of a fortnight between courses.

Praziquantel has also been used either alone or with albendazole. Some cases will still need surgery, but it is best to wait until after a trial of albendazole and/or praziquantel.

Prevention of infection in dogs is an important public health measure, and consists of regular deworming of dogs. The importation of offal for use as pet foods and for the preparation of canned pet food should be under close supervision of the health inspectorate.

Schistosomiasis

Next to malaria, schistosomiasis is one of the most widespread of the parasitic infestations of man. It occurs in most countries of tropical Africa, the Middle East, Central and South America, the Caribbean, and in the Far East. It is estimated that there are 200 million persons in the world affected with the parasite, and that amongst Egypt's 37 million people, 20 million have the disease. Developments involving major irrigation projects have resulted in an increase in the infection since the parasite and its intermediate host are able to spread along irrigation canals to village communities which were far from it before.

There are three main species. S. haematobium, which is found in the vesical venous plexus of man (occurs in Africa and the Middle East); S. mansoni which is found in the colonic venules (common in Africa and Central and South America) and S. japonicum also found in the colonic venules (occurs in the Far East). The adult worms are found in the vesical or colonic venules according to the species concerned. Eggs pass through the vessel wall into the urine or faeces of the host as the case may be. On reaching the outside the eggs must find another host, the freshwater snail in which they undergo many changes before emerging into the water as infectious cercariae. Man is infected by contact with surface water during washing or bathing or even wading through infected pools.

Schistosomiasis is one of those curious infections where many people get infected, some develop symptoms and only few have complications and die. The development of symptoms depends upon the worm load, the number of eggs being laid including the time over which the process has been continuing and the reaction of the tissues to the worm load. In the highly endemic areas virtually everyone is infected at some time in life. Community surveys have revealed infection rates of 100 per cent in children at the age of ten years. It is not unusual to find an egg output of 800 eggs of S. haematobium per 10 ml of urine in the endemic areas. Infection occurs at an early age and the egg output increases progressively until the age of twelve when it falls off. In spite of widespread infection only between 10–30 per cent of the population show heavy infection and will go on to develop symptoms since pathology is closely related to tissue response of the host to the worm's eggs.

Animal experiments have shown that infection with Schistosoma gives immunity against reinfection. This is known as premunition which means that the host can resist reinfection as long as some degree of infection by the parasite persists and it ceases soon after cure. The fall in egg output as age advances in the case of the infected individual may be due to such premunition or due to decreasing incidence of water contact. Coexisting malnutrition predisposes to schistosomal liver disease. Longitudinal studies in children have shown that in those with poor nutrition the enlarged livers did not regress spontaneously.

S. mansoni infection presents with diarrhoea and blood in stools and is often difficult to distinguish from ordinary diarrhoea and dysentery without careful microscopic examination of the stools. Salmonella infections are relatively frequent in persons affected with S. mansoni. In S. haematobium infections, the patient usually presents with haematuria and proteinuria. Long-standing infections can cause fibrosis and calcification of the bladder wall. Involvement of the ureteric orifices in the fibrotic process can lead to vesico-uretic reflux progressing to hydronephrosis even in comparatively recent infections. Many of these lesions are reversible with early treatment.

As the eggs are being laid, many get swept away along the blood stream to other organs. The liver is most commonly involved and granuloma or fibrosis may be seen in liver tissue surrounding the eggs. In advanced cases, there is portal hypertension and fibrosis associated with splenomegaly. Occasionally, the eggs travel beyond the liver and become lodged in the pulmonary circulation causing pulmonary hypertension and cor pulmonale. Schistosoma granuloma have been described in association with the venules of the spinal cord causing pressure on the cord and paraplegia. Similar granuloma have also been reported in the introitus in females.

Treatment

The treatment of schistosomiasis has been revolutionised by the introduction of new, more effective and less toxic drugs like praziquantel, oxamniquine, metriphonate, and several others.

Praziquantel is effective against all human schistosomes given as a single oral dose of 40 mg/kg (60 mg/kg in three divided doses on one day for S. japonicum infections).

Oxamniquine is effective against S. mansoni infections only. The dose varies from 15mg/kg as a single dose to a total of 60mg/kg over two to three days. It is important to bear in mind that occasionally it can cause epileptic fits.

Metriphonate is effective against S. haematobium infections only. It is given by mouth in three doses of 7.5 mg/kg at intervals of two weeks.

All these drugs achieve cure rates in excess of 75 per cent. In those patients who are not completely cured there is up to 80 per cent reduction in egg counts.

Because of their low toxicity, single dose or short duration of treatment, and high degree of efficacy these drugs provide exciting opportunities for control of schistosomiasis. The strategy of control comprises a reduction in the reservoir of the disease by mass chemotherapy combined with breaks in the pathway of transmission. All successful programmes have used multipronged approaches like treatment of water sources with molluscicides, reducing man-water contact, and intensive health education combined with periodic mass treatment.

Further reading

Amoebiasis
  Casemore D P. Foodborne protozoal infections.
  Lancet 1990; 336: 1427–32.
Ravdin J I. Entamoeba histolytica: pathogenic mechanisms, human immune response, and vaccine development.
  Clin Res 1990; 38: 215–25.

Cryptosporidiosis
  Current W L, Garcia L S. Cryptosporidiosis
  Clin Micro Rev 1991; 4: 325–358.

Strongyloides
Genta R M. Global prevalence of strongyloidiasis: critical review with epidemiologic insights into the prevention of disseminated disease.
Rev Inf Dis 1989; 11: 755–765.

Schistosomiasis
Jordan P, Webb G. (Eds). *Schistosomiasis: the St. Lucia Project*. Cambridge: Cambridge University Press, 1985.

General
World Health Organisation. *Prevention and control of intestinal parasitic infections*. Geneva: World Health Organisation, 1987. Technical Report Series No. 749.

Section VI

Care of the Newborn

22 Perinatal priorities in developing countries

The last decade has witnessed major developments in perinatal medicine. A better understanding of the biology of the newborn and of the birth process has led to the development of various methods of monitoring the vital physiological functions in the neonate. The care of the mother in pregnancy and puerperium as well as the day-to-day care of the small or the sick newborn has become more meaningful. A great impetus to the study of perinatal problems has come from national surveys and studies of maternal and infant mortality in several countries. Such studies have helped to identify areas in which further efforts can be more rewarding.

Definitions

Perinatal mortality is the sum of two mortality rates, namely, late foetal deaths (still-births) and neonatal deaths. Late foetal death rate is defined as deaths occurring in the foetus after the 28th week of pregnancy and before parturition, per 1000 births. Neonatal deaths are defined as deaths occurring in the newborn after birth and during the first week of life, per 1000 live births. Environmental, social and biological factors in the mother and the foetus contribute to these deaths, and the perinatal mortality rate is an indication of the health of women of child-bearing age in the community, as well as the effectiveness of the obstetric and neonatal services. In many affluent societies with well developed health services the perinatal mortality rates reported are under 25; these rates are less than half of those recorded 30 years ago in the same countries. In developing countries the picture is different, and perinatal mortality rates between 40 and 80 are quite common.

Perinatal mortality in developing countries

Adequate information on perinatal mortality is lacking in most developing countries. Wherever studies have been carried out it is found that the perinatal mortality may be as high as infant mortality and deserves the same amount of concern and attention. Hospital and field based studies in several countries of South-east Asia sponsored by the World Health Organisation revealed rates of between 80 and 100 per 1000 births. Low birth weight was found to be the underlying cause in at least a third of perinatal deaths. In a hospital-based study reported from Hyderabad, India, the perinatal mortality rate was 91.7 per 1000 births. In rural areas the figure is likely to be higher.

More recently, hospital-based data in Zaria, Nigeria where 40 per cent of all deliveries occur in hospital revealed an overall perinatal mortality rate of 86.4 per 1000. In babies with low birth weight (< 2.5 kg) the rate was 251.8 per 1000 compared with 59.3 per 1000 in babies who weighed 2.5 kg or more at birth. In this study 61 per cent of all perinatal deaths were still-births, once again emphasising the large contribution made by still-births to the perinatal mortality.

In recent years China has made considerable progress in improving the health of mothers and children. Perinatal mortality rates quoted from a maternity hospital in Shanghai show rates of 16.5 per 1000, which compares favourably with hospital data in Cardiff. The still-birth rate in Shanghai was 9.5 per 1000 compared to 12.6 in Cardiff. A striking feature of the Shanghai data was that only 4.7 per cent of the babies weighed less than 2501 g at birth.

It is often believed that reduction in perinatal mortality can be achieved only by means of intensive care units and similar other expensive methods of caring for the sick newborn and the infant born with a low birth weight. This is not true. Even in the affluent societies of Western Europe the dramatic fall in perinatal mortality has been due to a reduction of late foetal deaths and not so much to a reduction of neonatal deaths (figure 22.1).

In most developing countries late foetal deaths make up more than half the total perinatal mortality. An analysis of the factors contributing to these foetal deaths and resulting in relevant programmes of prevention should be the first priority in reducing perinatal mortality.

The classic triad: maternal age, parity and socio-economic class in perinatal mortality

Maternal age plays an important role in determining pregnancy outcome. A large proportion of perinatal as well as maternal mortality occurs in young mothers. For example, in the Nigerian study quoted above, 12 per cent of all maternal deaths occurred in mothers aged less than 16 years. In most rural societies marriages occur early and usually about the age of menarche (table 22.1). Childbearing commences soon after (tables 22.2 and 22.3).

In all societies the distribution of perinatal mortality by parity is very much similar to that by maternal age. The primipara is at risk and in the case of the very young mother the risk is greater. The risk in the case of the grand multipara is even greater. In many developing countries 40 per cent of mothers have four or more children and it is these who are at greater risk for both perinatal and infant mortality. Adequate spacing of children will allow mothers to recover from the accumulated deficit of successive pregnancies. For example, two years on a normal diet are needed to restore the 1000 mg of iron required for a single gestation. Often full lactation is the only effective means of increasing the birth interval in the rural society.

Besides maternal age, parity and the birth interval, perinatal mortality is also influenced by the personal and social characteristics of the mother as well as by the quality of medical and obstetric care she receives. Thus, in the British perinatal mortality survey it was possible to identify two broad categories. In one group it was obvious that death could have been averted by good obstetric care. Such cases formed 44 per cent of all perinatal deaths. The remaining 56 per cent were considered to be less amenable to obstetric care but were mainly related

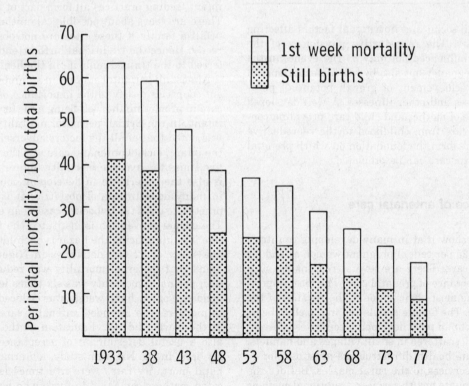

Figure 22.1   Trends in perinatal mortality in England and Wales 1933–1977

Table 22.1   Age at marriage in Java, Indonesia

Age (years)	Rural		Urban	
	Mojolama (No. = 777)	East Java (No. = 1225)	Surabaya (No. = 2664)	Semarang (No. = 1598)
10–14	18.1%	33.9%	20.4%	19.3%
15–19	58.0%	54.3%	58.3%	52.3%
20–24	20.9%	11.8%	16.4%	22.6%
25 and over	3.0%	–	4.9%	5.8%
Mode (years)	17	16	17	17

Table 22.2   Age at marriage in Hyderabad, India

Area	No.	Age (years)					
		<7	7–10	10–12	12–14	14–16	>16
Rural area 1	100	–	12	18	32	30	8
Rural area 2	300	9	69	141	67	12	2
Urban	100	–	4	2	16	46	18

Table 22.3   Age at first delivery in Hyderabad, India

Area	No.	Age (years)			
		<16	16–18	18–20	>20
Rural	100	28	44	20	8
Urban	100	10	48	22	20

to personal, social and nutritional factors affecting the mothers. The reproductive physiology of the mother is influenced not only by the events in the current pregnancy but also by her life experience of nutrition, achievement of growth potential, parasitic diseases and other illnesses. A well developed programme of mother and child care providing continuity of care from childhood to the reproductive phase of life form the foundation on which prenatal and obstetric care can be promoted.

Importance of antenatal care

Estimates show that in many developing countries only 20 to 25 per cent of pregnant women attend for antenatal care. There are several reasons for such a poor acceptance of prenatal care. The most important and the most obvious one is the rurality of the population. The female population in the child bearing age group in most developing countries is essentially rural, scattered in small villages and hamlets. An adequate health infrastructure must develop to carry the services to the rural masses. Besides the lack of adequate health services, traditional customs and practices prevent rural women from making use

of whatever services exist. Birth is an important event in the life of an individual and there are many 'rites of passage' related to the process. Dietary restrictions, beliefs regarding the 'evil eye', place and method of delivery, disposal of the placenta, isolation of the mother during the puerperium and infant feeding practices all form part of these rites. There are fears about possible calamities that may befall a family if these rites are not observed correctly. Hence the traditional birth attendant is preferred to the trained midwife in the health centre.

Almost all perinatal surveys in a number of different countries testify to the importance of antenatal care in promoting the well-being and survival of the infant. In the British perinatal mortality survey it was noted that of all the factors adversely affecting the infant, lack of antenatal care was the worst with five times the average mortality (figure 22.2). This is also the experience in developing countries and in many departments of obstetrics it is the usual practice to treat the unbooked case as an emergency. The earlier prevention is instituted the more effective it is in reducing the hazards of childbearing. In one study of 12 000 deliveries in Nigeria, it was found that maternal mortality was reduced fifteen fold, perinatal mortality was six times less and the incidence of low birth weight was reduced three fold in mothers who attended antenatal care compared to those who did not. Education of the mother is also a useful determinant of acceptance of health services. In the Nigerian study, maternal and perinatal mortality rates were five times less in educated mothers compared to those who had received no formal education.

The traditional birth attendant

Several countries are experimenting with new approaches for improving prenatal care in rural areas. The trained nurse or midwife is not culturally acceptable in many peasant societies. For example, it has been observed that the auxiliary nurse/midwife (ANM) in India delivers as few as 40 to 60 babies a year and almost all of them are within a radius of two miles from the health centre. It has therefore been suggested that the indigenous midwife or 'dai' should be given practical training in selection of cases for referral, in clean handling of the mother in labour and so on, and thus made a part of the overall MCH programme in the area. Such an approach has been successfully implemented in Sudan and Indonesia.

Priorities in perinatal care

A programme of perinatal care in developing countries should have its own specific priorities. The emphasis wil be more on the establishment of a basis for healthy motherhood and childhood rather than the diagnosis of abnormalities. As emphasised above, true prevention begins even before pregnancy through promotion of good growth, nutrition and physical and mental health. Preventive measures during pregnancy are to be considered as second line of defence. Measures at the time of delivery and in the newborn period, such as resuscitation and intensive care are increasingly rarely resorted to and are the least rewarding.

During pregnancy the first need is to ensure that all pregnant women have access to a basic level of health care. Higher skills and facilities should then be made available to those at high risk. The main reason for improvement in perinatal mortality rates in China is the extensive coverage with antenatal services using auxiliaries and 'barefoot doctors'.

The main objectives of antenatal care in developing countries are nutrition education, prevention and treatment of anaemia and eradication of the parasitic load. Several studies have emphasised the importance of maternal nutrition in ensuring adequate foetal growth. A significant correlation between maternal triceps skinfold thickness and the weight and length of the infant was found in South India. In Tanzania it has been observed that to have a baby weighing 3.1 kg a mother should consume 2200 calories daily and only 20 per cent of the women had as much. Many women in the low socio-economic group enter pregnancy after a childhood characterised by under-nutrition and recurrent illnesses. In Guatemala where several detailed studies on maternal nutrition in pregnancy have been conducted during the past several years it was noted

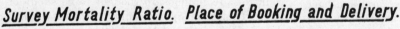

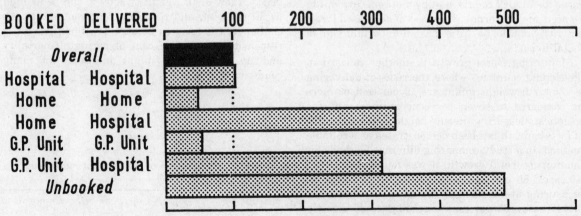

Mortality Ratios by Places of Booking and Delivery

Figure 22.2   Perinatal mortality in England and Wales – 1958. Importance of antenatal care
(Source: Butler and Bonham, 1963)

that the average maternal height was 149 cm which is 12 cm less than the average height for white women in the USA. Much of this low maternal height was accounted for by growth retardation during the first seven years of life. The average weight gain during pregnancy in Guatemala and in several studies reported from other developing countries was 7 kg, which is about half of that in well-nourished women in more affluent societies. Food supplementation studies in Guatemala revealed that increasing the caloric intake in pregnancy contributed to improved foetal growth.

Anaemia is also widespread in most developing countries. In one study of nutritional anaemia in pregnancy conducted in seven Latin American countries, 38.5 per cent of pregnant women studied were anaemic.

The village midwife can make a major contribution by providing nutrition education and by the distribution of iron and folic acid tablets to pregnant women. She can also help by carrying out primary selection on the basis of age, parity, stature, previous obstetric history and previous history of stillbirths or neonatal deaths, and persuading such women to deliver at the health centre.

Village midwives can be trained to identify problems and foetal risks during the course of a normal pregnancy. For example, close association has been demonstrated between foetal activity and foetal wellbeing. A 12-hour daily foetal movement count records ten movements in 12 hours in the case of most healthy infants. Reduction of movements below this level indicates impaired foetal welfare. It should be possible to identify such cases and refer them to the health centre or hospital early. In most cases foetal kick counts kept by mothers turn out to be accurate. Maternal awareness of decreased foetal activity can thus be utilised as an important sign of foetal hypoxia.

Monitoring foetal growth is another concern in developing countries where the risks of delivering a low birth weight infant are 19 per cent or more as compared to seven per cent in more affluent societies. Measuring uterine height as an indicator of foetal growth has been demonstrated as a reliable method. In a study comparing different methods for monitoring foetal growth, it was found that out of 44 cases, 86 per cent were diagnosed correctly by measuring uterine height. On the other hand, out of 147 cases, 69 per cent were diagnosed correctly using the biparietal diameter and out of 44 cases using urinary oestrogen level, 70 per cent were diagnosed (table 22.4). By comparison, ultrasound gave a 75 per cent correct assessment of foetal growth.

In all communities it should be possible to identify the 10th and 90th percentile of uterine heights at 26 weeks (6 months), 30 weeks (7 months) and 35 weeks (8 months) of pregnancy. Tape measures with appropriately coloured segments can then be used by village midwives to identify for referral, the mother in whom foetal growth appears inadequate.

Major associates of perinatal mortality: low birth weight, infection and congenital abnormality

Studies of perinatal mortality in several countries have revealed that intrauterine growth of the foetus and the subsequent weight of the baby at birth are closely related to the outcome of pregnancy. In general, the perinatal mortality rates in western countries are 30–35 times higher in infants weighing 2500 g or less at birth compared to those with higher birth weights. It has also been demonstrated that a difference of as little as three per cent in the number of live-born infants of low birth weight raises the perinatal and infant mortality rate by 5 per 1000. Thus low birth weight is undoubtedly an important factor associated with perinatal mortality.

It is estimated that about 22 million low birth weight babies are born each year, which is equivalent to one-sixth of total births. Only five per cent of these are in developed countries and are mostly pre-term. Of the remaining 21 million in developing countries, 16 million are thought to be small-for-dates. Thus in many developing countries the incidence of low birth weight (<2500 g) can be as high as 30 per cent, and therefore represents a serious challenge, the more so because low birth weight is responsible for 70 per cent of perinatal mortality and up to half the infant mortality in many countries.

Table 22.4 Comparison of methods for monitoring foetal growth

Method	No.	Diagnosed correctly	Undiagnosed
Uterine height	44	86%	14%
Biparietal diameter	147	69%	31%
Urinary oestrogens	44	70%	30%
Ultrasound	28	75%	25%

Infection

After the baby is born, an important factor in his survival is the availability of breast milk. In this matter, the establishment of successful lactation is as crucial as prenatal care and supervised labour. The way in which a pregnant woman's metabolism changes so that she lays down stores of nutrients to provide for lactation; the hormonal changes in pregnancy and at parturition culminating in the flow of milk; the physical changes in the mammary gland in response to the hormonal variations during pregnancy; the flow of immune substances in the mother's milk; and so on, all point to the fact that lactation is an integral part of the process of reproduction in which parturition is a milestone but not the end.

In quoting perinatal mortality figures, it is the usual practice now to consider the deaths occurring in the first week of life. For the developing countries it may be more useful to include also some of the late neonatal deaths. Such a practice would then take into account deaths due to neonatal tetanus and would provide a more correct picture of the hazards of birth in a traditional society. In a study of 11 villages in the Punjab in India, tetanus was found to be responsible for 20.3 deaths per 1000 live births. It was further shown that these deaths can be reduced by 66 per cent if the indigenous midwife can be taught clean cord-handling techniques and by administering tetanus toxoid to the mother during pregnancy. Thus another major contributor to perinatal mortality in developing countries can be tackled by relatively simple means.

Besides tetanus and diarrhoea, infection has been recognised as an important perinatal hazard, especially for babies of low birth weight. Mortality rates of up to 80 per 1000 births have been reported due to infection in studies from Africa, New Guinea and India.

Foetal malnutrition and maternal mortality

These are two priorities needing urgent attention. As we have seen rates of low birth weight (<2500 g) tend to be much higher in developing countries. In some societies between a third to a half of all newborns fall into this category. Most cases are due to undernutrition in the mother. Supplementation of pregnant women during the rainy season in the Gambia, when food supplies run low and there is heavy physical work to be done on the land, helped to raise average birth weight. The incidence of low birth weight fell from 28 per cent to five per cent.

Intrauterine growth is partly under intrinsic control (for example genetic and hormonal determinants), and partly dependent on the supply and transfer of nutrients as well as energy across the placenta. The nutritional status of the woman before pregnancy, nutritional demands of repeated pregnancies and diet during pregnancy all affect foetal growth. Socio-economic development, particularly when it benefits women, is associated with a reduction in the incidence of low birth weight as indeed has been the case in China, Sri Lanka, and the Indian state of Kerala. On the other hand the high rates of low birth weight in some developing countries indicate that in these countries a large proportion of individuals begin life with an experience of malnutrition, and that malnutrition is likely to remain a life long companion.

Growth retarded foetuses are prone to intrauterine asphyxia. Not only is placental gaseous exchange compromised, but also there are low reserves of cardiac glycogen so that the foetus is less able to cope with asphyxia. Other complications like recurrent apnoea, periventricular brain ischaemia and haemorrhage, hypoglycaemia and sepsis are also more frequent in low birth weight infants.

In foetal life maximum linear growth occurs at 20 weeks of gestation, and of body weight at 34 weeks. Growth retardation occurring largely in the third trimester results in asymmetrical growth from which 'catch-up' in late infancy is possible, particularly with breast feeding. Such catch-up is more difficult in symmetrically growth retarded babies in whom growth retardation has been prolonged and severe.

When born at term, growth retarded babies have only a slightly increased risk of major handicaps like cerebral palsy. But between 10 and 35 per cent may have minimal cerebral dysfunction like speech and language problems, attention deficits, learning problems, and minor neurological problems. In preterm *and* small for date babies the incidence of major handicaps is much higher than in their term born counterparts. In most cases it is the degree of prematurity which determines the outcome.

Maternal mortality

Studies initiated in a number of countries in the 1970s by the World Health Organisation revealed that world-wide about 500 000 maternal deaths occur annually, the majority in the developing countries. Maternal mortality rates are 200 times higher in the developing countries compared to Europe and North America. Since the average number of children borne is four to six in the less developed countries compared to one to two in the more developed countries the average life time risk of dying due to pregnancy related causes is also high. It varies from 1 in 50 to as high as 1 in 14 in some countries of sub-Saharan Africa. By comparison the average lifetime risk in the more developed countries is between 1 in 4000 and 1 in 10 000.

Every maternal death carries with it the risk of perinatal mortality for the infant. Hence reduction of maternal mortality is an important aspect of the overall programme for the reduction of perinatal mortality. The main causes of maternal deaths are haemorrhage, difficult labour, eclampsia, sepsis and anaemia. But the roots lie in deficiencies and discrimination women suffer since birth, and which continue throughout childhood and adolescence into adult life.

It is estimated that in some countries between 25 and 50 per cent of maternal deaths are due to illegal abortion, and that over 50 per cent of women worldwide do not have the assistance of a trained person during labour.

The immediate intervention needed for the reduction of maternal mortality is to bring the essential elements of obstetric care (good antenatal care; skilled assistance at the time of labour; care of obstetric emergencies; transfusion services; asepsis) as near as possible to the woman in labour. This is part of the Safe Motherhood Initiative launched by the World Health Organisation.

Prospects for better perinatal health in developing countries

There is little difference between the perinatal risks in the most advantaged groups in different countries including between developed and developing countries. The major determinant of the overall perinatal mortality rate in any nation is the proportion of the population at socio-economic disadvantage and the extent of the deprivation. In this respect care of the pregnant woman and provision of services need to be thought of as a social service. Lack of adequate prenatal care puts the mother and her infant at a considerable disadvantage.

Intensive care units and similar other highly technical and expensive services will have the least influence on reducing perinatal mortality as long as the bulk of the population is without basic services. Improved nutrition, prevention of anaemia, clean and hygienic methods of delivery are easy to provide and do not require highly trained personnel. In this respect the experience of several countries with

training traditional birth attendants has proved to be rewarding.

Infections in the neonatal period including tetanus are preventable and should be provided for even in the most elementary services. Establishment of adequate lactation in all mothers helps to maintain the life-line of the infant in the critical months after birth. These measures are simple and within the reach of all modest health budgets in rural districts.

Further reading

Alberman E. Prospects for better perinatal health. *Lancet* 1980; i: 189–92.

Butler N R, Bonham D G. *Perinatal mortality*. The first report of the 1958 British Perinatal Mortality Survey. Edinburgh and London: Livingstone, 1963.

Butler N R, Alberman E. (eds.) *Perinatal problems*. The second report of the 1958 British Perinatal Mortality Survey. Edinburgh and London: Livingstone, 1969.

Chalmers I. Better perinatal health, Shanghai. *Lancet* 1980; i: 137–9.

Chamberlain G. Background to perinatal health. *Lancet* 1979; ii: 1061–3.

Chiswick M. Intrauterine growth retardation *Brit Med J* 1985; 291: 845–848.

Crosby W M. Studies in foetal malnutrition. *Am J Dis Childh* 1991; 145: 871–876.

Ebrahim G J. Practical Mother and Child Health in Developing Countries. London: Macmillan Press Ltd. 1991 (4th Ed.).

Editorial. Maternal Health in Sub-Saharan Africa. *Lancet* 1987; i: 255–257.

Fleming A F. Tropical Obstetrics and Gynaecology. 1. Anaemia in pregnancy in tropical Africa. *Trans Roy Soc Trop Med Hyg* 1989; 83: 441–448.

Harrison K A. Better perinatal health – Nigeria. *Lancet* 1979; ii: 1229–32.

Kramer M S. Determinants of low birth weight: methodological assessment and meta analysis. *Bull Wld Hlth Org* 1987; 65: 663–737.

Mahler H. The Safe Motherhood Initiative. *Lancet* 1987; i: 668–670.

Manglacas A M, Simons J. *The potential of the traditional birth attendant*. Geneva: World Health Organisation, 1986.

Royston E, Armstrong S. *Preventing maternal deaths*. World Health Organisation, 1989.

Sterky G, Mellander L. (eds.) *Birth weight distribution – an indicator of social development*. Report from a SAREC/WHO Workshop No. R:2 1978. Uppsala: Swedish Agency for Research Co-operation with Developing Countries, 1978.

World Health Organisation. *The prevention of perinatal morbidity and mortality*. Geneva: World Health Organisation 1972; Public Health Paper No. 42.

World Heath Organisation. *Maternal care for the reduction of perinatal and neonatal mortality*. Geneva: World Health Organisation, 1986.

23 *Illness in the newborn – diagnosis and management*

Several maternal conditions in pregnancy are known to be associated with poor foetal growth or with difficulty in adjustment of the newborn to extrauterine life. Any of the following circumstances should alert the physician, and the baby should be kept under close observation for the first two to three days of life.

History

A history of previous perinatal deaths or illnesses or abnormality in infants. These may result from

(1) Lack of antenatal and obstetric care.
(2) Poor social and hygienic conditions in the home.
(3) Ignorance of the mother regarding care of the newborn.
(4) Failure of lactation.
(5) Genetically determined disease.
(6) Conditions which are not genetically determined but may recur in subsequent pregnancies, for example small-for-date infants, or tetanus.

Lack of antenatal care

Any existing complication of pregnancy will have remained undiagnosed and not treated, with the result that it may have reached an advanced stage with serious effects on the foetus. In many of such unbooked cases, the family will have decided to deliver the mother at home in the traditional way, but when things go wrong or complications are suspected, the mother is brought to hospital. Hence all unbooked cases should be considered as emergencies and the baby should be admitted to the observation nursery for 48 hours.

Complications of pregnancy

These can affect foetal growth because of their effect on placental function or indirectly through the effect of drugs used for treatment. The complications to be looked for are

(1) Toxaemia or hypertension in which foetal growth is affected so that the baby is born small-for-dates. Treatment with drugs such as chlorthiazide and Serpasil (reserpine) can also adversely affect the foetus.
(2) Polyhydramnios and oligohydramnios. Both these conditions are known to be associated with congenital abnormalities in the baby.
(3) Antepartum haemorrhage.
(4) Malpresentation.
(5) Prolonged rupture of the membrane which can lead to chorio-amnionitis and sepsis in the newborn due to ascending infection from the birth passages.

Medical conditions

Medical conditions in the mother existing before the pregnancy or which may have developed during the course of the pregnancy, for example,

(1) Diabetes. The baby is born large for dates and is at risk of developing respiratory distress syndrome or hypoglycaemia.
(2) Sickle cell anaemia. The baby is at greater than average risk of perinatal asphyxia.
(3) Tuberculosis, leprosy or other illnesses in the mother.
(4) Psychiatric illness in the mother or a known social problem in the family.
(5) Drugs administered to the mother during the pregnancy. Table 23.1 lists such drugs and the effect produced on the foetus.

Table 23.1 Effects of drugs on the foetus

Drug	Effect in the foetus or newborn
Anaesthetic	Respiratory depression
Streptomycin	Neonatal deafness
Tetracycline	Staining of deciduous teeth
Sulfonamides	Coagulation defects
Quinine	(In heavy doses may cause abortion
	(Deafness
	(Thrombocytopaenic purpura)
Antimitotics	Foetal death or malformation
Thiazides	Thrombocytopaenia
Progesterone	Masculinisation
Pyridoxine	Pyridoxine-dependent convulsions
Morphine	Respiratory depression
Vitamin D	Infantile hypercalcaemia
Phenobarbitone	Coagulation defects

A history of abnormal liquor – blood or meconium-stained or foul-smelling

Whenever possible the placenta should also be included in the examination. In many instances the presence of gross pathology in the placenta can provide additional information about events leading to the disorder seen in the newborn. Thus, in some cases of unexplained birth asphyxia there is a firm adherent retroplacental clot indicating that antepartum haemorrhage had occurred and led to partial separation of the placenta. Infarcts are common in toxaemia and may be the cause of birth asphyxia especially when they are large; they occur on the maternal surface of the placenta and are centrally situated. Offensive smell in the placenta associated with a cloudy appearance of the membranes is a sign of chorio-amnionitis due to ascending infection from the birth canal and usually occurs in cases of prolonged rupture of the membranes. Examination of the placenta is most useful in arriving at a diagnosis of foetal haemorrhage, which is commonly mistaken for antepartum haemorrhage at the time of delivery, and in cases of the twin transfusion syndrome, when dissection of the placenta may reveal communication between the two circulations.

Acute emergencies

Life-threatening situations can arise at different times in neonatal life. Soon after birth an emergency may occur due to failure of establishment or maintenance of respiration. In the first few days of neonatal life emergencies are commonly due to congenital defects incompatible with extrauterine existence or due to low birthweight. Emergencies in late neonatal life are either of metabolic origin or secondary to birth trauma or due to infections. In the newborn, prompt treatment of any disease process is important because deterioration can be very rapid and therefore alertness in noting any deviation from the normal is necessary.

Failure to cry at birth

Failure to cry at birth is a common emergency and needs prompt resuscitative measures. In most cases it will be the midwife who has to resuscitate the baby and so should be conversant with the procedure.

Certain obstetric situations are commonly associated with asphyxia of the newborn, and so difficulties should be anticipated when such conditions occur, and resuscitation equipment should be at hand. These conditions are

(1) Maternal states such as
   (a) Age over 35 years.
   (b) Grand multiparity.
   (c) Diseases like diabetes or toxaemia.
(2) Obstetric factors such as
   (a) Prolonged second stage of labour.
   (b) Prolonged rupture of membranes.
   (c) Prolapse of the cord or cord entanglements.
   (d) Difficulty with the delivery of shoulders.
(3) Foetal distress as manifested by
   (a) Meconium-stained liquor.
   (b) Tachycardia of more than 160 per minute or bradycardia of less than 100 per minute.
(4) Drugs or anaesthetics administered to the mother.

The basic principles of resuscitation are to establish and maintain an airway and to secure adequate ventilation and circulation.

(1) Establishment of the airway – all mucus in the mouth should be cleansed and the oropharynx should be sucked out with a mucus catheter. The drainage of secretions is helped by a head low position of the baby. In the collapsed patient the tongue tends to fall backwards and blocks the air passages. An airway should be inserted to prevent this.
(2) Oxygen administration – even with a feeble gasping respiration, the newborn can take in more oxygen than during vigorous artificial respiration. As soon as an adequate airway has been established, oxygen should be administered either by a funnel (flow rate 4

litres/minute) or by a nasal catheter (flow rate 1 litre/minute).

(3) Naloxone, a narcotic antagonist is of use if respiratory depression is known to be due to morphine or its analogues given to the mother. Its indiscriminate use in all cases of asphyxia is dangerous because it may cause depression of the respiratory centre. (Dose – 60 µg/kg intravenously or 200 µg intramuscularly as a single dose.)

(4) Intermittent positive pressure by mouth-to-mouth breathing is an effective way of ventilating the lungs of a baby who has failed to establish respiration. Endotracheal intubation provides better access to the lungs but requires skill. It has the added advantage that the cords can be inspected before intubation and any mucus or meconium is aspirated under vision. After insertion the endotracheal tube is connected to a supply of 40 per cent oxygen flowing at a rate of 2 litres/minute, and a pressure of not more than 30–35 cm of water. By using the Y-adaptor and intermittently occluding the other limb of the Y, the lungs can be inflated intermittently. Alternatively, the attendant blows on the endotracheal tube using only the cheek muscles, at a rate of 30–40 per minute.

A number of devices for mask and bag ventilation are available on the market. For effective action the face mask should have a pneumatic rim to obtain a tight seal on the infant's face. The bag should have a volume of at least 500 ml and should be fitted with a blow off valve. A better approach is to attach a T-piece to the face mask and the other end to an oxygen cylinder, with oxygen flowing at a pressure of 20 to 30 cm of water. Intermittent occlusion, with a finger, of the open end of the T-tube provides the intermittent pressure for ventilation.

(5) If the baby is limp, pale, or cyanosed and with low or absent heart rate, external cardiac massage should be commenced before intubation and continued during resuscitation. In doing cardiac massage the heart is compressed rhythmically between the sternum and the vertebral column (rate 80–100/minute).

(6) A baby who has experienced severe apnoea with limpness, cyanosis and bradycardia develops acidosis rapidly and should be given alkali as soon as adequate respiration has been established. 10 ml of 8.4 per cent sodium bicarbonate should be administered through an umbilical cannula, followed by 5 ml or 20 per cent dextrose given slowly. In one study involving 1668 patients, foetal acidaemia (pH 7.25 or less) occurred in 45 of the 295 patients who showed clinical signs of foetal distress. Foetal tachycardia was the presenting sign in 33 of these 45 patients.

When dealing with respiratory difficulties in the newborn it is important to remember the following general rules

(1) Infants who have experienced difficulty in establishing respiration will invariably show difficulty in maintaining respiration. Hence those who needed resuscitation at birth should be kept under observation for a minimum period of 24 hours and checked for cyanotic spells, apnoea, irregular respirations or tachypnoea.

(2) Respiratory difficulties in the low birth weight baby are never benign and an early chest X-ray should be taken to help establish the diagnosis.

(3) In the first hours of life, mild tachypnoea may occur, but if a baby of low birth weight shows a respiratory rate of over 50 per minute in the second hour of life, he should be watched for the development of the respiratory distress syndrome.

(4) If meconium has been passed in utero due to foetal distress, it may be inhaled and give rise to chemical irritation of the tracheobronchial tree.

Congenital malformations of the gastro-intestinal tract

A large proportion of babies requiring emergency surgery in the first few days of life do so because of congenital abnormalities in the gastro-intestinal tract. The final outcome in such babies depends largely upon the rapidity of diagnosis and corrective surgery before complications set in. Presence of certain warning signs should alert the obstetrician, and the baby should be kept under observation. These signs are

(1) Polyhydramnios: in about 75 per cent of such babies there is obstruction of the upper small intestine.

(2) Presence of only two vessels in the umbilical cord.

A baby with intestinal obstruction develops abdominal distension, vomiting, and fails to pass meconium in the first 24 hours. Sometimes with high intestinal obstruction a mucoid grey stool may be passed and create confusion. When the above triad of symptoms occurs a stomach tube should be passed and the stomach emptied. If at the first emptying more than 40 ml of fluid is obtained and especially if there is presence of bile, obstruction should be suspected and the following studies should be carried out

(1) Repeated physical examination for intestinal patterns of the abdominal wall, or distension of abdomen.
(2) Digital examination of the rectum, for example, empty rectum in Hirschsprung's disease.
(3) Examination of the contents of the rectum. Blood may be passed per rectum in volvulus of the small bowel.
(4) X-ray studies – plain views of the abdomen in the erect position, postero-anterior and lateral; also a plain view of the abdomen in the supine position.

The presence of air, fluid levels and the delineation of part of the bowel with air will show whether there is obstruction and its level. In most cases contrast studies are not needed, but if undertaken, lipiodol or hyapaque should be used instead of barium.

The baby with intestinal obstruction due to a congenital anomaly does not look ill and it is therefore necessary to investigate any vomiting in the first few days of life, especially if bile-stained. By the time the baby begins to look ill, pathological changes in the bowel are far advanced.

Delay in diagnosis and treatment may lead to the following complications: electrolyte imbalance; aspiration pneumonia; perforation of the gut due to enterocolitis; strangulation and gangrene due to obliteration of blood supply.

The baby with *oesophageal atresia* shows excessive salivation, has drooling from the mouth and will have been reported as 'mucusy'. In some cases there is also respiratory distress. Attempts at feeding will result in choking and respiratory distress. It is important to make a firm diagnosis before any feeds are offered in order to avoid aspiration and lung infection.

Diagnosis is established by attempting to pass a stomach tube, when an obstruction is felt at the site of the atresia. A soft catheter will get curled up in the upper oesophageal pouch and give the false impression of the tube passing into the stomach. Hence the contents should be aspirated and tested with litmus paper for acidity. A small quantity of lipiodol is injected into the tube and an X-ray taken to outline the site of the atresia, together with any fistulous connections to the respiratory tract.

A *diaphragmatic hernia* is suspected in cases of respiratory distress at birth which fail to respond to early resuscitative measures. Physical examination will reveal signs of mediastinal shift to the opposite side. On suspicion, X-ray of the chest should be taken to confirm the diagnosis. An early X-ray is often difficult to interpret because air may not have reached the bowel, so the loops of the intestines are not outlined well.

Both oesophageal atresia and diaphragmatic hernia not uncommonly present with signs of respiratory distress rather than symptoms and signs indicating pathology in the gastro-intestinal tract.

Some of the other malformations requiring early management or emergency surgery are exomphalos, open meningocele, Pierre Robin syndrome and choanal atresia.

Haemorrhage

Any obvious bleeding in the newborn should be treated with utmost care. The total blood volume of the newborn is 350 ml and a loss of as little as 15–30 ml (½–1 oz) is tolerated poorly. The commonest cause of bleeding is a slipped ligature from the umbilical stump or oozing from it. In a baby who is well wrapped up in clothing, such bleeding may go unnoticed for several hours. Other causes of acute blood loss in the newborn are incision of the placenta during a Caesarean section, tear of the umbilical cord during a difficult delivery, and an anomalous connection of the cord with the placenta.

A large cephalhaematoma may cause an appreciable loss of blood, and there is also an added threat of jaundice as the breakdown products of haemoglobin get absorbed into the circulation. For all practical purposes, cephalhaematomas are best left alone because of the danger of introducing infection, unless the baby is in danger of hyperbilirubinaemia.

Subaponeurotic haemorrhages can be severe and cause exsanguination. It has been observed that such haemorrhages are more common after vacuum deliveries, and are very often associated with an underlying haemorrhagic tendency in the newborn.

Bleeding in the gastro-intestinal tract is a frequent symptom in the newborn period. Swallowed maternal blood may appear as malaena or as blood-stained vomitus but can be excluded by Apt's test for foetal haemoglobin. This test depends on the fact that adult haemoglobin is denatured by 1 per cent sodium hydroxide, whereas foetal haemoglobin remains unaffected. If the test shows the presence of foetal haemoglobin, the baby should be given an injection of 1 mg vitamin K1 and the haemoglobin checked at repeated intervals for signs of severe anaemia. As mentioned above, volvulus of the gut can present with intestinal bleeding; hence all babies with malaena or passing of blood per rectum should be observed carefully and in cases of doubt a plain X-ray of the abdomen should be taken.

Bleeding may be concealed, as when a baby bleeds into the maternal circulation, or when one twin bleeds into another. On the other hand, haemorrhage from the baby might have been mistaken as antepartum haemorrhage or as maternal blood loss during labour. In such cases, the baby is found to be ill soon after delivery. There is pallor or grey colour; air hunger and tachycardia also occur. Anaemia is confirmed by haemoglobin estimation and urgent blood transfusion may be required. In the case of one twin bleeding into another, the recipient twin will also be in danger because of the overloading of his circulation.

Concealed haemorrhage may occur some time after birth, into an internal organ, and cause sudden collapse. Thus, haemorrhages in the liver, kidneys, lungs or the brain are found at autopsy and are the cause of sudden and unexpected death in otherwise healthy newborns.

Transfusion in the newborn

In an emergency, blood transfusion can be commenced using uncross-matched blood of the same ABO and Rh groups as of the baby while the results of cross-matching are awaited. Samples of blood and serum should be obtained from both the baby and the mother. If the baby's blood group is O, the blood used for transfusion should also be of group O which has been cross-matched against the mother's serum. If the baby's blood group is A, B or AB, the blood used for transfusion should be of the same ABO group as the baby and cross-matched against the baby's serum.

Any available peripheral vein can be utilised for transfusion using the scalp vein needle or a cut-down. If the umbilical vein is patent and the cord stump is clean the umbilical route may be found to be the most convenient.

The quantity of blood infused at any one time should not exceed 10 ml/kg body weight in 24 hours and should be infused as slowly as possible, never to exceed four to five drops per minute.

Twitching and fits

It is often difficult to distinguish between normal and abnormal behaviour in the newborn and this is particularly true in respect of abnormality of movements. A normal newborn may show momentary

jerks, especially on waking, or tremors of the jaw during crying. On the other hand, generalised tonic – clonic convulsions are rare in the newborn period, though neonatal fits may have some tonic and clonic movements. The commonest form of presentation of neonatal fits are eye blinking or rolling, jerking movements at a rate of one to three per second, 'jitteriness', jerky nystagmus and chewing movements.

The incidence reported in different studies varies from 8.6 to 14.6 per 1000 births. There are two peak periods when fits occur – within the first 48 hours and after 120 hours of birth. The earlier fits are most likely to be associated with cerebral birth injury while fits occurring later are usually due to metabolic disturbance. In all instances it is important to control the fits by means of injected paraldehyde at a rate of 0.2 ml/kg or injected phenobarbitone at a rate of 3 mg/kg body weight. Phenytoin should be avoided in the newborn period because of the possibility of damage to the rapidly developing cerebellum of the baby.

The common causes of fits in the newborn period are

(1) Prenatal conditions, for example, malformation of the brain or intrauterine infections such as toxoplasmosis, rubella, or cytomegalovirus infection.
(2) Factors operating during birth causing hypoxia or cerebral injury.
(3) Metabolic conditions operating after birth, such as hypoglycaemia, hypocalcaemia, electrolyte disturbances and rarely inborn errors of metabolism.
(4) Sepsis, as in meningitis and tetanus.
(5) Withdrawal of drugs, as in the case of pyridoxine.

The effects of hypoxia and birth trauma are usually self-limiting and gradual recovery takes place over a few days. The diagnosis of rubella, toxoplasmosis and other intrauterine infections may be suspected from the antenatal history, from the involvement of other organs such as the heart and the liver and occasionally from cerebral calcification seen on skull X-ray. Serological studies are necessary to confirm the diagnosis. Hypoglycaemia as a cause of fits is diagnosed when at least two consecutive blood sugar estimations show levels below 40 mg/100 ml in the baby with average birth weight and lower than 20 mg/100 ml in the baby with low birth weight. The Dextrostix is an easy and reliable method of monitoring blood sugar in the newborn and should be used for regular blood sugar estimations in conditions where hypoglycaemia is known to occur, for example, in the baby with low birth weight, especially if small-for-dates, maternal diabetes, birth asphyxia, and haemolytic disease of the newborn. Experience has shown that in all these states, hypoglycaemia can be prevented by early feeding of infants. It responds well to glucose administration and is usually short-lived. Rarely, hypoglycaemia may be due to an inborn error of metabolism as in leucine sensitivity, fructose intolerance, galactosaemia and glycogen storage disease, or a pancreatic cell tumour. In all these conditions, hypoglycaemia is persistent and does not respond to early feeding. On the other hand, in leucine sensitivity, galactosaemia and fructose intolerance hypoglycaemia persists on milk feeding and disappears when the baby is kept on oral glucose.

The brain cells are dependent upon a constant supply of glucose in the blood stream for normal functioning and it is now generally accepted that hypoglycaemia per se can lead to neuronal damage in the newborn. On confirming the diagnosis, therapy should commence immediately with 50 per cent glucose, 1–2 ml/kg, given intravenously and followed by infusion of 15 per cent glucose in N/5 saline at the rate of 75–100 ml/kg in 24 hours. Oral feeding with breast milk should be commenced immediately except in the rare case of a contraindication to milk feeding.

Jaundice in the first 24 hours of life

During foetal life, the placenta plays an important role in the excretion of bilirubin by the foetus. It transfers unconjugated bilirubin from the foetus to the maternal circulation for excretion by the maternal liver. At birth, the total bilirubin level is below 3 mg/100 ml in all normal newborns. If excessive haemolysis occurs in foetal life, the placenta is swamped with large quantities of bilirubin and cannot clear all its load, with the result that the baby is born with high levels of bilirubin in the blood or is clinically jaundiced. Soon after birth, the baby's liver has to take over the function of conjugation and excretion of bilirubin. The normal newborn produces an average of 8.5 mg/kg of bilirubin per day, which is twice the rate in the adult (3.8 mg/kg per day), and is due to the relatively larger red cell mass in the newborn and shorter life span of the cells in neonatal life. If the production of bilirubin is excessive, as happens during a haemolytic process, the blood bilirubin level rises and clinical jaundice is seen. Thus, any jaundice occurring within the first 24 hours of life is usually caused by a haemolytic process in the baby. The newborn is at

risk not only because of acute and severe anaemia but also due to the toxic effects of unconjugated bilirubin accumulating in the body tissues, especially in the brain cells. The risk of such a complication arises when bilirubin levels approach 20 mg/100 ml. Hence serum bilirubin should be estimated at regular intervals in all babies with clinical jaundice appearing in the first 24 hours of life. If at the first estimation the bilirubin level is above 12 mg/100 ml, and if there are daily increments of more than 4 mg/100 ml, further tests should be carried out to ascertain the cause and to arrange for an exchange transfusion. The commonest cause of haemolytic jaundice in the newborn is incompatibility between the blood types of the baby and the mother. Haemolysins and antibodies in the mother's serum, which may be pre-existing as in ABO incompatibility or may be produced in response to sensitisation as in Rh incompatibility, traverse the placenta into the baby's circulation and cause haemolysis of red cells. The purpose of the exchange transfusion is to remove the sensitised red blood cells of the baby and to replace them with compatible normal cells from the donor, and to 'wash out' the bilirubin and antibody in the baby's circulation by replacing his blood plasma with normal plasma in the donor blood.

In Western Europe the commonest cause of haemolytic jaundice in the newborn is incompatibility in the Rhesus blood groups. In tropical Africa and in many countries of Asia this condition is relatively rare, the proportion of people who are Rhesus negative comprising one to three per cent of the population as compared to 15 per cent in Western Europe. Hence, incompatibility in the ABO blood groups is more often the cause of neonatal jaundice. In several countries, deficiency of the red blood cell enzyme G–6-PD is common in the population and can give rise to jaundice in the newborn. Kernicterus due to haemolytic jaundice occurring in newborns with deficiency of the enzyme G–6-PD has been reported in West Africa, in the Middle East and amongst the Chinese in South-east Asia.

Exchange transfusion

The type of donor blood should be carefully selected. If the exchange is performed for rhesus sensitisation, group O Rh-negative blood is used. With ABO incompatibility, group O Rh-specific blood may be used. Since naturally occurring haemolysins are present in group O blood, all such donor bloods should first be screened for haemolysins. Fresh blood is preferred to stored blood since the latter may give rise to electrolyte disturbances.

The volume of donor blood to be used at any one exchange is in the range of 150–200 ml per kg body weight and should not exceed 300 ml per kg body weight. In a baby weighing 3 kg an exchange transfusion with 500 ml of blood will accomplish a 40–50 per cent exchange.

The infant should be well sedated, and a feeding bottle with five per cent dextrose should be available as a pacifier if necessary.

Exchange transfusion is a major procedure, the success of which depends upon attention to every little detail. A team of three carries out the procedure and a fourth 'observer'maintains close watch on the baby's condition, respiration and pulse rate and also maintains a record of the volume put 'in' and taken 'out'.

All precautions should be taken to prevent air embolism which can be immediately fatal. The catheter needs to be introduced into the umbilical vein only as far as necessary to get a free flow of blood; if the tip of the catheter rests above the diaphragm, air may be sucked in during negative pressure in inspiration. The catheter should be watched for air bubbles and all apparatus should be leak-free.

The other dangers of exchange transfusion are congestive cardiac failure, electrolyte disturbances, sepsis introduced through the umbilical stump, transfusion reactions from mis-matched blood and a spreading thrombophlebitis in the portal tract as a late complication.

Problems in the first week of life

The newborn period is one of transition from intrauterine existence, in which the foetus is dependent upon the maternal organism for life support, to extrauterine life. In doing so, several of the baby's vital physiologic systems take over independent function. Thus, the placenta serves as the organ for gas exchange, nutrition intake and excretion of waste products in foetal life. Soon after birth, the various physiologic systems of the baby begin to take over these functions. For example, at birth the placental circulation is disconnected and the pulmonary circulation opens up so that important anatomic and functional changes occur in the heart and the lungs. The gastro-intestinal tract begins the function of digestion and absorption of nutrients which will provide the energy needs of basal metabolism, maintenance of body temperature and growth. The kidneys take over the secretion of urine, excretion of metabolic waste and maintenance of homeostasis. The endocrine system produces

hormones required for the metabolic function of tissues. The baby comes into a new physical environment which is much cooler than the body temperature of the mother so that temperature regulation becomes important.

Several factors can interfere with the process of adjustment. Events in prenatal life including intrauterine infection, inadequate nutrition, medical illnesses and abnormalities of pregnancy in the mother, exposure to drugs and chemicals, etc., can interfere with the growth of the foetus and give rise to abnormalities of development or function in the various organ systems of the baby and thus cause difficulties in the process of adjustment at birth. The process of labour itself and drugs administered to the mother during delivery often depress the physiologic reflexes of the foetus so that vital acts like initiation of respiration, or suckling and swallowing, become delayed or inefficient.

Certain disease processes are peculiar to the newborn period and ideally every newborn should be observed for at least 48 hours. Presence of any symptoms requires early and urgent management because the physiologic reserves of the newborn are small, and life-threatening situations can arise rapidly. Hence such symptoms are designated as 'danger signals' signifying their threat to the baby's survival. The common danger signals to be watched for in the newborn are discussed below.

Cyanosis, respiratory distress or apnoea

In the normal newborn, the peripheral circulation is sluggish and there may be a blue discoloration of the hands and feet, especially when exposed to cold. Some newborns may show circumoral cyanosis after a feed, the etiology of which is not understood. On the other hand, central cyanosis indicates poor oxygenation of blood and requires immediate investigation and treatment. Any generalised cyanosis with respiratory distress is nearly always due to lung pathology such as inadequate expansion of the lungs, extensive pneumonia, pneumothorax or a diaphragmatic hernia. X-ray of the chest is necessary to arrive at a definite diagnosis. Generalised cyanosis without respiratory distress and gross lung pathology is usually due to cardiac malformation with a right to left shunt. A murmur is not always present. On the other hand many cardiac malformations known to be associated with cyanosis, like Fallot's tetralogy, do not give rise to cyanosis in the first few weeks of life. Cyanosis with poor respiratory effort occurs when respiratory centres are depressed, either because of drugs or due to cerebral birth trauma.

Respiratory distress presents in various ways. The respiration may be irregular or gasping in character with spells of apnoea. On the other hand it may be very rapid. Costal recession or grunting may also be present. In the case of all newborns who are under observation for respiratory difficulties, the rate of breathing should be recorded at regular intervals. The trend of the respiratory rate is a useful guide to prognosis. A high mortality rate has been reported in those who show a steadily rising rate in the first few hours of life, especially if the heart rate is below 100 per minute.

The causes of respiratory distress in the first week of life are

(1) Extra pulmonary conditions
   (a) Lesions of the central nervous system: intracranial haemorrhage or anoxia; congenital malformations.
   (b) Congestive cardiac failure.
   (c) Oesophageal atresia.
   (d) Diaphragmatic hernia.
(2) Pulmonary conditions.
   (a) Hyaline membrane disease.
   (b) Massive aspiration syndrome.
   (c) Atelectasis.
   (d) Pneumonia.
   (e) Pneumothorax.
   (f) Congenital malformation of the upper respiratory tract.

The frequency with which the above conditions are diagnosed will vary from one place to another and with facilities available for diagnosis. In an analysis of 100 consecutive cases of respiratory distress in Dar-es-Salaam, Tanzania it was found that pneumonia and aspiration syndromes were more common than the hyaline membrane disease. In a study reported from the Hospital for Sick Children, Toronto, Canada, it was found that of 1981 babies admitted to the neonatal unit during 1960–61, 430 had respiratory distress occurring within the first 48 hours after birth. Of these, 228 died. The main causes were hyaline membrane disease in 142 (67 deaths), extrapulmonary conditions in 63 (28 deaths), pulmonary pathology other than hyaline membrane disease in 109 (54 deaths) and cardiac conditions in 100 (76 deaths).

Clinical diagnosis is possible in most instances. When the cause is cerebral a diminution of the respiratory drive is more common. Irregular respiration or spells of apnoea should raise the suspicion of intracranial pathology. There may also be a bulging fontanelle or a cerebral cry. An association of the triad of tachycardia, tachypnoea and hepatomegaly occurs in congestive cardiac failure. Diaphrag-

matic hernia is usually on the left side and is diagnosed without difficulty by means of a chest X-ray.

Apnoeic attacks are serious in the ill newborn. They are most commonly seen in preterm babies and in those who have respiratory distress due to any cause, and nearly always indicate poor prognosis. Other causes of apnoea are regurgitation of feeds, any handling of an ill or a small baby, cerebral birth injury, hypoglycaemia, septicaemia and meningitis. When apnoea is reported in a baby, oxygen should be administered by funnel or a hood, and handling should be minimum except to provide stimuli for respiration. The blood glucose should be examined to rule out hypoglycaemia and swabs should be taken from the nasopharynx and the umbilical stump to rule out sepsis. Besides oxygen administration management consists of treatment of the underlying condition.

Pallor, bleeding and echymoses

See also haemorrhage in the newborn (acute emergency in the newborn period) above (page 236).

All normal newborns have low levels of coagulation factors which are dependent on vitamin K for synthesis. The concentration falls still lower during the first few days of life and it is at its lowest on the third day. It then rises slowly towards adult levels which are reached at a few weeks of age. In about one per cent of babies this physiologic and transient deficiency is sufficiently exaggerated to cause spontaneous bleeding. Commonly it occurs from the mucosa of the stomach and intestine or from the cord stump as slow oozing; rarely there may be echymoses or petechiae on the skin as well. Due to the increased tendency for bleeding any trauma during delivery can cause a large haemorrhage in the form of a cephalhaematoma, caput succeedaneum, or as subaponeurotic bleeding. Pre-term babies are particularly prone to bleeding because the deficiency of coagulation factors is greater than in the case of full-term infants, there is increased capillary fragility and platelet function is also inadequately developed. Response to vitamin K 1 mg given intravenously is often dramatic.

A study of 3000 full-term infants has shown that haemorrhagic disease of the newborn is typically a disease of otherwise healthy breast fed infants who did not receive vitamin K. Prophylactic vitamin K given to the baby will prevent bleeding. It has been demonstrated that vitamin K administered to the mother before or during labour does not protect the baby and also that parenteral administration in the baby is preferable to oral drops. In a busy obstetric unit it may not be possible to give injections of vitamin K to all newborns because of economic and administrative difficulties. In such a case prophylactic vitamin K should be offered to all those who are at risk, such as those with low birth weight, those born after a difficult or instrumental delivery, those with a maternal history of illness or a complication of pregnancy, and those who are under observation for any illness peculiar to the newborn period.

A severe form of bleeding due to disseminated intravascular coagulation is encountered at times in the very ill infant. The diagnosis is suspected when the bleeding does not respond to injected vitamin K and is confirmed by low platelet counts and sub-normal levels of fibrinogen in the blood. Infections especially with Gram-negative organisms and herpes virus, hypoxia and acidosis as seen in the hyaline membrane disease and severe illness act as triggering mechanisms for disseminated intravascular coagulation. This complication occurring on top of the underlying illness makes the prognosis very poor. Several maternal conditions also have been known to be associated with bleeding and thrombotic episodes in the newborn. These are toxaemia of pregnancy, placenta praevia, abruptio placentae and renal disease, and their presence should warn the paediatrician to observe the baby closely.

Jaundice

Jaundice is relatively common in the first week of life. Not only is bilirubin produced in large quantities, as mentioned above, but also the liver enzyme required for the conjugation of indirect bilirubin and its conversion to bilirubin glucuronide for excretion is poorly developed. The result is that in all newborns the blood level of serum bilirubin tends to be high. When it exceeds 5 mg/100 ml clinical jaundice occurs. Such jaundice makes its appearance usually after the first day of life and with improvement in enzyme function begins to fade before the week is over. It is referred to as 'the physiologic jaundice of the newborn', implying thereby that any jaundice appearing during the first 24 hours of life or persisting after the first week requires investigation of its cause.

Certain drugs are excreted by the liver after conjugation with glucuronic acid utilising the same pathway as bilirubin. Hence they compete with bilirubin for excretion so that jaundice is aggravated when they are administered to the baby and the physiologic jaundice tends to persist longer. Examples of such drugs are sulphonamides, novobiocin, vitamin K analogues and salicylates. On the other hand in the pre-term baby enzyme function is immature in keeping with other biologic functions, so that there is a higher incidence of jaundice as well as a tendency for the icterus to persist. As a rule it is advisable to investigate the etiology of jaundice in any baby with a serum bilirubin level greater than 12 mg/100 ml.

Hyperbilirubinaemia can be prevented in several ways. It has been observed that the incidence of jaundice is much less on a regime of early feeding of infants. Hence mothers should be encouraged to put their babies to the breast soon after birth, and particularly so in the case of the baby with a low birth weight. Secondly, in recent years it has been shown that exposure to daylight lowers the levels of serum bilirubin, probably by oxidising bilirubin, and in this respect blue light has been demonstrated to be most effective. Phototherapy cannot counter rapid rises of serum bilirubin as occurs in Rhesus incompatibility, but there have been several reports of its usefulness in conditions like ABO incompatibility and G-6-PD deficiency where the haemolysis is less severe. In such cases it may be possible to avoid exchange transfusion, which even in experienced hands carries a mortality risk of five to ten per cent. There are minor side effects of phototherapy, for example increased insensible water loss and skin reactions, but the main danger is due to delay in the recognition of meningitis and septicaemia which may be the underlying cause of jaundice.

Jaundice observed for the first time in the second week of life needs investigation. Such jaundice is due to biliary atresia or the inspissated bile syndrome in the large majority. Other causes are hepatitis due to congenital syphilis, intrauterine infection with rubella, cytomegalic virus or toxoplasmosis, endocrine deficiency as in cretinism, or metabolic disorders like galactosaemia and tyrosinosis. In all such cases the bilirubin is of the conjugated type and the enzyme levels are raised.

Fits

See also acute emergency in the newborn (page 237).

In developing countries a common cause of fits in the newborn period is tetanus. It is seen predominantly in babies delivered outside the hospital, but also at times in babies who were born in hospital and had to be discharged early because of overcrowding. In the latter there is almost always a history of home brews and pastes being applied to the umbilical stump. The mortality in neonatal tetanus is very high and those who survive are at risk of brain damage due to recurrent risk of hypoxia during the fits. The prevalence of tetanus in the community is high and in almost all developing countries neonatal tetanus is the next most common cause of death in the newborn after low birth weight. Hence its prevention by means of injections of the toxoid to the pregnant mother is a high priority in all antenatal clinics. In addition, the need for cleanliness in handling the cord stump should be emphasised in all health education classes. The treatment of neonatal tetanus is described on page 243.

Other causes of fits are brain damage and metabolic disturbances such as hypoglycaemia and hypocalcaemia. Convulsive episodes in the first four days of life are commonly due to brain damage and those occurring after this period are metabolic in origin. This observation is derived from several follow-up studies of neonatal fits. In one such study it was found that the mortality rate was four times as great in convulsions during the first four days of life and severe handicap in survivors six times as great as with convulsions occurring after this period. After the first week of life meningitis is a frequent etiologic factor.

The common metabolic causes of convulsions, namely, hypoglycaemia and hypocalcaemia, are largely preventable. Early feeding of all infants and particularly of those with low birth weight, those who have suffered hypoxia at birth and those at risk of illness due to causes in pregnancy or the birth process, is important in preventing falls in blood sugar levels. Hypocalcaemia, on the other hand, is common with feeding on cow's milk because of its high phosphate content. Insistence on breast feeding by all mothers in the maternity wards will not only reduce the incidence of this complication but also that of infective diarrhoea in the nursery.

Convulsions in the newborn are serious. In a follow-up of 112 infants with convulsions in the first 28 days of life, 105 survived the neonatal period. Out of the 83 available for follow-up at the age of one year, 14 (17 per cent) were detected as having a motor handicap, a further convulsion or an intelligence assessment below 85.

Failure to pass meconium in the first 24 hours after birth

Meconium is normally passed within the first 24 hours after birth. In cases of foetal distress and asphyxia meconium may be passed in utero and stains the amniotic fluid. In which case it may be aspirated by the foetus during the gasping movements resulting from anoxia, and give rise to chemical pneumonitis. Alternatively, the viscid meconium may cause obstruction in an air passage and result in atelectasis or pneumothorax.

Meconium may not be passed in the first day after birth. Such delay in passing meconium is seen in the small baby, the very ill infant and in the baby whose mother has been treated with large doses of antihypertensive drugs. In some babies, a plug of very thick meconium gives rise to signs of intestinal obstruction with vomiting and abdominal distension. The plug is passed spontaneously or after a rectal examination and normal bowel movements follow.

Failure to pass meconium occurs in imperforate anus and in intestinal obstruction, though some babies with high obstruction will pass meconium in the early stages. Such meconium may be abnormal in amount or consistency but not always so, and the baby may be considered normal. In all cases, where there has been a failure or delay in passing meconium a rectal examination should be performed, and a plain X-ray of the abdomen should be taken in the erect and lying down positions and in each position the anterior and lateral views should be obtained. The air swallowed with the onset of respiration passes down the intestinal lumen and marks out the gut contours so that sites of obstruction and fluid levels are outlined.

If intestinal obstruction is diagnosed all oral feeding should be withheld, a gastric tube should be passed and stomach contents should be aspirated every 15 minutes and an intravenous infusion should be commenced to prevent dehydration or electrolyte imbalance. Referral for surgical relief of obstruction should be arranged urgently.

Failure to pass urine in the first 24 hours

In the normal newborn urine is passed within a few hours after birth. Failure to pass urine is rarely a serious problem. Small quantities may have been passed and not noticed or urine may be passed together with meconium and mistaken to be the latter. In all such cases, the genitalia and the external urethral meatus should be examined to exclude any malformation. The abdomen should be palpated for the presence of a mass and if one is felt an IVP should be performed to exclude hydronephrosis, renal anomaly or a distended bladder. If urine only dribbles and is not passed as a strong stream, posterior urethral valves should be suspected and excluded by means of a cysto-urethrogram.

Infections

Gonococcal infection

The infection is acquired at the time of birth. Inflammation and a purulent discharge are usually evident within a few days of birth. In rare instances colonisation of the pharynx, rectum or septicaemia can occur.

Systemic penicillin (benzyl penicillin 30 mg/kg daily) in two divided doses for three days is required in addition to penicillin eye drops instilled every five minutes for two hours; then every 15 minutes for 12 hours, and half hourly for the next day. Penicillin resistant cases need treatment with spectinomycin.

Chlamydia trachomatis

Chlamydia infection is transmitted by direct inoculation into the neonate's eye or by inhalation of infected material during birth. Up to 30 to 50 per cent of infants born to infected mothers are likely to develop eye disease and 10 to 20 per cent pneumonia. The eye infection becomes apparent one to three weeks after birth and varies from a mild conjunctivitis to severe ophthalmia. The condition usually resolves on its own, but in rare instances can progress to conjunctival scarring. The lung infection usually presents one to three months after birth with low grade fever, paroxysmal cough, tachypnoea and failure to thrive. Chest X-ray shows diffuse infiltrates. There is usually accompanying conjunctivitis or a history of it.

Neonatal chlamydia infection (including conjunctivitis) should be treated with systemic erythromycin 50 mg/kg daily for two to three weeks.

Syphilis

Unlike gonorrhoea and chlamydia, syphilis is a prenatal infection. When the mother has a primary or secondary disease the infectivity is virtually 100 per cent. Penicillin given during pregnancy produces complete cure.

The clinical signs of congenital syphilis appear after about three weeks, and include snuffles (due to infection of nasal bone and cartilage), eczema around the mouth with fissures, hepatosplenomegaly, skin rash, failure to thrive, and fever.

Early treatment with penicillin (30 mg/kg daily in two divided doses) is essential to avoid permanent damage, and should be continued for 10 to 14 days.

Neonatal tetanus

In spite of mass campaigns of immunisation with tetanus toxoid in women of child bearing age, and during pregnancy cases of neonatal tetanus are still being reported in many countries.

In a proportion of cases of neonatal tetanus there may be additional sepsis, and even septicaemia. If facilities are available local swabs and blood samples should be taken for culture.

With regard to treatment the spasms must be controlled with injection paraldehyde 0.3 ml/kg intramuscularly and sedation (phenobarbitone 5 mg/kg six hourly alternating with diazepam 1–2 mg/kg six hourly and chlorpromazine 2 mg/kg six hourly). A nasogastric tube is passed for feeding. Injection penicillin 30 mg/kg daily in two divided doses is given for five days to eliminate any *Clostridia tetanii* present. Another antibiotic may have to be added depending on culture results. Injection ATS 5 000 units is administered intramuscularly as a single dose.

Mortality from neonatal tetanus continues to remain high. Intensive nursing care, effective control of spasms, and control of infection are factors which determine survival.

Neonatal herpes

Infection is acquired during passage through the birth canal, and infection can occur if the mother has active herpes at the time of delivery, either with lesions or without (asymptomatic shedding of the virus). The risk to the newborn is greater from primary than from recurrent episodes in the mother.

Neonatal herpes can be fatal within the first few weeks or result in permanent brain damage in the survivors. In all instances of suspected herpes infection in the mother, the delivery should be by caesarean section.

Congenital virus infection

A number of viruses are able to cross the placenta and infect the foetus. Rubella virus, cytomegalovirus, human immuno-deficiency virus, hepatitis B virus, and human T cell lymphotrophic virus are known to cause perinatal infection.

The effects of rubella in pregnancy are well known. If acquired in the first trimester it almost invariably affects and damages the foetus. Congenital defects occur less frequently (roughly 15 per cent of cases) when maternal infection occurs between 13 and 16 weeks of gestation, and much less after infection at between 17 and 20 weeks.

In contrast with rubella, cytomegalovirus infection in the pregnant woman goes clinically unnoticed. Transplacental transmission occurs less frequently (30 to 40 per cent cases), and 10 per cent of infected foetuses are severely damaged. But damage can result from infection occurring at any stage of pregnancy. Congenital cytomegalovirus infection is still the most common microbial cause of mental retardation.

HIV infection in the mother is transmitted to the foetus in 30 to 40 per cent of cases, the higher figure being in women with more advanced or recently acquired disease. Some 25 to 40 per cent of infected infants die before their second birthday.

Sclerema

This is a condition in which there is abnormal firmness of soft tissues. It is best felt by palpation of the trunk and the extremities. When present, the limbs lose their normal softness and take the consistency of firm rubber. Sclerema is often seen in low birth weight infants who have become hypothermic or as a terminal event in Gram-negative septicaemia. When present it heralds a grave prognosis. The treatment is that of the underlying causative disease.

Further reading

Avery G B. *Neonatology, pathophysiology and management of the newborn.* (2nd ed.) Philadelphia: J. B. Lippincott Co., 1981.

Davies P A. Low birthweight infants: immediate feeding recalled. *Arch dis childh* 1991; 66: 551–553.

Davies P A, Gothefors L A. *Bacterial infections in the foetus and newborn infant.* Philadelphia: W. B. Saunders, 1984.

Ebrahim G J. Care of the newborn in developing countries. London and Basingstoke: Macmillan, 1979.

Kadam S B, Daga S R, Daga A S. Quality of survival on conservative neonatal care. *J Trop Ped* 1991; 37: 250–253.

Milner A D. Resuscitation of the Newborn. *Arch dis childh* 1991; 66: 66–69.

Robertson N R C. *A manual of neonatal intensive care.* (2nd ed.) London: Edward Arnold, 1986.

Whittle M J. Rhesus haemolytic disease. *Arch dis childh* 1992; 67: 56–68.

Section VII

Systemic Diseases

24 Diseases of the respiratory system

The respiratory passages and the alveoli of the lungs constitute a system over which air is rhythmically moved in order to provide oxygen to the blood and to remove carbon dioxide from it. The movement of air in and out of the lungs is achieved by the work of the muscles of respiration, which overcome the resistance of the air passages, and the elastic recoil of the lung tissue.

A large proportion of particulate matter is filtered out of the inhaled air by the mucous membrane of the upper air passages. Laryngeal and airway reflexes initiate cough or bronchoconstriction to limit the entry of foreign particles and ciliary action helps to remove those which may be deposited. When such particulate matter contains infectious organisms, contact between them and surface cells is prevented by the intervening mucous blanket covering the respiratory epithelium. The movement of the ciliated epithelium keeps the mucous blanket moving so that the time of contact between the invading organisms and the individual cells is not long enough for penetration and active infection to occur. When the mucus ceases to move, penetration and invasion of surface cells becomes possible. The effective maintenance of the cilia-propelled mucous blanket is an important defence mechanism of the respiratory tract.

Defence mechanisms in the respiratory system

The respiratory system is the most extensive of all body tissues coming into direct contact with the environment. It is continually exposed to infectious agents, environmental pollutants and particulate matter which are potentially harmful. At the same time a number of mechanical, phagocytic and humoral defence mechanisms exist to guard against infection and injury.

The nose and the nasopharynx help to filter out large particles. Inhaled smaller particles are cleared up the tracheo-bronchial tree by the mucociliary transport system. Ciliated cells are the most common cells in the trachea and bronchi, with approximately 200 cilia per cell. Smoke and virus infections are two common agents affecting ciliary function.

The alveolar macrophage is the first line of defence against inhaled matter reaching the alveoli. These macrophages comprise up to 90 per cent of the effector cells present in the lung parenchyma. Besides ingesting and degrading foreign matter and transporting it out of the lung they also enhance or modulate lymphocyte responses, and secrete a variety of cytokines.

Chemotactic factors released by macrophages or from other sources can attract neutrophils from the pulmonary circulation into the lung parenchyma. Because of the large number of receptors on their surface neutrophils are able to tackle a greater variety of microbes than the macrophages. They also have a better bactericidal capacity. Macrophages, however, can act as scavengers and remove products of neutrophil activity which are damaging to the lung tissue.

Besides the hilar and other lymph nodes, lymphocytes occur in the bronchus-associated lymph tissue (BLAT), the interstitial lymph nodules and as free lymphocytes in the parenchyma and the air space. In these alveoli 73 per cent of the lymphocytes are T cells and about six per cent of them are activated. They secrete lymphokines which regulate the traffic and function of other effector cells. About eight per cent of the alveolar lymphocytes are B cells. Of these 0.1 per cent to 0.3 per cent are actively secreting immunoglobins.

A variety of humoral substances like immunoglobins, complement, lysozyme, fibronectin and so on can be identified in fluid obtained by alveolar lavage. They all have specific anti-microbial roles.

The ease or otherwise with which the lungs are able to expand during inspiration is called the 'compliance of the lung'. Diseases which cause stiffness of the lung, for example, asthma, bronchiolitis, lung oedema, etc., decrease the compliance of the lungs and thereby increase the work of respiration. In the healthy adult the work of breathing is about 0.3 kg m/min. In conditions like mitral stenosis and emphysema it is known to increase tenfold.

Cardio-pulmonary relationship

Lung function is closely related to the work of the heart. Pulmonary disease causing hypoxia will lead to vasoconstriction in the pulmonary vasculature. Presence of acidosis and carbon dioxide retention makes the vasoconstriction worse. If the underlying cause of the hypoxia is short-lived and can be corrected, pulmonary hypertension is reversible. In progressive lung disease in which there is a destruction of alveolar walls, as well as diffuse fibrosis and destruction of the pulmonary vasculature, pulmonary hypertension can be severe. It is then also non-reversible and eventually leads to cor pulmonale.

In the very young infant, acute pulmonary infection is often associated with right-sided heart failure. This is common in bronchiolitis and is also seen in some cases of bronchopneumonia. In both these conditions, inflammation of the lung tissue results in increased blood flow to the lungs; in addition, any existing hypoxia will cause pulmonary hypertension and overloading of the right ventricle, resulting in failure.

Upper airway obstruction as a cause of reversible cor pulmonale has been described in the literature. Most of the cases described fall within the age range of three months to nine years, with a peak in the age-group two to four years. Hypertrophied tonsils and adenoids are the usual cause of obstruction in the upper airway. The affected child has noisy breathing due to the obstruction in addition to the clinical signs and symptoms of congestive cardiac failure. In some of these children there may also be evidence of pulmonary oedema on X-ray examination.

Respiratory disease in the community

Mortality from respiratory disease has a characteristic age pattern, being highest in children under one year of age and declining as the age increases. Mortality has declined sharply in Western Europe since 1940 and in the case of infants under the age of one year, this decline was most noticeable between 1940 and 1955. In the case of children in the age group 1 to 14 years, there has also been a gradual and continuous decline. One of the reasons for this reduction in mortality from respiratory disease is the improvement in living and working conditions. Improved socio-economic status also plays a role. Health and vital statistics show a generalised improvement and the decline in mortality from respiratory disease is part of this overall improvement. The introduction of antibiotics has additionally contributed to this reduction.

Several studies have been carried out to determine the epidemiology of respiratory illness in the general population, including inter-regional and global studies by the World Health Organisation (WHO). All these studies indicate that acute respiratory illnesses are amongst the most common afflictions of mankind and are responsible for more than half of all acute illnesses.

In the global study of respiratory disease carried out by WHO it was found that 61 per cent of the total number of deaths associated with respiratory illness were caused by acute infections. Also, acute respiratory infections in the form of viral and bacterial pneumonia were responsible for 6.3 per cent of deaths from all causes.

In the 1980s collaborative studies on the epidemiology of acute respiratory infection in 10 countries showed incidence rates of 12.7 to 16.8 new episodes per 100 child-weeks of observation. Rates of lower respiratory tract infection ranged from 0.2 to 3.4 new episodes per 100 child-weeks of observation. Children spent from 21 per cent to 40 per cent of observed weeks with acute respiratory infection, and from one per cent to 14 per cent of observed weeks with lower respiratory infection. Case fatality rates ranged from 3.2 per cent to 15.8 per cent being higher in children less than one year old. The incidence rate was higher in children less then 18 months of age. Viral agents were recovered more frequently than bacteria, the most common virus isolated being RSV. Amongst the bacterial agents isolated, the most common were *S.pneumonia* and *H.influenzae*. Young mother, her level of education, nutritional status of the child, overcrowding in the home, and presence of a smoker in the household were common risk factors.

In a search for causative organisms laboratory data were compiled from 13 studies of children with pneumonia. Organisms had been cultured from lung aspirates and blood. In the more developed countries viruses were more common, in particular the RS virus, parainfluenza and influenza, and adenoviruses. In the less developed countries bacteria predominate, the most common being *S.pneumoniae* and *H.influenzae B*. These two groups of organisms accounted for more than two-thirds of all bacterial isolates. Often bacterial infection was super-imposed on viral. In 20 per cent of confirmed cases of acute lower respiratory infection, a bacterial superinfection was also demonstrable by culture of blood or lung aspirates.

In children lung infection is often caused by inhalation of infected nasopharyngeal secretions into the lungs. Aspiration of secretions is not uncommon especially during sleep. If the nasopharynx has been colonised by pathogens even small amounts of aspiration can deliver a heavy inoculum into the lungs, especially if the defence mechanisms have been affected by malnutrition, viral infection, smoke or other factors. A number of studies have isolated the same pathogen from culture of lung aspirates or blood and in the nasopharynx. Studies in birth cohorts in a number of countries have shown the high rates of colonisation with *S.pneumoniae* and *H.influenzae* early in life.

Respiratory infection very early in life may permanently affect respiratory function. Ventilatory function was found impaired at the age of five years in a group of children who had pneumonia or bronchitis in the first year of life. Early treatment and prevention of respiratory illness in young children is important for better health in adult life. In this respect parental smoking and early smoking by young school children are two areas where extensive health education is necessary.

Viral infections of the respiratory tract

Viral infections of the respiratory tract are responsible for a large proportion of respiratory illnesses, especially in infants, and contribute to many infant deaths. Thus, morbidity data from rural Punjab show that nasal discharge and cough were responsible for 97 and 45 symptom-days respectively per child in a year. In the UK there are approximately 3000 deaths per year from acute respiratory infec-

tions in children aged one month to one year and many of these are thought to have an acute viral origin.

A respiratory virus may involve the entire respiratory tract but causes maximum impact in a given region, and accordingly a characteristic clinical picture emerges. In a study of children admitted with respiratory symptoms to hospitals in Newcastle, five main categories of symptoms were found, namely upper respiratory infections, croup, bronchitis, bronchiolitis and pneumonia. Virologic studies give the results shown in table 24.1.

The RS virus is an important pathogen in children under the age of one year, and whereas the common respiratory viruses are present throughout the year, the RS virus shows a peak incidence at certain times of the year, indicating the occurrence of small epidemics in the community. Whether the same obtains in developing countries is not known. Geographic and environmental factors may play a role and require epidemiological studies.

Upper respiratory infections

Three respiratory syndromes are included under this heading, namely common cold, febrile nasopharyngitis and acute respiratory disease. They are characterised by varying degrees of nasal congestion and discharge, conjunctivitis, sore throat, cough and injection of the tonsillopharyngeal area. The etiology is usually viral, though infection with group A *Streptococcus* can also give rise to a similar clinical picture.

In the healthy individual, these infections are self-limiting. Occasionally in the malnourished child or in the small infant they may be followed by bacterial pneumonia, sinusitis or otitis media. Hence careful examination and follow-up care is necessary in children.

Antibiotics have no place in the primary management of acute viral infection of the respiratory tract.

Table 24.1   Results of virologic studies in various respiratory symptoms

Presenting symptoms	No. of cases	Virus isolated	No. positive
Upper respiratory infection	516	RS	178
		Influenza/Parainfluenza	178
		Adenovirus	90
Croup	117	Parainfluenza	74
Bronchitis	211	RS	120
Bronchiolitis	546	RS	499

Prophylactic antibiotics to prevent secondary bacterial infections have not been shown to prevent such complications and can be harmful because of alteration of the normal bacterial flora and the establishment of resistant forms.

Acute tonsillopharyngitis

Acute tonsillopharyngitis with either exudate or membrane is commonly due to streptococcal infection in older children. In the very young, however, a similar clinical picture may also be seen with viral infections. When acute tonsillopharyngitis occurs with vesicles or shallow ulcers on the tonsils, the causative agent is usually coxsackie A or herpes simplex virus. In practice, most cases of acute tonsillopharyngitis are without vesicles, ulcers, exudate or membrane formation, and the aetiology is in doubt. In the case of streptococcal throat infections, the drug of choice is penicillin. For complete eradication of the organisms it is necessary to maintain effective blood levels for at least ten days.

Sinusitis

Sinusitis is a common complication of respiratory infection in childhood, though in most cases there may be no symptoms pointing to this diagnosis. Fever, pain and tenderness over the involved sinus, the classical signs of sinusitis in the adult, are usually absent in the child. The diagnosis is considered when any of the following signs are present: (1) Persistent mucopurulent discharge in large quantities from one or both nostrils following acute rhinitis. (2) Long-standing cough. (3) A diffusely red pharynx with a thick mucopurulent discharge clinging to the posterior pharyngeal wall – the postnasal drip.

In acute sinusitis antibacterial drugs and manoeuvres to assist drainage are necessary. The invading organism is often a *Staphylococcus* which may be resistant to penicillin. Hence, if there is no immediate response, culture and sensitivity studies should be carried out, followed by appropriate therapy. When there is a chronic or recurring infection of the sinuses, the possible role of smouldering infection in the adenoids and the tonsils, allergy, or a deviated nasal septum should be thought of as possible causative factors. Acute frontal sinusitis is an especially serious situation because of the threat of spread of infection to the brain or the orbit. Any child who has acute pain, swelling or tenderness over the frontal sinus should have an X-ray of the sinuses taken in the upright position. The presence of a fluid level in the area of the frontal sinus is an indication for drainage, regardless of whether or not the symptoms are subsiding.

Otitis media

Normal eustachian tube function may be disrupted by swollen adenoids, drainage from infected sinuses or inflammation of the mucous membrane. A simple obstruction of the tube causes serious otitis. If there is an associated entry of pathogenic organisms, suppurative otitis media may follow. The usual causative organisms are *Pneumococcus, Haemophilus influenzae* and group A *Streptococcus*. Infection of the eustachian tube can occur without a history of ear pain or pulling at the ear, and in the absence of fever. Hence careful examination of the ear drum is essential in all cases of acute respiratory infections in children. A red tympanic membrane without alteration of the land-marks or the light reflex does not necessarily mean bacterial otitis media. But when the ear drum is bulging, and there is loss of light reflex or the landmarks are obliterated, suppuration in the middle ear is likely.

The management consists of treating the source of infection in the nasopharynx with antibiotics, and drainage of the accumulated pus by myringotomy, if necessary. If the child fails to respond adequately to penicillin therapy by the third day of treatment, infection with *H. influenzae* should be suspected and the antibiotic therapy appropriately modified. Perforation of the ear drum indicates that there has been occlusion of the blood supply to the central vascular area of the tympanic membrane as well as pressure due to accumulation of fluid in the middle ear. Hence the treatment of a draining ear has to be vigorous to avoid this sequel. The duration of therapy is determined by the appearance of the drum, and so careful follow-up is essential in both non-draining and draining otitis media. A draining ear should be treated until it is dry and the drum has returned to normal. If the drainage persists after two weeks of antibiotic therapy, the child should be seen by an otologist.

Acute epiglottitis

Acute epiglottitis is characterised by fever, a barking cough, drooling from the mouth on account of painful swallowing, respiratory distress with stridor and a red swollen epiglottis. The typical 'croupy cough' may be absent if there is severe obstruction to air entry or if the child is too exhausted to cough. The most common etiologic agent is *H. influenzae* type B. Occasionally bacteraemia is associated with the infection of the epiglottis and the child may be very ill.

Children with viral croup have a history of runny nose, sometimes with sore throat and mild fever for one or two days before the onset of cough, hoarseness of voice and stridor. In contrast a child with *H. influenzae B*, epiglottitis presents with a history of a few hours of increasingly painful sore throat and difficulty in breathing. There is high temperature, the child prefers sitting upright to lying down, may be unable to talk or drink and is drooling saliva. Absence of a croupy cough in a child with acute stridor and fever is suggestive of acute epiglottitis.

Because of the high mortality, vigorous therapy and careful nursing are necessary. The emergence of resistance to ampicillin has led to intravenous chloramphenicol 50 mg/kg daily as the preferred treatment. The child should be under close observation for respiratory obstruction. Intubation or tracheostomy may be needed in half to two-thirds of the cases. Both are life saving and should not be unduly delayed once the diagnosis is made and signs of respiratory obstruction are present. The response to treatment is rapid. On the other hand, in staphylococcal tracheolaryngitis antistaphylococcal drugs like flucloxacillin are needed, and intubation will have to be continued for several days for the secretions to settle.

Acute laryngotracheobronchitis

Clinically, this syndrome resembles acute epiglottitis except that examination of the pharynx reveals a normal epiglottis. The child presents with inspiratory stridor, cough, fever and hoarseness of voice. There is marked respiratory effort, and in severe cases, exhaustion of respiratory muscles. There is marked irritability and restlessness due to anoxia and clinical examination may be difficult. The common causative organisms are parainfluenzae 1, 2 and 3 and influenza A2 and B viruses. In various reported series, bacteria have been isolated in less than 20 per cent of the cases.

Recurrent or spasmodic croup without fever or coryzal symptoms is usually associated with atopy. Hyperreactivity of the upper airway is the underlying mechanism.

Bacterial tracheitis (commonly due to *Staphylococcus aureus, H. influenzae* or Streptococcal infection) results in copious purulent secretion and mucosal necrosis. The child is toxic with high fever and signs of progressive airway obstruction. The croupy cough and absence of drooling help to distinguish the condition from acute epiglottitis.

The child with croup should be under careful observation to detect any increase in the obstruction of the respiratory passages. Sedatives should be avoided, since restlessness is an important indicator of anoxia. Oxygen therapy may help to overcome anoxia, and a humid environment keeps the secretion from drying up. Adequate hydration can usually be achieved by encouraging small frequent drinks. Children with severe dyspnoea may need intravenous fluid. Not all children with croup need oxygen, but it helps those with dyspnoea. Adrenaline delivered by a nebuliser via a face mask (5 ml of 1:1000 solution) helps those with severe obstruction and can be repeated every two to four hours. Those who have no improvement or require more frequent inhalation require intubation. The value of corticosteroids is not established, and they are best avoided. Intravenous antibiotics either as chloramphenicol or ampicillin and flucloxacillin are needed for seven to ten days in bacterial tracheitis, which is potentially fatal and requires vigorous treatment. About two to five per cent of children admitted with croup require an artificial airway. Increasing tachycardia, tachypnoea, chest retraction or the appearance of cyanosis, exhaustion or confusion are indications for intubation or tracheostomy. Thorough tracheal suction and adequate oxygenation should be carried out after the procedure. Children with an endotracheal tube need intensive nursing care and observation to avoid potentially fatal complications like blockage or displacement. Any pus aspirated either at the start or later should be sent for culture.

Bronchiolitis

Bronchiolitis frequently occurs in epidemics and mainly affects infants and young children. The clinical features consist of coryza lasting from one to several days followed by rapid progress to acute illness with fever of variable degree, rapid respiration, a harsh cough, an expiratory wheeze, and the presence of fine rales on clinical examination. Chest X-ray may reveal pulmonary distension in most cases and linear areas of collapse in some. Clinically, hyperinflation of the chest with costal retraction is of special diagnostic importance. Bronchiolitis should be suspected in infants presenting with a clinical picture of asthma with fever and signs of exhaustion.

The Respiratory Syncytial (RS) virus is the most common causative organism though influenza A, the rhinoviruses, the adenoviruses and the parainfluenza viruses have all been isolated from infants admitted to hospital with a clinical picture of bronchiolitis. The severity of the illness is determined chiefly by the presence or otherwise of the RS virus and the age of the patient.

On admission, the infant is acutely ill with anoxia, hypercapnoea and dehydration. All handling should be minimal and oxygen should be administered by mask at a rate of 4.0 litres/minute. Intravenous infusion of one-fifth saline in five per cent dextrose should be commenced to provide one and a quarter of the normal maintenance requirement per day. Because of the severe dyspnoea there may be difficulty with feeding and tube-feeding is necessary. The very severely ill infant is acidotic. If facilities for measuring the base deficit are available sodium bicarbonate should be administered intravenously using the formula $0.25 \times$ body weight in kg $\times$ base deficit = m eq of $NaHCO_3$ required. A large proportion of infants respond satisfactorily to this line of treatment. In the severely ill, four clinical patterns will emerge as the disease progresses: (1) progressive respiratory difficulty culminating in severe respiratory failure; (2) peripheral circulatory collapse; (3) recurrent apnoeic attacks; and (4) generalised convulsions. Digoxin should be administered to those with increasing tachycardia (heart rate above 180/minute) and an enlarged liver. Hydrocortisone may be required for those showing poor peripheral circulation. Increasing respiratory rate in excess of 60/minute, drowsiness and cyanosis are signs of respiratory failure and are seen in about three per cent of all infants under the age of two years admitted to hospital with acute lower respiratory tract infection. If facilities are available, such infants can be helped with mechanical ventilation for two or four days to tide them over the difficult period, after which many are able to make a good recovery. In a large proportion of cases it is not possible to exclude bacterial etiology. If available ampicillin 50 mg/kg per day and cloxacillin 50 mg/kg per day are administered to provide a broad antibiotic cover.

Bronchopneumonia and pneumonia

The classical signs of consolidation, described in the adult, are often absent in the child. Instead there is diminished air entry and localised or widespread fine rales over the affected lung tissue. Chest X-ray shows lobar involvement in the typical case of pneumococcal pneumonia, and infiltration extending and spreading from the hilar regions in the case of bronchopneumonia (figure 24.1). In many cases it is not possible to distinguish bronchopneumonia from bronchiolitis clinically.

The vast majority of previously healthy infants, especially if breast fed, will have a lower respiratory infection of mild to moderate severity, which clears within a week with treatment. One child in 50 requires hospitalisation. Of these three per cent to seven per cent are severely ill with respiratory failure, and one per cent die.

Figure 24.1   Lobal pneumonia (R) side

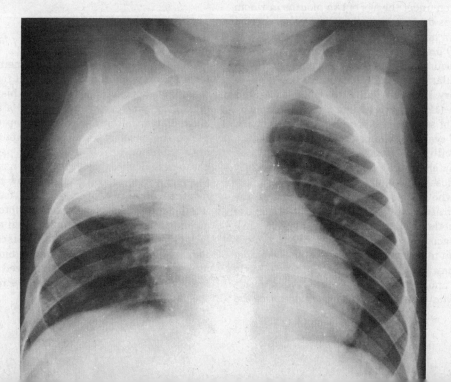

In children presenting with acute respiratory infections three main groups may be identified as follows

(1) Those with severe pneumonia or other severe disease needing antimicrobial treatment and referral for in-patient care.
(2) Respiratory infections requiring antimicrobials but treated as out-patients.
(3) No pneumonia, but simple cough and cold, wheezing, bronchitis and so on.

The protocol for case management at primary care level as proposed by the World Health Organisation is to distinguish cases of pneumonia from other cases of acute respiratory infection and to provide appropriate treatment. The protocol takes into account two presenting signs viz. cough and difficulty in breathing. Respiratory rate is next taken as the distinguishing criterion. A rate ⩾ 50 per minute in children two to 11 months old, and a rate ⩾ 40 per minute in those one to four years old is taken as a predictor of pneumonia and an indication for antimicrobial therapy. In children less than two months old, the critical rate is ⩾ 60 per minute for the diagnosis of pneumonia. In all cases, the protocol recommends confirmation of respiration rate by a second reading ten minutes later.

If in addition to increased respiratory rate there is also in-drawing of the chest wall a diagnosis of severe pneumonia is made and the child admitted to hospital. Presence of other signs like inability to drink, undue drowsiness, convulsions or malnutrition indicate severe cases and urgent admission to hospital is necessary.

All children under the age of two months in whom pneumonia is diagnosed are at high risk and must be treated in hospital.

The WHO protocol recommends out-patient treatment of pneumonia with inj. procaine penicillin (intramuscularly 300 mg), co-trimoxazole (240 to 480 mg every 12 hours orally according to age) or amoxycillin (125 mg every eight hours by mouth). In the case of severe pneumonia (inability to drink, presence of cyanosis) the protocol recommends inj. benzyl penicillin (10–20 mg/kg daily in four divided doses) or inj. chloramphenicol (50–100 mg/kg daily in divided doses) and oxygen.

Infants who develop bacterial infection of the lower respiratory tract respond satisfactorily to standard methods of treatment with oxygen, antibiotics and good nursing care. About five to ten per cent may fail to respond. In such cases, the infecting organism may be a *Staphylococcus*, or there is early circulatory and/or respiratory failure. *Staphylococcal pneumonia* (figure 24.2) is more common in the young infant and in the malnourished child, and here a high index of suspicion is necessary. The onset is insidious, but there is rapid progression of the illness to cause pneumothorax, emphysema, pyopneumothorax, lung abscess or tension cysts. All of these complications can present as emergencies requiring urgent resuscitative measures. Mortality from staphylococcal pneumonia is high, ranging from 12–50 per cent in various series. Death is usually due to overwhelming sepsis or respiratory embarrassment caused by a tension pneumothorax.

Treatment should be commenced with flucloxacillin by injection (intravenously 65 – 125 mg if less than two years old; 125 – 500 mg if two to ten years old; or intramuscularly 60 to 125 mg every six hours), then continued by mouth 60 to 125 mg according to age every six hours. Empyema and pneumothorax should be treated by draining with an underwater seal. If the immediate life-threatening complications are controlled and suitable antibiotics are administered, the prognosis for recovery is good.

Rapidly progressive pneumonia culminating in respiratory failure

The main cause of respiratory failure is obstruction of the smaller airways by viscid mucus. The child is cyanosed with poor air entry in spite of marked respiratory effort. Drainage of the lower airway by positioning and by nasotracheal intubation, if necessary, should be instituted early in the management of such cases.

Pneumonia presenting with circulatory failure

Unlike the usual forms of bronchopneumonia where respiratory symptoms are prominent from the onset, some infants present with a short history, a minimum of respiratory symptoms, and a sudden onset of circulatory failure. A state of collapse occurs even before the onset of signs and symptoms that can draw attention to the lungs as the primary site of pathology. Such a presentation is usually seen in the very young infant, usually below the age of six months. Lethargy, stupor, refusal to feed, pallor and mottled cyanosis are associated symptoms. Oliguria or anuria is an important early sign of circulatory failure and should be looked for in all cases. Laboratory investigations show a raised blood urea and altered electrolytes. Such infants need resuscitative measures for the circulatory failure in addition to specific antibiotic therapy.

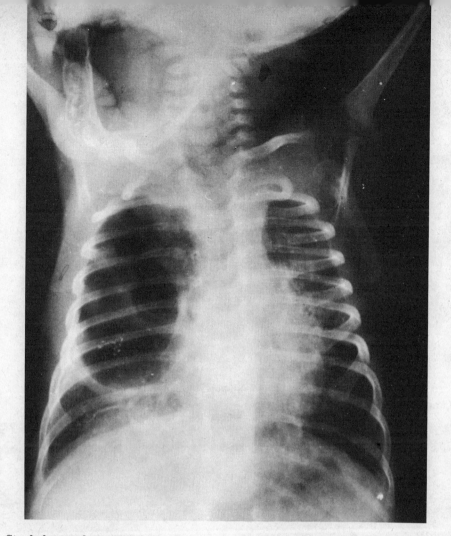

Figure 24.2 Staphylococcal pneumonia

Risk factors

A high mortality from pneumonia occurs in young children. In several studies around the world 20 to 30 per cent of all deaths from respiratory infections were reported in children less than five years old, and particularly in those less than two months old. Besides age, other risk factors are prolonged duration of illness, severe changes on X-ray, cyanosis, inability to feed, severe chest in-drawing or grunting respiration. Malnourished children are at high risk particularly when there is no febrile response to lung infection.

Suppurative lung disease

Abscess

Abscess formation in the lung (figure 24.3) may occur as a complication of pneumonia due to Staphy-lococcus, *Klebsiella* or rarely *Pneumococcus*. The most likely etiology is an overwhelming infection, with lack of drainage leading to necrosis of alveolar walls and coalescence of multiple small cavities. The condition is commonly encountered in small infants and in malnourished children. Culture and sensitivity studies on the sputum, if possible, are helpful in planning therapy. Pending such studies, or in their absence, the child should be treated with a wide spectrum of antibiotic therapy in the form of a combination of methicillin and gentamicin. Any underlying condition such as malnutrition, anaemia or bronchiectasis should also be treated.

Bronchiectasis

Bronchiectasis (figure 24.4) may be congenital but, more commonly, is due to the destruction of the walls of the bronchi as a complication of obstructive pneumonia with impaired bronchial drainage or due

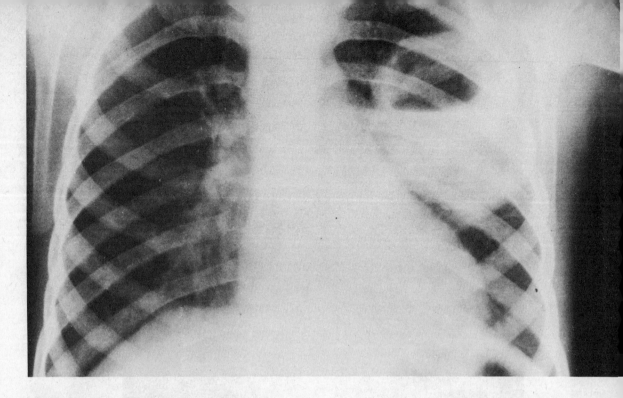

Figure 24.3   Lung abscess

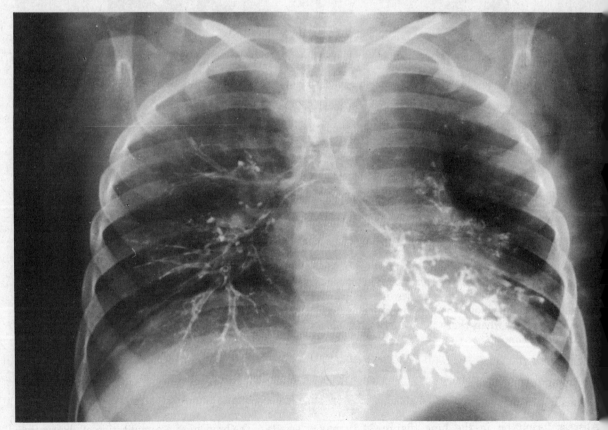

Figure 24.4   Bronchiectasis

to a necrotising pyogenic infection. It can also occur as a complication of measles, whooping cough or primary tuberculosis. Hence the key to the prevention of chronic suppurative disease in children rests in the first five years and probably in the first three years of life.

The clinical picture of bronchiectasis is one of a chronic cough with the expectoration of large quantities of purulent sputum especially on rising in the morning, repeated haemoptysis and recurrent chest infections. Chronic chest infection often leads to parenchymal fibrosis, hypoxia with cor pulmonale and congestive failure. In addition, bronchiectasis is usually associated with generalised airways obstruction which often responds to bronchodilators.

The management consists of bronchial hygiene through postural drainage and specific antimicrobial therapy for acute exacerbations of chest infection. Whatever the underlying cause of the bronchiectasis the common infecting organisms are *Haemophilus influenzae* and *Streptococcus pneumoniae*. Infection with *Staphylococcus aureus* is an ever present risk. Most patients respond satisfactorily to regular postural drainage and antibiotics early in an infective exacerbation. Surgery is indicated only when medical treatment fails to control the production of purulent sputum or when recurrent haemoptysis becomes a risk to life.

Asthma, hay fever and wheezy bronchitis

Respiratory allergy and its various clinical manifestations are another group of common clinical problems in paediatric practice. Asthma and bronchospasm are the usual modes of presentation, which can vary from the very mild to the severe forms. Longitudinal studies of children suffering from different manifestations of respiratory allergy have helped to identify the characteristic features of each type.

Broadly speaking asthmatic children can be divided into three groups. About three quarters have infrequent acute episodes of wheezing, usually associated with viral infection of the upper respiratory tract. The episodes vary in intensity and duration, but usually lung function returns to normal in between attacks. Eighty per cent of such children will stop wheezing before adulthood.

About a quarter of asthmatic children have more frequent and prolonged wheezing triggered by infective, allergic, emotional and physical stimuli. Their asthma begins at a younger age. In between attacks the peak flow may return to normal, but signs of airflow obstruction persist.

A small third group, about one to three per cent, have severe wheezing which continues throughout childhood. They are mainly boys; symptoms start before the age of two years, and many also have eczema and rhinitis. Usually there is a strong family history of atopy. Many become underweight, and develop chest deformity. All have abnormal lung function between attacks, and the majority continue to have attacks in adult life.

In severe asthma the onset is early, usually before the age of two years, with a high frequency of attacks in the first year of onset. There is clinical and laboratory evidence of airway obstruction in between attacks in a large proportion of such children and many go on to develop a chest deformity in the form of a barrel or pigeon chest, or Harrison's sulcus. They continue to suffer from asthma in adult life. In contrast, the milder forms have an onset in later childhood and the attacks are of an episodic nature, with no evidence of airway obstruction in between attacks. In many cases, the attacks subside before the child is ten years old. In the average child who is being followed up regularly it is usually possible to determine the severity and chronicity by the time he is seven years old.

Characteristically, the asthmatic child shows a high incidence of all features of allergy. Thus hay fever, eczema and urticaria are more common amongst asthmatics than in matched controls, and the high frequency as well as increased severity of these conditions are most common in children who suffer from severe forms of asthma. This is also reflected in results of skin tests for allergy. By the age of 14 years, almost half the children with mild asthma and practically all with chronic asthma react to skin tests with commonly occurring antigens. Those with more severe asthma react to a wider range of allergens.

There is much more to asthma than allergy, though atopy plays a very major role. For example, it has been demonstrated that in the susceptible person asthma can be aleviated and also precipitated by suggestion. The bronchi of asthmatic subjects are hyper-sensitive to exercise even in the case of subjects who may not have wheezed for as long as 20 years. It is a common observation that attacks of asthma are often precipitated by infections with viruses, especially the rhino, parainfluenza and RS viruses. All these are examples of factors which can trigger attacks of asthma in the susceptible person.

The role of house dust in causing respiratory allergy has been known for some time. In recent years it has been demonstrated that this allergy is due to the presence of the mite *Dermatophagoides* in house dust. A close parallel between reactions in patients allergic to house dust and to *D. pteronyssinus* has been demonstrated using skin, nasal and bronchial provocation tests. The mite feeds on human skin scales and likes warmth, so that its common habitat is bed linen, eiderdowns, blankets and pillows.

Management

An important part of management consists of steps to reduce exposure to house dust. In the overcrowded homes of many developing countries this may not be possible; on the other hand feather pillows, eiderdowns and mattresses are never seen in rural homes and the single sheet or mat which is spread on the floor for the child to sleep on can be washed at frequent intervals.

Bronchodilators like salbutamol administered at the first sign of an attack help to abort asthma and should be used prophylactically. When administered by inhalation the onset of action is fast, and the effect lasts from four to six hours. Oral treatment requires 20 times the inhaled dose for a similar effect, and so side effects are more common. Several types of inhalers are now available, and it is essential that the technique is checked until the patient is able to use the inhaler correctly. Children under the age of two are unable to use inhalers, and a nebuliser is necessary. Parents should be warned that whereas bronchodilators are valuable for prophylaxis, once a full-blown attack has set in adrenaline 1:1000 may be necessary.

For the persistent asthmatics and for those who are prone to severe attacks, two recent therapeutic advances have been found useful. Disodium cromoglycate, given by inhalation, is known to prevent the release of histamine from the mast cells in the lungs and is proven to be a useful prophylactic. The drug is inhaled in a powder form with a device known as the 'spinhaler', which releases the powder from a capsule. It is ineffective in an established attack of asthma and its only use is for prophylaxis. Experience with disodium cromoglycate has shown that a large proportion of severe perennial childhood asthmatics can now be adequately controlled without requiring systemic steroids. There are, however, about 25 per cent of such children in whom disodium cromoglycate is ineffective. Such children can now be helped with beclomethasone aerosol spray. This synthetic steroid derivative has a high level of topical anti-inflammatory activity and little systemic effect. It is inhaled from a metred aerosol delivering 50 μg per dose and the average requirement is 300 to 600 μg per day. Like disodium cromoglycate it is a preventive agent and must be taken regularly. During an established attack it may fail to reach the bronchioles and oral or systemic corticosteroids should be used in such cases. The chief advantage of disodium cromoglycate and beclomethasone lies in the fact that long-term therapy with oral steroids is no longer necessary and the side-effects can therefore be avoided.

Status asthmaticus

Status asthmaticus is a medical emergency and an indication for immediate hospitalisation. The first sign of the development of the status attack is that the patient is unable to obtain relief from the usual bronchodilators like salbutamol and epinephrine. it should be stressed upon all parents that if the child's condition is not responding to the usual measures, a change in treatment is necessary. Clinical examination reveals a distressed child with thoracic overinflation, tachycardia and pulsus parodoxus. The ability to continue conversation is a good guide to the degree of severity, for example, mild – frequent pauses between speech; moderate – monosyllabic speech; and severe – too dyspnoeic to speak. Hypoxaemia is usually present and in the very ill patient hypercapnia may occur as well.

Treatment is commenced with salbutamol (0. 25–1 ml of respirator solution according to age diluted in 3–4 ml of 0.9 per cent saline) by nebuliser using oxygen at 6–8 1/min. If the patient responds the treatment is repeated after every two to four hours. Oral prednisolone 1–2 mg/kg in 24 hours is now added to the treatment.

If symptoms continue to persist nebulised ipratropium bromide is added to the treatment. If there is no improvement intravenous aminophylline 0.9 mg/kg/hour is added to the treatment, provided the patient has not been given theophylline in the past 24 hours.

If a nebuliser is not available, treatment is commenced with aminophylline 4 mg/kg, after ascertaining that the drug or theophylline have not been administered in the past 24 hours. Aminophylline needs to be given slowly and well diluted. Half the calculated dose is administered through the drip over a period of 10 minutes or longer, and the remainder is added to the container of the intravenous fluid to run slowly over 12 hours. Intravenous salbutamol is also useful in place of aminophylline. If there is no improvement, or if in a previous attack the patient needed corticosteroids, hydrocortisone may be given intravenously in a dose of 4 – 5 mg/kg every 12 hours. On recovery from the attack corticosteroids should be continued orally for several days before tapering the dose.

Prevention

Approximately 10 000 children die from pneumonia every day, which is more than the number dying from diarrhoea or measles. In the majority of cases the infecting organisms are *S.pneumoniae* and *H.influenzae B*. In addition to a rational approach to case management, there is a need for effective vaccines. Both the organisms have a polysaccharide capsule, and immunity is primarily dependent on the presence of antibodies to the capsular polysaccharide. The antibody response is largely independent of cell mediated immunity, and young children make little or no antibody to T cell independent antigens. Moreover, each different serotype carries a different polysaccharide. Young children under two respond much better to vaccines in which the polysaccharide is conjugated to a protein. Field testing of several pneumococcal vaccines is currently in progress. With regard to *H.influenzae* type B, four conjugated vaccines have been licensed and extensively field tested. It is a matter of time before vaccination against *H.influenza* gets included in the national immunisation programmes of several countries.

Further reading

Bale J R. (Ed). Etiology and epidemiology of acute respiratory tract infection in children in developing countries. *Rev Inf Dis* 1990; Supplement 8.

Bulla A, Hitze K L. Acute respiratory infections: a review. *Bull Wld Hlth Org* 1978;56: 481–98.

Colley J R T. The epidemiology of respiratory disease in childhood. In: Hull D, (ed). *Recent advances in pediatrics*. p. 224. Edinburgh: Churchill Livingstone, 1976.

Grossman M, Klein J O, McCarthy P I, Schwartz R H, McCracken G H, Nelson J D. Consensus: management of presumed bacterial pneumonia in ambulatory children. *Ped Inf Dis* 1984;3:497–500.

Milner A D. Changing concepts in asthma. *Archs Dis Childh* 1978; 53: 525–6.

Murphy S. Florman A L. Lung defences against infection: a clinical correlation. *Pediatrics* 1983;72: 1–13.

Phelan P D, Stocks J G. Management of severe viral bronchiolitis and severe acute asthma. *Archs Dis Childh* 1974; 49: 143.

Royal College of Physicians of London. *Smoking and health now*. London: Pitman Medical, 1971.

Selwyn B J. The epidemiology of acute respiratory tract infection in young children: comparison of findings from several developing countries. *Rev Inf Dis* 1990;12:S870–887.

Shann F. Etiology of severe pneumonia in children in developing countries. *Ped Inf Dis* 1986;5: 247–252.

Simpson H, Mathew D J. *et al*. Acute respiratory failure in bronchiolitis and pneumonia in infancy. Modes of presentation and treatment. *Br med J* 1974;2: 632.

Warner J O. Asthma: a follow-up statement from an international paediatric asthma consensus group. *Arch dis childh* 1992;67: 240–248.

World Health Organisation. *Technical bases for the WHO recommendations on the management of pneumonia in children at first-level health facilities*. Geneva: World Health Organisation WHO/ARI/91.20.

25 *Diseases of the cardiovascular system**

Rheumatic fever

Rheumatic fever is one of the commonest causes of acquired heart disease in children and young adults in developing countries. It is a systemic illness affecting the connective tissue and characterised by fever, inflammation and pain in the larger joints of a 'fleeting' nature, skin manifestations in the form of rashes and nodules, cardiac involvement, and in some cases neurologic manifestations. An important step in the understanding of the natural history of rheumatic fever was the demonstration of its relationship to infection with group A β haemolytic *Streptococcus*. The evidence for such a relationship was derived from epidemiologic studies showing a correlation between attacks of rheumatic fever and antecedent streptococcal infection, identical seasonal and age incidence for streptococcal infection and rheumatic fever, and in some instances, almost simultaneous occurrence of epidemics of streptococcal infection and acute rheumatic fever in crowded areas. This knowledge of the role of streptococcal infection in the etiology of rheumatic fever has important implications on prevention, especially of recurrences. It has been estimated that recurrent episodes of rheumatic fever make up 15 per cent of all cases.

As regards streptococcal infections, further studies have shown the following

(1) the duration of throat carriage of group A *Streptococcus* is important. Failure to eradicate the organism during three to five weeks of infection gives a high attack rate. Adequate treatment with penicillin commenced as late as one week after the onset of streptococcal infection has been shown to reduce the incidence of rheumatic fever.
(2) The degree of immune response of the host also contributes to the occurrence of the illness. For example, attack rates tend to be high in those who show strong immune responses.

* By P. Vichitbandha, Siriraj Hospital, Bangkok 7, Thailand, and G J. Ebrahim.

Epidemiology

The past few decades have seen a rapid decline in the incidence of rheumatic fever in many of the affluent societies of the West. This decline began even before the days of antibiotics and has been largely due to improvements in the socio-economic conditions and a possible change in the natural history of the disease, or both. The development of medical services and the advent of antibiotics have contributed further to this decline, so that rheumatic fever has now become relatively uncommon.

Rheumatic fever is essentially a disease of poverty. Its incidence in the developing world is related to overcrowding, nutritional deficiency, bad housing and poor environmental conditions. In many industrial cities, it is three to four times as frequent in the poorer children of shanty towns as in the children of the well-to-do.

There are very few studies on the epidemiology of rheumatic fever in the developing countries. Surveys on the prevalence rates indicate that its prevalence varies from 1–1.5 per 1000 individuals below 20 years of age. In Soweto, Johannesburg, 12 050 African children were examined over a period of five months. The overall prevalence rate of rheumatic heart disease was 6.9 per 1000, with a peak rate of 19.2 per 1000 children of seventh school grade. Ninety two per cent of the children were asymptomatic and in 82.5 per cent, rheumatic heart disease was diagnosed for the first time during the school survey. Group A β haemolytic *Streptococcus* was isolated from the throats of 52 per 1000 children. The carrier rate was highest during the winter months and dropped dramatically with the approach of warm weather. There was a significant correlation with the number of people sharing the child's bedroom. A similar survey on random samples of 33 361 subjects in Chandigarh, India, showed a frequency of rheumatic heart disease equal to 1.62 per 1000 population.

In all such surveys, the most consistent predisposing factors in the etiology of rheumatic fever are overcrowding in the home and inadequate treatment of streptococcal throat infections. Both are widespread in the crowded cities and poor rural homes of the developing countries. In the absence of properly organised basic health services diagnosis is delayed and treatment is inadequate so that the throat carriage of *Streptococcus* is inevitably prolonged. High frequency of streptococcal infection is suggested by community surveys of ASOT (antistreptolysin-O-titre) in several countries.

Several other factors are important in the etiology and epidemiology. For example, rheumatic fever is more common in children from the lower socio-economic groups. Those living in the slum areas of the large cities have a higher incidence. In the rural areas children with rheumatic heart disease tend to be underweight and show other signs of malnutrition. Familial disposition appears to play an important role. This may be partly due to genetic and constitutional factors or because of sharing the same environment.

Clinical picture

A history of antecedent sore throat due to streptococcal infection can be obtained in a large majority of children occurring four to six weeks before the onset of present illness.

The signs and symptoms of rheumatic fever are grouped into major and minor manifestations for purposes of diagnosis. Presence of two major and one minor, or one major and two minor manifestations confirms the diagnosis.

The major manifestations are carditis, polyarthritis, chorea, subcutaneous nodules and erythema marginatum.

The minor manifestations include fever, arthralgia, history of previous rheumatic fever, evidence of streptococcal infection and abnormal laboratory tests such as raised ESR and ASOT levels.

The list of diagnostic criteria has been modified to take into account atypical forms of presentations as follows

Chorea In many instances chorea is the sole manifestation of rheumatic fever.

Insidious or late onset carditis There may be a vague history or no history of rheumatic fever. The patient presents with heart failure, and physical examination or investigations reveal valvular heart disease. Other forms of myocarditis must be excluded. On the other hand signs of active inflammation like raised ESR and C-Reactive protein must be sought to confirm the diagnosis of rheumatic fever. Infective endocarditis must be excluded in all such cases.

Rheumatic recurrence In patients with established rheumatic heart disease who have not been adequately treated, the presence of one major criterion or fever, arthralgia or elevated levels of C-reactive protein or of ESR suggests a presumptive diagnosis of rheumatic recurrence. Additional evidence of preceding streptococcal infection, for example raised ASOT should be looked for.

Arthritis and fever are the two most frequent symptoms of acute rheumatic fever. In a typical case, the larger joints are affected and the pain is of a fleeting nature so that after a day or so of acute pain in one joint, the pain subsides somewhat and another joint becomes involved. The affected joints show signs of inflammation and are acutely painful.

Carditis occurs in 45–55 per cent of children with first attacks of rheumatic fever. The main danger of rheumatic fever stems from its effects on the heart, and as far as prognosis is concerned what really matters is the extent of cardiac involvement. Carditis can present with a pericardial friction rub, as myocarditis with changes in heart rate and rhythm, muffled or altered heart sounds and acute distress, or as endocarditis with murmurs. As a general rule a murmur is almost always present in rheumatic carditis. Hence a knowledge of the patient's cardiac signs before the illness is useful. If carditis has been present at the time of the first attack, it is likely to become more severe in subsequent episodes. Chronic rheumatic heart disease seldom develops in patients who present only with arthritis or chorea without carditis at the first attack of rheumatic fever. The worst results are seen in those with severe carditis.

Large series of cases of mitral stenosis in young children have been reported from the Middle East, India and South-east Asia. At Siriraj Hospital in Bangkok, 13.2 per cent of cases of mitral stenosis requiring surgery are below the age of 16 years (figures 25.1 and 25.2). It has been suggested that rheumatic fever tends to run a more malignant course in many developing countries because of poor nutritional status of the patients, crowded living conditions and inadequately developed health services.

About 85 per cent of patients with rheumatic fever tend to suffer a recurrence within eight years of the first attack, if they are not protected from further streptococcal infections. Patients with existing rheumatic heart disease are particularly susceptible to recurrences.

Various studies indicate that mortality during the acute attack is higher in the tropics. In Johannesburg, four per cent of African children died in the acute stage due to cardiac involvement, whereas in American and British children the first year mortality is in the region of one per cent. In a Jamaican study 11 per cent of children with acute rheumatic

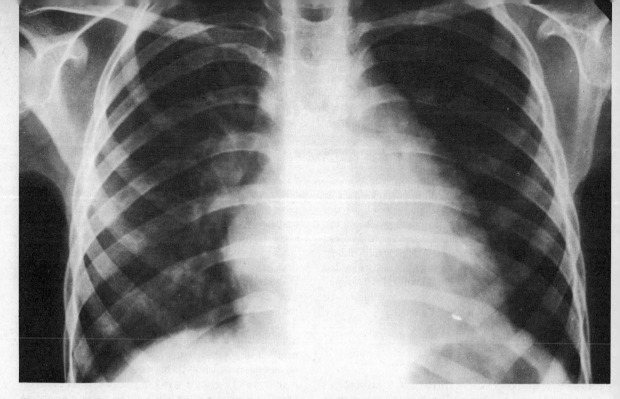

Figure 25.1   Mitral stenosis with enlarged (L) atrium and pulmonary congestion

Figure 25.2   Mitral stenosis with enlarged (L) atrium and pulmonary congestion (lateral view)

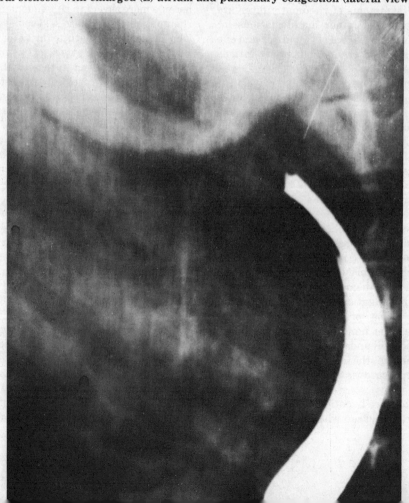

fever died within a few weeks of the onset of illness due to progressive pancarditis and a further 11 per cent within one to three years, mainly from cardiac failure. Thus if rheumatic fever in the tropics is different when compared to that in temperate climates, then the difference is because it tends to affect younger age groups and is more severe.

Treatment

The aim of treatment is to prevent carditits and damage to the heart, and to make the patient as comfortable as possible. Bed rest is necessary until all rheumatic activity has ceased, as demonstrated by normal ESR and pulse rate.

Penicillin is administered to eradicate streptococci from the throat. It is given either as intramuscular injection 600 000 units daily for ten days or by mouth 250 mg four times a day for two weeks.

Salicylates are prescribed for the relief of pain in doses of 120 mg/kg body weight to begin with and then reduced according to severity of illness to 60–75 mg/kg body weight. Salicylates are continued for about six weeks. The guide to dose in any individual case is clinical and often the dose has to be sufficiently high to cause mild intoxication. In children, the first sign of such intoxication is often over-breathing. The response of arthritis and fever is dramatic to the administration of salicylates but there is no conclusive evidence that salicylates influence rheumatic activity or carditis in any way. Certainly when there is clinical evidence of cardiac involvement, corticosteroids are preferred to salicylates, and administered in doses of 25 mg of prednisone twice daily for four to six weeks, depending on the individual response.

Prevention

Preventive intervention is based on the evidence first presented in 1940 that streptococcal infections and recurrent attacks of rheumatic fever can be prevented by small doses of sulfonamides. It was later shown that patients with proven streptococcal pharyngitis treated with sufficient penicillin to eradicate the organisms from the throat were much less likely to develop rheumatic fever compared to untreated individuals.

All children who have suffered from rheumatic fever should receive prophylactic antimicrobial agents throughout childhood. Such therapy can be in the form of sulfadiazine 0.25 g daily, oral penicillin 500 mg daily, or benzathine penicillin by intra-muscular injection 600 000 units once a month. Patient compliance is important, and therefore in cases who have suffered carditis administration by injection is preferred. In patients with rheumatic heart disease, prophylactic antimicrobial therapy is desirable throughout life.

Endomyocardial fibrosis

Endomyocardial fibrosis (EMF) is a disease of unknown etiology, endemic in the wetter parts of the tropics. It is characterised by scarring and fibrosis of the endocardium and the gradual obliteration of the cavity of one or both ventricles. It is a disease of children and young adults, and in endemic areas its prevalence rate is almost the same as that of rheumatic fever. The pathologic process, once established, remains active and progressive and is possibly recurrent.

The natural history of the disease has been described by workers in Nigeria. Careful enquiry in their patients revealed that in many cases there were initial episodes of fever. Malaise, anorexia and pyrexia lasting weeks or months gradually merged with signs and symptoms of cardiac involvement. The usual mode of presentation, however, is with established heart lesion or carditis in the acute stage. In the typical patient there may be several such episodes of acute illness with fever and cardiac involvement needing hospital admission. Such a history indicates that there is a recurrent inflammatory process with fresh necrosis in the heart tissue each time. There is thus a strong analogy with rheumatic fever in the mode of onset, recurrent episodes of illness and in the predilection of the disease for younger age groups.

The progress of the disease process is relentless. In a study of case records of 46 patients at the Mulago Hospital, Kampala, the mean survival time was found to be two years, with a range of 12 days to 12 years. The cause of death was either myocardial failure associated with pulmonary events such as broncho-pneumonia and pulmonary oedema, or a sudden unexplained death.

Pathology

The heart has a limited response to injury so that the fibrosis in EMF must be a result of non-specific injury. Fibrin gets deposited on the damaged endocardium, followed by thrombus formation. During the healing process the thrombus gets incorporated into the endocardium, producing an area of scarring.

At necropsy, fibrosis is seen in three main sites. These are: (1) the apex of the right ventricle; (2) the apex of the left ventricle; and (3) the posterior wall of the left ventricle. Though a predominantly right or left ventricular pathology can occur, biventricular EMF is the usual picture. The fibrotic process involves mainly the endocardium and inner third of the myocardium. When fibrosis is extensive, the papillary muscles and chordae tendinae of the valves get caught up in it, resulting in free communication between the atrium and the ventricle. This commonly happens on the right side, so that a very much enlarged right atrium is a typical finding.

The more recent scars are found covered by a soft thrombus, but in chronic and long-standing disease the endocardial lesions are hard and sometimes even calcified. Thus the evolution of the lesion proceeds from fibrinous deposits overlying the damaged endomyocardium to adherent thrombi followed by dense fibrosis and a contracted ventricle. Unlike rheumatic fever, the valves do not show signs of inflammation. However, they often get involved in the fibrous tissue being laid on the endocardium underneath and become incompetent.

Epidemiology

EMF has been described mainly from countries of tropical Africa, but there are also reports of cases from Sri Lanka, south India, Thailand, Malaysia, Brazil and Colombia. It has also been reported in Europeans who have lived in endemic areas for long periods.

EMF is an important cause of cardiac illness in the endemic areas. Its prevalence rate is almost the same as that of rheumatic heart disease in Uganda and about half the number of patients are children below the age of 15 at the time of first presentation.

Many workers have stressed that the etiology of the condition lies in the environment, and several hypotheses have been advanced to specify these environmental factors. At necropsy, in many cases the hearts examined show simultaneous occurrence of endomyocardial fibrosis and rheumatic lesions. The frequency of occurrence has been found to be five times more than would be expected if there was no association between the two conditions. Both are a form of pancarditis involving the connective tissue. There is a similarity in age and sex distribution. In their natural histories, both show a tendency for recurrences and for several family members to be affected.

When antibodies to heart tissues were assayed in one series of cases, it was found that these were frequently present in those who also showed high titres of malarial antibody. It is likely that some form of immunologic mechanism is involved in the pathogenesis.

In Ibadan, Nigeria, it was observed that most patients came from the forest region rather than the savannah where the city is located, and it was suggested that filarial infestation, especially *Loa loa* which is common in the forest zone, was involved in the etiology. Free microfilariae of *Acanthocheilonema perstans* have been demonstrated in the pericardial effusion on tapping in some cases. Filaria antibodies have also been shown in those Europeans who have developed the disease after a prolonged period of residence in the tropics.

Most patients with EMF show eosinophilia in the acute stage, and it has been suggested that the eosinophils may be responsible for endomyocardial damage in the same way as it happens in some cases of eosinophilic leukaemia.

Clinical picture

Approximately half the cases, and especially children, present with pericardial effusion. Typically, there are symptoms of increasing weakness and exercise intolerance with puffiness of face, periorbital oedema and an enlarged firm liver. Clinical examination shows signs of pericardial effusion such as increased area of precordial dullness, distant heart sounds and a large pear-shaped heart shadow on X-ray (figure 25.3). The pericardial effusion is rich in protein and lymphocytes which may lead to a false diagnosis of tuberculous pericarditis.

In endemic areas EMF should be suspected in any patient presenting with congestive cardiac failure and trivial precordial signs to explain the cause of the failure. When the disease process involves predominantly the right ventricle, there is raised jugular venous pressure, and massive ascites with absence of peripheral oedema. An important clinical sign of right ventricular disease is parasternal pulsation along the left upper margin of the sternum due to a hyperactive right ventricle. Chest X-rays may show right atrial enlargement which in some cases may be aneurysmal.

When the disease is predominantly left ventricular, pulmonary congestion and oedema are the more important features. On auscultation an early systolic murmur of mitral incompetence can usually be heard.

Disturbances of rhythm are common and usually occur as terminal events.

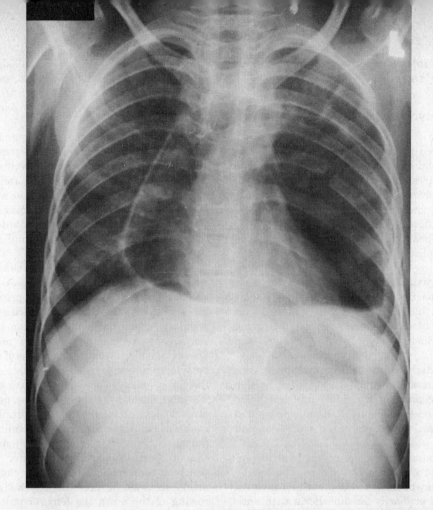

Figure 25.3 Pericardial effusion in EMF and after air insufflation following tapping. Note the thin pericardium

Treatment

Treatment is unsatisfactory. Prolonged bed rest, high protein diet and large doses of vitamin supplements have been tried with no demonstrable benefit. Congestive cardiac failure requires treatment with digitalis and diuretics.

Cardiac beri-beri

Infantile beri-beri continues to exist in many countries of South-east Asia. South Vietnam, Laos, Thailand, Burma and the Philippines are the principal areas from where this disease has been regularly reported.

The infant, apparently in good health and entirely breast fed, is abruptly seized with a cry, its body stretches, the pulse becomes thready and the face ashen grey or even cyanotic. This state may last for about half an hour and spontaneously disappear only to reappear with increasing frequency and severity. Death occurs during one of the episodes. The aphonia of beri-beri is characteristic. The child is apparently crying but no sound is heard. The infant is usually dyspnoeic with enlargement of the heart and liver. Oedema is rare. There is tachycardia with gallop rhythm. X-ray shows cardiac dilation and in the electrocardiogram there is increased Q-T interval, inversion of T waves and low QRS voltage.

Injection of thiamine (vitamin B_1) produces a dramatic response in a matter of hours.

Infantile beri-beri is due to deficiency of thiamine in the milk of a mother who is herself deficient due to a diet of polished rice. In countries where rice is a staple diet, cardiac beri-beri also may be encountered in older children and adults. It is useful to bear the condition in mind, especially when confronted with an infant in heart failure without a murmur in a rice-eating area.

Diphtheritic myocarditis

A toxin produced by the diphtheria bacillus causes degeneration and necrosis of the myocardium. The fibres lose their striations and present a swollen granular appearance. The pathological lesions are patchy and only short segments of individual muscle fibres may be affected. The toxin also causes cardiac arrhythmia or heart block.

Cardiac complications usually arise towards the end of the first week or in the second week of illness. A common early sign is disturbance of rhythm. This is followed by partial or complete heart block or by bundle branch block. In other cases there is an abrupt fall in blood pressure with accompanying tachycardia. Such early collapse has a bad prognosis.

Late myocardial involvement occurs during convalescence. There is sinus tachycardia, gallop rhythm, enlargement of the heart and low pulse pressure. The onset of heart failure is suggested by breathlessness, pallor, precordial oppression and vomiting.

Presence of bundle branch or complete atrio-ventricular block is a bad prognostic sign. The bundle branch block may be transient or persist for months.

Treatment is primarily for diphtheria with anti-diphtheritic serum and penicillin injections. Bed rest and sedation with good nursing care and proper diet are essential. High doses of corticosteroids have been suggested in the management of diphtheritic myocarditis.

Primary arteritis of the aorta and its main branches (Takayasu's arteritis)

Although true coarctation of the aorta is said to be less common in many developing countries, a chronic inflammatory disease involving the main branches of the arch of aorta and other medium sized arteries has been widely reported from several countries, especially in South-east Asia. This condition was first reported by a Japanese ophthalmologist and is named Takayasu's arteritis after him. There are several synonyms according to the presenting signs and symptoms such as pulseless disease, acquired coarctation of the aorta, atypical coarctation of the aorta, primary arteritis, primary aortitis, the middle aortic arch syndrome and so on. The etiology of this disease is unknown. Some

relationship with syphilis, tuberculosis, rheumatoid disease, and rheumatic fever has been suspected. Several authors have postulated that an auto-immune mechanism triggered by one of these illnesses is in operation.

There is marked intimal fibrosis and fibrous scarring of the media together with degeneration of the elastic fibres, accompanied by chronic inflammatory cell infiltration. This process most often involves the arch of aorta and its major branches so that several segments and the entire aorta may be involved. There may be partial or complete obliteration of the renal artery by hyperplastic intimal plaques causing hypertension of renal origin.

The clinical manifestations of the disease vary from no symptom to serious illness according to the sites and severity of the disease process. There is local pain over the affected arteries in the neck, shoulder, chest, back and abdomen together with some general symptoms such as malaise, fever, anorexia, nausea, vomiting and loss of weight. Later on symptoms and signs of inadequate circulation in the cerebrum, eyes, abdomen, kidney and extremities occur, such as dizziness, syncope, headache, impaired vision, abdominal pain, intermittent claudication in the upper and lower extremities. Deficit of pulsation of major arteries may be found on routine examination. Some patients suffer hypertension which is presumed to have been caused by renal artery stenosis. In some cases with significant narrowing of the aorta the femoral pulse is weak or absent and the blood pressure in the legs is lower than in the arms. Left heart failure may occur in severe hypertension.

Laboratory tests may reveal elevated ESR, increased serum globulin levels with reversed albumin to globulin ratio. LE cell preparations may show the presence of LE cells in a proportion of cases.

Retrograde aortography can help to outline the site and the length of the involved segments in the aorta and its branches.

Corticosteroids have been tried with some beneficial effect in the early and acute stage of arteritis. Surgical excision of the stenotic segment may be performed if localised. There is temporary symptomatic relief but symptoms soon recur because of the progressive changes in the inflammatory process affecting the aorta and its branches.

Prognosis in general is poor. At the onset of Takayasu's arteritis almost all patients begin to deteriorate progressively but some patients may be slightly improved owing to the development of collateral circulation with the basic condition remaining unchanged.

Kawasaki syndrome

A form of vasculitis occurs in the *Kawasaki syndrome*. Most patients are under the age of five and present with an abrupt onset of persistent high fever followed by conjunctival infection, and sometimes anterior uveitis. Then follow the characteristic features of the illness viz. reddening of the mucous membrane of the mouth, the pharynx, and the lips with fissuring; a strawberry tongue; erythema and swelling of the hands and feet. Within five days of onset of the fever a rash appears over the trunk and limbs. About a fortnight after the onset the skin peels over the fingers and toes, and sometimes over the palms and hands as well. All these signs are observed in over 90 per cent of the patients. Another diagnostic feature is cervical lymphadenopathy (hence the previous name of mucocutaneous lymph node syndrome) which is seen in 50 to 75 per cent of the cases.

The major complication of the Kawasaki syndrome is its cardiac effects. These occur in between 16 to 20 per cent of the cases. They include aortic or mitral incompetence, myocarditis, and pericarditis with effusion. The main problem, however, is coronary artery aneurysms in about 15 to 20 per cent of the cases. Adjacent to the aneurysms are stenotic lesions leading to myocardial infarction, usually within the first year of the illness. The more severe the symptoms at onset the more likely are the coronary abnormalities. Nodular enlargement of other arteries, for example brachial artery may be detected by palpation.

Laboratory findings are not specific. There is mild to moderate anaemia with leucocytosis. The platelet count is raised and so are levels of ESR and C-reactive protein.

The treatment consists of aspirin by mouth, and daily infusion of gamma globulin (400 mg/kg) for four days. The latter may not be possible in many developing countries due to costs and availability.

Congenital heart disease

Incidence

The true incidence of congenital heart disease in many of the developing countries is not known. In a postal enquiry involving 12 countries, mostly from South America, it was found to be 2.2 per cent in over a million children examined. The enquiry covered 42 different cities, and the nature of the cardiac defect was determined by catheterisation and angiocardiography, at surgery, or at necropsy. The ten

Table 25.1 Per cent frequency of common congenital heart defects

Country	Ibadan*, Nigeria	Kampala†, Uganda	Singapore‡	Colombo§, Sri Lanka
Number of cases studied	260	60	411	555
Ventricular septal defect	27	20	23.1	18
Patent ductus arteriosus	18	7	11.4	15
Atrial septal defect	14.2	25	–	32
Pulmonary stenosis	12.3	–	8.0	13
Fallot's tetratology	12.3	3	8.0	8
Transposition of the great vessels		–	5.1	1
Coarctation of aorta		8	4.6	1
Eisenmenger's complex		–	3.9	–
Truncus arteriosus		–	2.9	6
Atrio-ventricularis communis		–	2.9	–

* Combined clinical and necropsy study of 260 cases. *Source*: Antia A U. Congenital heart disease in Nigeria. Clinical and necropsy study of 260 cases. *Archs Dis Childh* 1974; 49: 36.

† Post-mortem records of 60 cases out of a total of 9432 necropsies performed between January 1951 and March 1968. *Source*: Wood J B, *et al*. Congenital heart disease at necropsy in Uganda. *Br Heart J* 1969; 31: 76.

‡ Post-mortem records of 411 patients out of a total of 19 415 necropsies performed between 1948 and 1957. *Source*: Muir C S. Incidence of congenital heart lesion in Singapore. *Br Heart J* 1960; 22: 243.

§ Prospective study of 555 cases of congenital heart disease. *Source*: Wallooppillai N J, Jayasinghe M de S. Congenital heart disease in Ceylon. *Br Heart J* 1970; 32: 304.

most common malformations in a descending order of frequency were as follows

Ventricular septal defect
Patent ductus ateriorsus
Atrial septal defect
Tetratology of Fallot
Pulmonary stenosis
Coarctation of the aorta
Aortic stenosis
Transposition of the great vessels
Tricuspid atresia
Ebstein's anomaly.

The data from several regions are summarised in table 25.1

Etiology

In a small number of cases direct causal relationship with intrauterine infection (for example rubella) or drug administration during pregnancy can be established. In a large majority there is no such history and the malformation must be presumed to be due to genetic factors. No single gene or chromosome is known to influence the development of the heart and the malformation is considered to be due to the interaction of several genes. There is usually a strong family history in such cases. For example, brothers, sisters and offspring (that is first degree relatives) of the index case are affected 30–50 times more often than the general population. When a couple has two offspring with the same malformation, the risks to subsequent offspring are much higher and limitation of the family on genetic grounds becomes necessary. An easy rule of thumb for predicting the risk for a given defect in first degree relatives of the index patient is to obtain the population frequency (for example, by examining newborns, infants in clinics, pre-school and school children) and to calculate its square root, which will be the risk factor. For example, if the population frequency of a defect is one per cent (written as .01) the risk to first degree relatives of the index patient is $\sqrt{.01} = 0.1$ or 10 per cent.

Diagnosis

Congenital anomalies differ from the acquired form of heart disease in that they tend to cause pure forms of right-sided or left-sided heart failure. In about 90 per cent of cases, congestive heart failure due to a malformation occurs before the end of the first year, and usually within the first few months of life, when diagnosis can be difficult.

In the small infant, congestive heart failure presents in an unusual form. For example, the only indication of dyspnoea may be difficulty with feeding. Suckling is the common form of physical exertion in early infancy, and because of reduced exercise tolerance the infant tires easily and will give up after a few mouthfuls at every feed. Hence there is poor weight gain and the infant is brought for growth failure. Similarly, there can be difficulty with sleeping. The infant is uncomfortable and breathless in the lying down position and will cry continuously. Breathing is improved when he is picked up and he stops crying, so that the family will think the baby is 'spoiled' and demands attention all the time. In some babies, dyspnoea takes the form of cough and wheezing.

Most of the severe forms of congenital heart disease are not associated with loud murmurs, and many malformations normally associated with murmurs do not show them immediately after birth. On average, only about 20 per cent of affected babies have murmurs in the first month of life. The heart sounds, especially if loud and abnormal, and the presence of ejection click are better guides to the presence of serious cardiac defects. Similarly, tachycardia and gallop rhythm should alert the physician to the presence of a cardiac problem. Increased respiratory rate, of more than 50 per minute, should always be taken seriously and repeated examination, including radiography, should be carried out to determine the cause.

Tachycardia, tachypnoea and hepatomegaly are the classical triad of congestive heart failure. However, in pure left-sided failure the liver is not always enlarged, so that there can be diagnostic difficulties.

Reduced amplitude of arterial pulse, absent pulsations or a bounding pulse are important clinical findings. In all infants with a suspected cardiac condition, the clinical examination is incomplete without blood pressure readings in the upper and lower extremities taken under sedation, if necessary.

The chest X-ray is a useful diagnostic aid. It may reveal abnormal shape of the cardiac contour, generalised enlargement, or the enlargement of a chamber. There may be congestion or decreased pulmonary vascular shadows in the lungs, and occasionally abnormal compression of the oesophagus or trachea may be seen on X-ray.

If facilities are available, an electrocardiogram (ECG) is a useful aid. Most serious cardiac malformations will produce an abnormality on the ECG.

Echocardiogram with doppler can provide valuable information with two dimensional imaging.

Management

In many cases of congenital cardiac defects intensive care is required. The infant with such a diagnosis should be referred to the nearest centre where specialist care and facilities for investigation are available. The presence of cyanosis or an episode of congestive cardiac failure are danger signals and major indications for proceeding with diagnostic studies.

When congestive failure is present, the cardiac glycosides remain the major therapeutic agents. Digoxin is the most commonly used preparation and is given in a dose of 40–60 μg/kg body weight for initial digitalisation, over 24 hours. Therapy is commenced with half the calculated dose, and the remainder is administered in three equal portions over the next 24 hours. Therapeutic treatment is continued with a maintenance dose of 4–7 μg/kg body weight in two equal amounts daily. Diuretics play a useful role in the treatment of congestive failure. Frusemide, 1–3 mg/kg body weight per day, or organic mercurials in the form inj. mersalyl 0.25 cc intramuscularly are helpful in reducing congestion in the pulmonary or systemic circulations. As the infant's condition improves, thiazide diuretics may be used for maintenance.

Other supportive measures

The infant should be nursed in an inclining position or in a 'cardiac chair' in order to promote pooling of blood in the dependent parts of the body and to ease breathing.

Sedation may be necessary in the very restless baby. Feeding with a nasogastric tube helps to ensure adequate milk intake. In the dyspnoeic and restless baby oxygen should be administered to overcome poor oxygenation in the lungs caused by congestion or a sluggish circulation.

In the case of patent ductus arteriosus, septal defects, aortic stenosis and several others, there is an ever present danger of subacute bacterial endocarditis. Hence the infant should be examined carefully at regular intervals to look for petechiae, changes in quality of heart sounds and murmurs, presence of splenomegaly, etc. A sudden and unexplained change in the general state of the infant can be due to subacute bacterial endocarditis. It is an indication for commencing intensive antimicrobial therapy after taking blood for culture. In the same way during minor illnesses adequate anti-biotic cover is essential as prophylaxis against this most dangerous complication.

Corrective surgery for a number of congenital heart defects is now possible.

Bacterial endocarditis

Infective endocarditis is the second most common complication of heart disease after congestive failure. It affects the damaged endocardium of acquired or congenital heart disease, and is characterised by infection of the vegetative lesions which form on a diseased valve after rheumatic disease or on the endocardium in congenital heart defects. Once the infection is established it can spread along the blood stream giving rise to bacteraemia. In addition, the infected vegetation on the endocardial surface is friable, and breaks off from time to time, seeding the blood with infected emboli.

Infection of the undamaged endocardium has been described in the literature. In undernourished and debilitated individuals such a process is part of a generalised septicaemia. It should be actively looked for in families of vagrants, neglected individuals and drug addicts, who seem to be specially prone to overwhelming infection.

Typically, infective endocarditis occurs on the damaged endocardium. The primary infection may be obvious, for example, an upper respiratory infection, or it may be a small focus of sepsis in the form of an infected tooth, a boil on the scalp, or infected 'jiggers' on the feet.

The infected vegetations shower the blood with emboli from time to time. In the classical case, they cause splinter haemorrhages under the nail, or subconjunctival and retinal haemorrhages, or petechiae. Any of the vital organs of the body may be involved. Emboli to the spleen cause an enlarged and tender spleen. Renal emboli are responsible for haematuria and in some cases may cause renal abscess. Neurological complications are frequent, being present in between 10–20 per cent of cases of infective endocarditis and varying from mental confusion or coma to acute hemiplegia.

Clinical presentation

The classical presentation is that of a child known to have rheumatic or congenital heart disease presenting with fever, anaemia and toxaemia. Clinical examination shows finger clubbing, petechiae, splinter haemorrhages, and splenomegaly. Subconjunctival or retinal haemorrhages may be noted. Freshly voided urine shows microscopic haematuria and blood cultures are positive.

Pyrexia of unknown origin is the more common way of presentation. The child is brought for fever of several days' duration. A murmur is audible in the precordium and there is usually anaemia. No previous history of rheumatic or congenital heart disease is present and the only clue to the diagnosis is a positive blood culture. Other causes of prolonged pyrexia such as tuberculosis, enteric fever and urinary infection should be excluded in the differential diagnosis.

Intractable and congestive cardiac failure is occasionally the only clue to infective endocarditis. A child with a known cardiac lesion and who is well compensated will suddenly go into congestive failure. On auscultation, there may be a change in the character of the murmer and heart sounds. The diagnosis should be suspected when there are sudden changes in the general condition of the patient and when congestive failure shows little response to treatment with digoxin and diuretics.

Neurologic complications due to emboli are not unusual. The commonest form is hemiplegia but other forms of neurologic deficits and meningitis can also occur. Finally, in some cases the only presenting sign is anaemia for which no obvious cause can be found. To complicate matters, the cardiac signs may be equivocal and the murmur may be thought to be of haemic origin due to anaemia. Several blood cultures are needed before the diagnosis can be confirmed.

Management

Infective endocarditis is a serious illness requiring intensive and vigorous therapy. Bed rest is essential, and the nutrition should be maintained with a palatable and adequate diet. Other supportive measures, such as treatment of congestive failure, may be indicated in severely ill patients.

The infection should be treated with bactericidal antibiotics selected according to the sensitivity studies on blood culture, and should be continued for at least six weeks. *Streptococcus viridans* is the commonest etiologic agent and is sensitive to penicillin, which should be administered by intramuscular injection in a dose of one mega unit of the crystalline form, four times daily. In the case of penicillin resistant or Gram negative infections other antibiotics such as ampicillin (60–200 mg/kg four times daily), cloxacillin (60–250 mg as single dose four times daily) and gentamicin (2.5 mg/kg three times

daily) will be necessary. Many of these antibiotics are expensive and may not be easily available in all district hospitals. When clinical diagnosis is not in doubt, but blood culture studies are not available or have been negative, treatment should be commenced with a combination of crystalline penicillin as above together with gentamicin 2.5 mg/kg/day for six weeks.

Prevention

Infective endocarditis results from transient bacteraemia which occurs during minor operations like extraction of teeth, tonsillectomy, etc. Any child with a congenital or valvular heart disease should be given an antibiotic 'cover' starting on the day before such a procedure and continued for two days afterwards. A mixture of crystalline and procaine penicillin, 400 000 units daily by intramuscular injection, is usually satisfactory for such prophylaxis.

Congestive heart failure

Congestive heart failure is a condition associated with disease in which the heart is either unable to supply the body with the requisite amount of blood or dispose adequately of the venous return or a combination of the two.

Left sided failure is characterised by weakness, fatigue, cough, dyspnoea on exertion, orthopnea, cardiac asthma, pulmonary oedema, moist sounds in the lungs, accentuated pulmonary closure, gallop rhythm and pulsus alternans.

Right sided failure is identified by increasing systemic venous pressure, enlargement of the liver, increased pulse and respiratory rates, oedema, ascites and oliguria.

Cardiac enlargement is present in both left sided and right sided failure. 90 per cent of cases of congestive failure due to congenital heart disease occur within the first year of life. Congestive failure associated with rheumatic heart disease usually does not occur before the age of four years and its presence during acute rheumatic fever indicates active rheumatic process.

Chronic rheumatic heart disease in most developing countries is usually encountered in an advanced state, with gross valvular involvement, cardiac enlargement and severe incapacity.

Anaemia, paroxysmal atrial tachycardia, hypertension from acute glomerulonephritis and myocardial disease are relatively common causes of congestive heart failure in childhood.

During the first week of life hypoplastic left heart syndrome, transposition of the great arteries and coarctation of the aorta are the commonest causes. In the period between one week and one year, the common lesions are transpositions of the great vessels, coarctation of aorta, ventricular septal defect, ductus arteriosus, endocardial fibroelastosis, total anomalous pulmonary venous drainage, atrioventricular communis, and paroxysmal tachycardia. In the rice-eating countries of South-east Asia, infantile cardiac beri-beri is a common cause.

Treatment

Treatment consists of rest in a propped up position. Sedation may be necessary in very distressed patients.

Digitalisation using digoxin is necessary. The oral dose for children less than two years of age is 0.06–0.1 mg/kg/day. For children older than two years the dose is 0.1 to 0.3 mg/kg/day. Daily maintenance dose is 25 per cent of the digitalising dose. In acute cases rapid digitalisation with parenteral digoxin is necessary. The parenteral dose is 75 per cent of the oral dose.

To avoid digitalis intoxication a careful history about previous medication is necessary before administering digoxin.

The indices of therapeutic effectiveness are slowing of the pulse, decreasing size of the liver, disappearance of the pulmonary rales and oedema, diminishing respiratory rate and improvement of colour, appetite and disposition, as well as weight loss.

In most cases diuretics are necessary to get rid of extra fluids. However, before commencing treatment with diuretics it is important to ensure a salt free diet. There is no point in administering diuretics if salt intake is not restricted. Frusemide (1–2 mg/kg) is given by injection. If diuresis is not produced within two hours a repeat single dose of up to 4 mg/kg may be tried. Frusemide can then be continued orally (1–3 mg/kg daily). Alternatively chlorthiazide is given orally (2 mg/kg daily not to exceed 50 mg/day).

The effectiveness of diuretic therapy can be monitored by keeping a weight chart for the patient. These potent drugs may produce severe potassium depletion. Increased potassium intake should be promoted by offering all patients on diuretic therapy orange juice, tomato juice, banana or potassium chloride by mouth. Serum electrolytes should be periodically checked.

Treatment of the underlying disease is essential for permanent relief of symptoms. Rheumatic mitral stenosis and many cardiac malformations can be treated surgically, and arrangements should be made for transferring the patient to a centre where facilities are available. Steroid therapy may be life-saving in rheumatic carditis. Similarly, infants with beri-beri can be saved with thiamine. Severe anaemia resulting in congestive cardiac failure caused by heavy hook-worm infection responds well to treatment with gratifying results.

Vasodilator therapy is a relatively new approach in the management of hypertensive heart failure. A number of vasodilators are available for paediatric use. The preferred treatment at present is intravenous labetalol (1–3 mg/kg/hour) and/or nitroprusside (1–8 microgram/kg/min) for a controlled and gradual reduction of blood pressure over the first 96 hours of admission.

Hypertension in children

High blood pressure may have been discovered by chance, may be iatrogenic, for example indiscriminate treatment with corticosteroids, or because of associated illness, for example renal disease, or because of symptoms like failure to thrive, headache, or neurological symptoms. Organs like the heart, eyes, or the kidneys may have been damaged by the time the condition is diagnosed. A severe form of hypertension is nearly always secondary to some underlying condition, and in 90 per cent of the cases is due to *renal disease*. In diagnosing the cause full investigation of the renal system is advisable. *Coarctation of the aorta* is usually associated with congestive failure, and absent femoral pulse, or disparity in blood pressure readings in the upper and lower extremities. *Endocrine causes* are rare. Besides treatment with steroids they include neuroblastoma, excess mineralocorticoid activity due to tumour, an inborn error of metabolism, or pheochromocytoma.

Investigation and treatment are best carried out at a specialist centre. In an emergency hypertension may be controlled by a combination of a vasodilator like nitroprusside (1–8 microgram/kg/min adjusted according to response) and a ß-blocker (labetalol 1–3 mg/kg/hour intravenously).

Further reading

Rheumatic fever

Back E H, de Pass E E. Acute rheumatic Fever in Jamaican children. *W Indian Med J* 1957; 6: 98.

Berry J N. Prevalence survey of chronic rheumatic heart disease and rheumatic fever in Northern India. *Br Heart J* 1972; 34: 143.

Koshi G, Benjamin V, Cherian G. Rheumatic fever and rheumatic heart disease in rural south Indian children. *Bull Wld Hlth Org* 1981; 59: 599–603.

World Health Organisation. *Rheumatic fever and rheumatic heart disease.* Geneva: W.H.O. 1988; Technical Report series No. 764.

Endomyocardial fibrosis

Ive F A, Willis A J P, Ikeme A C, Brockington I F. Endomyocardial fibrosis and filariasis. *Q J1 Med* 1967; 36: 495.

Oakley C M, Olsen E G J. Eosinophilia and heart disease. *Br Heart J* 1977; 39: 233.

Parry E H O, Abrahams D G. The natural history of endomyocardial fibrosis. *Q J1 Med* 1965; 34: 383.

Patel A K, D'Arabela P G, Somers K. Endomyocardial fibrosis and eosinophilia. *Br Heart J* 1977; 39: 238–241.

Somers K, D'Arabela P G, Patel A K. Endomyocardial fibrosis. *In*: Shaper A G, Kibukamusoke J W, Hutt M S R, (eds). *Medicine in a tropical environment.* London: British Medical Association, 1972: p. 348.

World Health Organisation. *Cardiomyopathies.* Geneva: W.H.O. 1984; Technical Rep. Ser. No. 697.

Cardiac beri-beri; diphtheritic myocarditis, primary arteritis of the aorta and its main branches.

Morales A R, Vichitbandha P, Chandruang P, Evans H, Bourgeois C. Pathological features of cardiac conduction disturbances in diphtheric myocarditis. *Archs Path* 1971; 91: 1.

Nakao K, *et al.* Takayasu's arteritis. Clinical report of 84 cases and immunological studies of 7 cases. *Circulation* 1967; 35: 1141.

Sukumalchantra Y, Tanphaichitr V, Tongmitr V, Jumbala B. Serial electrocardiographic changes in cardiac beriberi. *J Med Ass Thailand* 1974; 57: 80.

Vichitbandha P, Honghthai A, Somboonvitaya V, Prachuabmoh C, Bukkavesa A. The electrocardiogram in diphtheritic myocarditis. *Israel J Med Sci* 1969; 5: 938.

Vinijchaikul Kamolwat. Primary arteritis of the aorta and its main branches (Takayasu's arteriopathy). A clinicopathological autopsy study in eight cases. *Am J Med* 1967;43: 15.

Bacterial endocarditis.

Hughes P, Gould W R. Bacterial endocarditis: a changing disease. *Q JI Med* 1966; 35: 511.

Lerner P I, Weinstein L. Infective endocarditis in the antibiotic era. *New Engl J Med* 1969; 274: 199, 259, 323, 388.

Steiner I, Patel A K, Hutt M S R, Somers K. The pathology of infective endocarditis. *Br Heart J* 1973; 35: 159.

Congestive cardiac failure

Dreyer W J. Heart failure. *In* Garson A, Bricker J T, Macnamara D G. *The Science and practice of pediatric cardiology.* Philadelphia: Lea and Fabiger, 1990.

Keith J D. Congestive heart failure. Review article. *Paediatrics.* 1956; 18: 491.

General

World Health Organisation. *Community prevention and control of cardiovascular system disease.* Geneva: W.H.O. 1986; Tech. Rep. Series No.732.

26 *Haematological disease in the tropics**

Haematological diseases in the tropics are similar to those found in the temperate countries but their distribution, incidence and severity differ. The commonest haematological condition seen in the tropics is anaemia. Other conditions such as acute leukaemia, idiopathic thrombocytopenic purpura, haemophilia are reported but on the whole are rare.

Some of the conditions present in ways different from those described in standard textbooks. Others inevitably are seen in late stages. Many may be misdiagnosed due to lack of adequate laboratory facilities. Some of the conditions occur in association with other tropical diseases and so the clinical presentation may be complicated.

Anaemia

Definition

Anemia is defined as a state in which there is a low oxygen-carrying capacity of the blood. In measurable quantities there is low haemoglobin, and/or reduced number of red cells, as well as reduced packed cell volume (PCV).

The normal values vary with the age of the child. The haemoglobin of the normal newborn, for example, is 16–18 g per cent in affluent societies and the red cell count is 5–6 millions per cu mm. These high values are useful in carrying oxygen in utero where the oxygen tension is low. A newborn baby whose haemoglobin is 15 g per cent or less is considered anaemic.

An infant of 8–12 weeks has a normal haemoglobin of 11–12 g. This represents a large drop from the value at birth, almost halving the haemoglobin concentration. This brief period of fall in haemoglobin value is referred to as 'physiological anaemia'. At birth 75 per cent of the body stores of iron averaging about 290 mg is in the form of circulating haemoglobin. During the early months of life the iron contained in the haemoglobin is redistributed

*By N. Bwibo, Kenyatta National Hospital, Nairobi, Kenya.

to the growing tissues. Resumption of erythropoiesis begins at about seven weeks after a full term delivery.

The main mechanisms causing anaemia in the new born period are

(1) Blood loss – haemorrhage
(2) Blood destruction – haemolysis
(3) Decreased blood formation – hypoplasia and aplasia of bone marrow.

Any of these mechanisms may occur in the same patient, causing anaemia with complex haematological features. These multiple factors must be identified and treated simultaneously for a good response to occur.

Bleeding in the newborn period

Newborn babies may bleed and become anaemic because of haemorrhagic disease of the newborn, bleeding from the umbilicus or cephalhaematoma. Blood loss by itself accounts for five to ten per cent of severe anaemia in the newborn.

Rarely does a newborn bleed in utero, into the mother's circulation or into another foetus in the case of identical twins or into retroplacental space. A cut placenta at the time of Caesarian section or failure to ligate the maternal end of the umbilical cord of identical twins causes severe bleeding at the time of birth.

Bleeding from the cord

The commonest cause of bleeding from the cord is loose ligature, or untied cord as occurs in many cultures.

Urgent blood transfusion is life-saving. It is usually difficult to estimate the amount of blood lost but small children can easily bleed to death. Others are brought to hospital exsanguinated and in shock.

271

The blood volume of a newborn is 100 ml/kg. A three kg child therefore has 300 ml of blood. A loss of blood in the quantity of 100 ml is a large amount of blood in such a neonate.

Cephalhaematoma

This bleeding is common in the tropics and may be associated with trauma during delivery. It occurs after birth usually from the second to the fourth days of life but not at birth. In some cases there is no history of trauma, thus supporting the possibility that it is caused by coagulation defect.

The bleeding occurs usually over the parietal bone below the periosteum. The haematoma is limited by suture lines. The amount of bleeding may be very large causing severe anaemia. The cephalhaematoma resolves by itself with time. Aspiration is dangerous as it can introduce infection and give rise to sepsis. Haemolysing blood of the haematoma often causes severe neonatal jaundice requiring blood transfusion.

Subaponeurotic haemorrhage

Unlike cephalhaematoma, this occurs into the soft connective tissues of the scalp rather than in the sub-periostal space. It is not limited by suture lines. The bleeding occurs commonly after vacuum extraction in full term infants. Cases have been reported from Africa and from Singapore. Some children become very anaemic and severely jaundiced and require exchange blood transfusion. Subaponeurotic haemorrhage is said to be more common in the African infant, compared to the European. The reason for the racial difference in incidence is not known.

Haemorrhagic disease of the newborn

Haemorrhagic disease of the newborn is a syndrome of spontaneous external bleeding associated with defect in coagulation mechanism. It occurs between the second and fifth days of life. Bleeding usually occurs from the rectum, mouth, nose and umbilical stump. Rarely, the bleeding occurs on the skin.

The bleeding causes varying degrees of anaemia. The deficient coagulative factors are: prothrombin, factors V, VII, IX and X. These are vitamin K-dependent factors. All of them are at the lowest level from 48–96 hours of age, and are more reduced in non-white compared to white new born infants in South Africa where haemorrhagic disease of the

newborn is three times as frequent in the non-white as in the white infant.

Such cases have also been seen in East Africa. In Tanzania and at the Mulago Hospital in Kampala, Uganda severely affected infants were seen regularly in the maternity unit. Administration of vitamin K to all newborns is recommended.

Intramuscular administration of 1 mg vitamin K stops the bleeding soon by correcting the coagulation defect. Fresh blood transfusion, 10 ml/kg, corrects the coagulation defect as well as the existing anaemia.

The condition should be differentiated from bleeding which occurs commonly in the premature neonates on account of tissue anoxia and also bleeding from an infected cord. It should also be distinguished from swallowed maternal blood in which bloody stools are passed but the child is not anaemic. This swallowed maternal blood is changed by alkali to a brown alkaline haematin compound whereas foetal blood which is resistant to alkalis remains red or pink.

Iron deficiency anaemia

Iron deficiency anaemia is one of the world's commonest nutritional disorders among infants. It is more common in the tropics than in temperate climates. It is brought about by two main mechanisms: dietary iron deficiency and hookworm infestations.

Dietary iron deficiency anaemia

This type of iron deficiency anaemia is common in infants and less so in older children. Infants are born with iron stores in the haemoglobin and in the tissues. Infants born of mothers who are deficient in iron and pre-term babies have low iron stores. In utero, the foetus accumulates iron at a rate proportional to increase in body weight and maintains a body iron content of 75 mg/kg. In the normal infant 75 per cent of the iron endowment is present as haemoglobin. Infants born with decreased red cell mass will have a decreased iron endowment. Such babies are likely to develop iron deficiency anaemia during infancy. It is estimated that the newborn has 300–400 mg of iron of which 75 per cent is in the form of haemoglobin and the rest in the tissues, the latter being 30 mg/kg in the full term and 6 mg/kg in the premature baby.

Infants on a cow's milk diet for a prolonged period, as in some pastoral societies, develop iron deficiency anaemia. Cow's milk is a poor source of iron. Besides, infants on whole cow's milk lose blood in the gut, causing iron deficiency.

Perhaps 'Bahima disease', described by several authors in Uganda, is due to such a mechanism. This is a form of dietary iron deficiency anaemia common in the Bahima of Western Uganda who live on a milk-based diet. Anaemia persits into adult life. As many as 20 per cent of the Bahima pre-school children suffer from anaemia. Besides the iron deficiency anaemia, these children have skull changes similar to those seen in chronic haemolytic disorders such as sickle-cell anaemia and thalassaemia.

Pre-term infants on formulae containing large amounts of polyunsaturated fat and receiving supplemental iron tend to develop a haemolytic anaemia unless the formula contains adequate amounts of vitamin E. Many commercial formulae have now corrected the proportion of linoleic acid, vitamin E and iron, but it is advisable to keep a watchful eye on all low birth weight infants, especially if they are not breastfed.

Babies born at term to iron-deficient pregnant mothers develop iron deficiency anaemia during infancy. But they have normal haemoglobin at birth. The iron stores with which they are born cannot cope with the increased demand of rapidly growing tissues of the infants.

Iron occurs in two main forms in the diet:

(1) Inorganic or non-haem iron loosely bound with proteins, amino-acids or organic acids. Prior to absorption, this form of iron must be split from its combination with organic substances and reduced to the ferrous form. This happens during acid-pepsin digestion in the stomach. Reducing substances such as vitamin C help in absorption but phytates form insoluble salts and prevent absorption.

(2) Haem iron as in haemoglobin and myoglobin. Its absorption is not affected by phytate or ascorbic acid. Haem iron is absorbed intact into the intestinal epithelial cells and the iron is split off from the haem moiety within the epithelial cell.

The amount of iron absorbed in the gut is regulated by two factors, iron stores in the body and the state of activity of the bone marrow. The absorbed iron is carried in the blood stream by transferrin which is a specific plasma protein of the ß-globulin group.

Blood levels of serum iron vary in childhood. In the zero to two years age group serum iron is more than 30 μg/100 ml. In the two to five years age group it is more than 40 μg/100 ml while above five years it is 60 μg/100 ml or more. For older children 75–100 μg/100 ml is normal. In adults, serum iron ranges from 100–150 μg/100 ml.

Infants with iron deficiency anaemia are prone to infections. The infections are accompanied by anorexia which contributes to reduced iron intake and to diminished iron absorption in the gut, thus leading into a vicious circle. The cause of increased tendency to infection is not known.

There is growing evidence that infants with iron deficiency anaemia tend to be more fretful, and perform poorly on psychomotor tests for mental development, for example Bayley Mental Development Index. In several studies, performance has been shown to improve after one to two weeks of oral iron therapy.

Iron deficiency anaemia of infancy and early childhood can be prevented by correction of anaemia of pregnancy, prevention of prematurity and early introduction of the staple, vegetables and meat in the diet of infants.

Hookworm anaemia

This is widespread under the insanitary conditions in the tropics and subtropics. The adult worm lives in the small intestine hooked into the mucosa by its hooks, but wanders from one site to another leaving the bruised mucosa bleeding. It is estimated that *Ankylostoma duodenale* sucks 0.015 ml of blood per worm per day while *Necator americanus* sucks 0.03–0.05 ml of blood per worm per day. The amount of blood lost from the gut determines the development of anaemia. The severity of this anaemia depends upon: worm load, the type of worm, the age of the child, the nutritional status of the child including his dietary iron intake. Children on an adequate iron intake may keep pace with blood loss so that anaemia does not develop.

Hookworm anaemia is the commonest form of iron deficiency anaemia in the tropics. Other parasitic diseases, such as schistosomiasis, also lead to blood loss and thus cause iron deficiency anaemia.

Clinical features

The clinical features of iron deficiency anaemia are the same irrespective of whether the anaemia is caused by dietary deficiency or hookworm infestation.

The patients present with pallor, irritability, fatigue, anorexia, weakness, breathlessness on exertion, palpitation, cardiac murmurs, gallop rhythm.

The severity of these symptoms and signs depends on the degree of anaemia. Those with severe anaemia may go into cardiac failure, of high output type, especially when there is an added strain such as infection. The cardiac failure is characterised by oedema, raised jugular venous pressure and warm extremities. Since the anaemia develops slowly over the months, the clinical features are of insidious onset. Those with slight or moderate anaemia may be found on routine physical examination. Those with hookworm infestation complain of vague abdominal pain and altered bowel habits. Their stool is usually dark, resembling the malaena stool, due to altered blood. It is not known whether any toxins produced by the worms contribute to the clinical features.

Laboratory findings

Haematological features of iron deficiency anaemia include the following: a low haemoglobin, low haematrocrit or packed cell volume (PCV), low reticulocyte count. The peripheral smear shows microcytic hypochromic red cells with anisocytosis and poikilocytosis. Mean corpuscular haemoglobin concentration (MCHC) is less than 28 per cent. It usually ranges from 15–25 per cent. Serum iron is low and total iron binding capacity (TIBC) is high, ranging from 400–450 mg per cent. Bone marrow shows normoblastic erythropoiesis with no stainable iron.

Stool examination for those with hookworm infestation shows dark stool with positive occult blood and varying degrees of ova of hookworms.

Management

Management of iron deficiency anaemia consists of administration of iron either orally or intramuscularly depending upon the severity of the anaemia. Where the haemoglobin is dangerously low, blood transfusion is life-saving. Those with hookworms should be dewormed.

Administration of oral iron should be continued on an outpatient basis or at home for about three to six months after normal haemoglobin values are reached so as to replenish iron stores in the tissues. The dosage is 5 mg/kg body weight, divided into three doses. Usually there is a good response with increasing reticulocyte counts and haemoglobin level. When there is no response, the patient may not be taking the drug or there may be systemic disease which should be looked for and treated. The

other reason for lack of response is wrong diagnosis. Thalassaemia major and minor cause microcytic and hypochromic cells. This anaemia does not respond to iron therapy.

Patients with moderately severe anaemia need intramuscular iron. The total amount of iron required is calculated using the following formula

Total iron requirement (in mg)= $2 \times$ weight in lbs $\times$ (14 – Hb in g/100 ml)

To get the amount of iron dextran (Imferon) needed, the above is divided by 50. (One millilitre of Imferon contains 50 mg of iron). Example: A five year old weighing 40 lbs with a haemoglobin of 4 g per cent will require $2 \times 40 \times$ (14–4 g) of iron = $2 \times 40 \times$ 10 mg of iron = 800 mg of iron or 800÷50 = 16 ml of Imferon.

Blood transfusion is given when the haemoglobin is less than 5 g per cent and when there is associated cardiac failure, so as to relieve hypoxia. The blood should be given slowly so as not to overload the circulation. As these patients have a high plasma volume, one should aim at giving packed red cells or sedimented red cells where packed cells are not available. One way of giving sedimented red cells is to run the drip slowly. Some authorities give diuretics and digoxin at the same time so as to minimise the risk of overloading the circulation and causing cardiac failure.

Intramuscular Imferon used on an outpatient basis in selected patients with severe anaemia is rapidly effective in raising haemoglobin, thus saving bed space and blood. Administration of Imferon at multiple sites has been suggested to reduce the patient's hospital visits.

Deworming is done using bephenium, pyrantel or mebendazole. (See page 220 for details.)

Haemolytic anaemias

The main mechanisms leading into haemolysis of red cells are firstly intracorpuscular defects when something is wrong with the red cells, and secondly extracorpuscular defects when the defects come from outside the red cells. The former comprise congenital defects of red cells such as red cell enzyme deficiency, haemoglobinopathies, and other defects in the synthesis of haemoglobin. Sickle-cell anaemia, G-6-PD deficiency, thalassaemia are examples of conditions brought about by this mechanism.

Extracorpuscular defects comprise factors invading the red cells from outside. They include infections such as malaria and Gram negative scepticaemias, drugs and other chemicals, transfusion reactions, circulating antibodies as in haemolytic disease of the newborn and other forms of acquired haemolytic anaemias. Clinically the patients present with anaemia, jaundice, enlarged spleen and the specific features of the causative factors.

Haematologically there is low haemoglobin, normocytic, normochromic red cells, elevated reticulocyte count, poikilocytosis, anisocytosis and many normoblasts in the peripheral blood. Red cell osmotic fragility is increased. Indirect Coombs test may be positive or negative. There is elevated serum bilirubin mainly indirectly reacting. The bone marrow is hyperactive.

Haemolytic disease of the newborn

Haemolytic disease of the newborn in the tropics is mainly caused by ABO blood incompatibility. Rhesus blood incompatibility is a rare cause because Rhesus negative individuals in the population are few – about four to six per cent compared to 15 per cent in Western countries. Where the incidence of G-6-PD deficiency is high, as in West Africa, Singapore and Hong Kong, it is the main cause of haemolytic disease of the newborn.

In all cases the mother's blood group is O and that of the baby is usually A but it can be B. The mother has naturally occurring anti A and anti B in her serum but this causes little trouble to the baby. It is thought that when the group A or B erythrocytes from the foetus pass into her circulation, she becomes sensitised producing immune anti A and anti B which on reaching the baby's circulation destroy his red cells.

ABO haemolytic disease of the newborn is more difficult to prove than Rhesus incompatibility as the Coombs test is usually negative.

Haemolytic disease of the newborn due to the Rhesus factor occurs to a lesser extent in East Africa but is severe. The few that the author has seen give rise to much lower levels of haemoglobin than in the case of ABO incompatibility.

Many babies are seen with severe haemolytic disease but who have no obvious blood incompatibility or other known causes of haemolysis. The etiology needs to be determined.

Haemoglobinopathies
Normal haemoglobin

The normal haemoglobin molecule is made up of haem portion which is an iron-containing constituent, and globin consisting of polypeptide chains. The globin is made up of two identical alpha (α) chains and two identical beta (β) chains. These four polypeptide chains are folded together to form a globular molecule. Normal adult haemoglobin A is structurally represented thus ($\alpha 2 \beta 2$). Alpha and beta chains consist of a sequence of 141 and 146 amino acids respectively. Two and a half per cent of normal haemoglobin is A_2. This variety of haemoglobin has delta (δ) chains instead of beta chains. Its formula is represented ($\alpha 2 \delta 2$). Foetal haemoglobin (F) is represented ($\alpha 2 \gamma 2$), having gamma (γ) chains instead of beta chains.

Foetal haemoglobin

Foetal haemoglobin (F) begins to form in foetal life at about three months of gestation. Its production decreases as that of adult haemoglobin increases. This is explained by the presence of a switch over mechanism from the synthesis of γ to β chains, thus enabling adult haemoglobin to be made.

At birth, there is as much as 50–80 per cent of foetal haemoglobin which falls rapidly to one per cent at one year of age. By adulthood, there is only 0.4 per cent of foetal haemoglobin left.

High levels of foetal haemoglobin occur in haemoglobinopathies, thalassaemia, and in 'hereditary persistence of Hb-F'. The latter is a Mendelian recessive condition in which the defect lies in the switch over mechanism so that the synthesis of γ chains continues leading to elevated foetal haemoglobin. The homozygous has 100 per cent foetal haemoglobin whereas the heterozygous has about 40 per cent foetal haemoglobin, the remainder being A and A_2. This condition has been described in Nigeria. The condition is asymptomatic and is discovered usually by chance on haemoglobin electrophoresis. The amount of foetal haemoglobin is estimated by 'one minute alkaline denaturation test'. The test depends on the property of Hb-F to resist alkaline denaturation whereas Hb-A or A_2 do not. The test measures the percentage of alkaline resistant pigment remaining after the exposure of the haemoglobin to standard alkali solution under defined conditions.

Abnormal haemoglobins

Abnormal haemoglobins are caused by abnormal

synthesis. The abnormality can occur in either the α or β chains. Commonly the abnormality is in β chains. The defect may involve just one amino acid in the chain but leads to a series of pathological changes. To have a homozygous child, the biological parents must both be heterozygous.

Change in the amino acid sequence of the globin chain also alters the electrical charge on the molecule. This feature is used in the diagnosis of haemoglobin-opathies by haemoglobin electrophoresis.

The most important abnormal haemoglobins are S, C, D, E, H and Barts. The others are rare, most of which are not of clinical significance. Haemoglobins Barts, beta, Hopkin 2, D and 1 are a result of defect in α chains, whereas in S, C, D, E the defect occurs in the β chain.

Sickle-cell anaemia

In sickle-cell disease, the abnormality is in the β chain so that the amino acid valine replaces glutamic acid in the sixth position of the chain from its N terminal.

When one chain is involved the patient is hetero-zygous (trait, AS). When both β chains are involved, the patient is homozygous (SS). Sickle-cell anaemia is widely spread in all countries of tropical Africa. It also affects people of African descent in the Caribbean and North and South America. Sickle-cell disease has been described in countries of the Middle East and in tribal groups in India.

Sickle-cell trait

The trait (AS) is usually asymptomatic. Flying in unpressurised aircraft can cause splenic infarctions in the heterozygote. Some may get haematuria due to vascular occlusion in the renal papillae or pelvis. Others have impaired concentration of urine.

The incidence of the trait varies from area to area. It may be as high as 12–40 per cent. In East Africa it varies from 0.8 per cent in the Masai to 45 per cent in the Bwamba. The high incidence is thought to be due to selective advantages of heterozygous where the AS protects an individual against the lethal effect of *Plasmodium falciparum* malaria. This hypothesis is based on the observation that the S gene is most common in an area where *Plasmodium falciparum* malaria is endemic. In the (AS) individual the proportion of haemoglobin (S) varies from 20–45 per cent. Sickle-cell trait may combine with another abnormal haemoglobin if either parent

is a carrier of such a gene. This gives rise to sickle-cell haemoglobin C (S—C) or sickle-cell haemo-globin D (S—D) disease or sickle-cell thalassaemia (S—TH).

Sickle-cell anaemia

This is a homozygous state resulting from the mating of traits. It produces a severe and chronic haemolytic anaemia. In infancy the disease mani-fests after six months of life when foetal haemo-globin declines and is less than 35 per cent, the rest being haemoglobin S. The presence of foetal haemoglobin protects the individual against the pathological effect of the sickling phenomenon. Indi-viduals and populations with higher foetal haemo-globin concentrations have fewer sickled erythro-cytes in their circulation and milder clinical disease. The main features of the disease in infancy are: swelling and pain of hands, fingers, feet and toes; pallor and, rarely, jaundice.

From the second year of life on, the disease is characterised by repeated attacks of fever, jaundice, anaemia, pain in the limbs and abdomen due to infarcts in the bones and mesenteric capillaries. There is normally hepatosplenomegaly. But the spleen shrinks with time due to repeated infarctions which heal by fibrosis. In long-standing cases the heart is dilated and has murmurs.

The clinical features are due to the abnormal hae-moglobin which forms crystals whenever there is lowered oxygen tension. The formation of such crys-tals alters the shape of the erythrocytes which are no longer globular but become sickled or half-moon in shape. The sickled cells are picked up and haemo-lysed by reticuloendothelial cells. This causes anae-mia and jaundice. Sickled cells tend to stick to the walls of capillaries, causing obstruction and infarc-tion. The above clinical features are punctuated by crises, usually haemolytic, but thrombotic, seques-tration, aplastic and mixed crises also occur. Infec-tions including malaria precipitate crisis. Exposure to cold and violent exercise too may precipitate a crisis. The main features of haemolytic crisis are anaemia, jaundice and fever. The features of throm-botic crisis are swelling, pain and fever, while those of aplastic crisis are mainly severe pallor without much jaundice. Sequestration is characterised by severe anaemia due to pooling of blood in the vis-cera, especially the spleen.

Patients with sickel-cell anaemia are prone to Gram negative infections, particularly *Salmonella*. It is thought that sickle-cell infarcts in the walls of the intestines encourage the systemic invasion by

Salmonella organisms. Osteomyelitis due to *Salmonella* is a particularly common complication.

Laboratory examination

Haemoglobin is usually about 7 g per cent. Red cells are normocytic and normochromic. Normoblasts and reticulocytes are abundant. There is marked poikilocytosis and anisocytosis.

A stained thin blood smear from a finger prick shows sickled cells in the case of homozygous (SS), and can be used for diagnosis. White blood cells are elevated. Sickle-cell preparation shows positive sickling for both AS and SS. Sickle-cell preparation is made using a freshly prepared 2 per cent solution of sodium bisulphite.

A drop of blood is sealed with petroleum jelly on a glass slide under a cover slip – a 'sealed drop test' – either by itself or with sodium bisulphite. The preparation is examined repeatedly under a microscope for the appearance of sickled cells. Early sickling indicates (SS) and late sickling indicates (AS). A preparation may be negative even in (SS) in as many as 20 per cent unless it is prepared well. Haemoglobin electrophoresis shows SS for sickle-cell anaemia and AS for the trait.

Diagnosis depends on clinical features and laboratory findings. In areas of high incidence of sickle-cell disease, the diagnosis is simple on clinical grounds. The disease should be differentiated from rheumatic fever, surgical abdomen, osteomyelitis and cerebral disease which it may simulate.

Management

Management is palliative and symptomatic. Blood transfusion is given for anaemia. Analgesics such as aspirin and pethidine are given for pain and the patient should have bed rest.

Painful crises are a result of vaso-occlusive episodes, and may be provoked by infection or dehydration. Young children suffer the 'hand foot' syndrome characterised by infarcts of the metatarsals and metacarpals, and painful swelling of the hands and feet. It is usually necessary to give intravenous fluids to those with severe pain or abdominal symptoms, whilst ensuring adequate oral intake. The haemoglobin concentration usually remains steady in a painful crisis. A falling haemoglobin value suggests sequestration in lung, spleen or liver.

Patients with sickle-cell disease are susceptible to infection because of hypersplenism, defective opsonisation, and other ill-defined reasons. The organisms to which they are particularly vulnerable are *H. influenzae, S. pneumoniae* and *Salmonella*. The risk of pneumococcus infection has been estimated to be at least 600 times that in the general population. The risk is greatest in the first three years of life. Continuous prophylactic penicillin in infants less than three years old reduces the infection rate by 80 per cent. The advent of an effective vaccine against *H.influenzae*, and similar developments in pneumococcal and other vaccines will go a long way to protect children with sickle-cell disease from infection. Parents should be counselled about the risk of infection and urged to bring their children to the hospital for assessment whenever they are febrile. Very young children should be treated with broad spectrum antibiotics when febrile, whilst a thorough search is made for a source of infection (in blood, lungs, urine, and in the meninges if indicated).

Splenic sequestration of erythrocytes is a major cause of mortality in the early years, and may be precipitated by infection. It leads to sudden anaemia. The clinical signs are sudden onset of pallor, breathlessness, abdominal pain, and splenic enlargement. The need for blood transfusion in most cases is urgent.

Minor episodes of splenic sequestration are predictive of life threatening severe episodes later. Sustained hypersplenism is also more common in those developing minor or major episodes of acute sequestration compared with those without such a history. Minor episodes of sequestration can be diagnosed by a sudden and unexplained fall in haemoglobin level by more than 2 g/dl together with evidence of marrow activity and an enlarging spleen. Recurrences can be avoided by splenectomy.

The most devastating complication of vaso occlusion is stroke, and is an indicator for acute exchange transfusion. The risk of recurrence is high, and a programme of regular transfusion as well as other prophylactic measures should be maintained for prevention.

Older children and adults get the chest syndrome characterised by lung consolidation on X-ray, and chest pain. The patient may deteriorate rapidly. Antibiotics should be given intravenously, after taking sputum and blood samples for culture. A blood transfusion is indicated if the haemoglobin concentration is falling.

Aplastic crises occur from time to time, characterised by temporary cessation of erythropoiesis and a fall in haemoglobin. In many instances the episodes are triggered by parvovirus infection. A blood transfusion is needed to tide the patient over the crisis.

Between crises, malarial prophylaxis and folic

Table 26.1 Schedule for malarial prophylaxis and folic acid between crises

Age in years	0–3	3–6	6–12	Above 12
Paludrine mg/day	25	25	50	100
Chloroquine mg/week	150	200	250	250
Folic Acid mg/day	2.5 alternate days	2.5	2.5	5.0

acid are given routinely. The schedule shown in table 26.1 is recommended.

Prognosis

The condition carries chronic haemolytic anaemia in which 80 per cent of the cases occur before two years of age. They die of severe anaemia or infections. Some patients die suddenly with no apparent cause. The survivors have physical and sexual growth retardation.

Other abnormal haemoglobins

Haemoglobin C

This predominates in Africans and their descendants and has been described in West Africa. It may occur as homozygous SC or C—thalassaemia. There is a varying degree of anaemia depending upon the combination. SC causes less severe disease than sickle-cell anaemia (SS).

Haemoglobin D

Both haemoglobin chains may have abnormalities. It is seen in India, the Mediterranean areas, Nigeria, Zaire, Turkey, Iran and Indonesia. It predominates in Africans and their descendents. Homozygous (DD) has mild disease while heterozygous (AD) has no symptoms. It may be associated with other haemoglobinopathies.

Haemoglobin E

This is a β-chain abnormality. The homozygous (EE) has mild disease. Heterozygous (EA) has no symptoms. It is found in Burma, Malaysia, India, Sri Lanka, Turkey and Egypt and Thailand where it is commonest. It may be associated with other abnormalities.

Thalassaemia

This is an inherited disorder in the synthesis of the haemoglobin molecule. It is inherited as autosomal recessive. The abnormal haemoglobin synthesis may occur either in the β-chain which is the commonest form or in the α-chain which is rare. The former is called β-thalassaemia and the latter α-thalassaemia. In both there is decreased formation of normal adult haemoglobin A $(\alpha_2\beta_2)$.

β-thalassaemia

When the abnormality occurs in one β-chain of haemoglobin, as for example in the heterozygous, the resulting disease is mild and hence called thalassaemia minor. When the abnormality occurs in both chains, as in the homozygous, the disease is called thalassaemia major because of its severity.

β-Thalassaemia major (Cooleys anaemia)

There is a defective synthesis of adult haemoglobin. Instead of β-chains, γ-chains and δ-chains are synthesised in increased amounts. The synthesis of α chains proceeds normally, hence the combination of α and γ chains leads to the formation of haemoglobin F. Similarly, the combination of α and δ chains leads to haemoglobin A_2. These patients thus have larger than normal amounts of haemoglobin F and A_2. Foetal haemoglobin ranges from 10–40 per cent. Their heterozygous parents have high levels of haemoglobin A_2.

β-Thalassaemia is widely distributed in the world, but the highest incidence is in the Mediterranean regions, the Middle and Far East. There is a low incidence in tropical Africa. In India, thalassaemia is frequent amongst the Punjabis. Some of the cases reported in India are heterozygous with other haemoglobinopathies, for example, thalassaemia—haemoglobin E disease; thalassaemia—haemoglobin D disease and so on.

Where sickle cell and haemoglobin C occur, the thalassaemia gene may combine to form sickle-cell – thalassaemia or haemoglobin C – thalassaemia, as has been reported from Ghana.

The disease is characterised by severe anaemia of hypochromic type. Anisocytosis poikilocytosis and target cells are present. Basophilic stippling of red cells and nucleated red cells are marked in the peripheral blood. Reticulocytosis and leucocytosis are also common.

At presentation the main problem is to identify the small proportion of patients with thalassaemia intermedia. In these cases the anaemia is milder than usual, and just compatible with life. Presentation after the age of two years, and a haemoglobin of more than 8g/dl are useful indicators of a mild form of disease.

Red cell survival is shortened. This gives rise to increased indirect serum bilirubin levels and marked siderosis in all organs. Hypertrophy of the haemopoietic tissue causes characteristic bone changes. The 'hair on end' appearance is seen on skull X-ray. The cortex of the long bones is thinned. There is deformity of maxilla and dental arch with protrusion of frontal teeth, leading to changes in facial appearance.

Congestive cardiac failure with arrhythmias and heart block is common, and is the cause of death in many of these patients. Pericardial effusion together with effusion in other body cavities is also seen. The other causes of death are severe anaemia and haemosiderosis. Diagnosis is based on the finding of hypochromic microcytic anaemia and raised A_2 and foetal haemoglobin. Lack of response to iron therapy in an individual presenting with haematological characteristics of iron deficiency should raise suspicion of thalassaemia minor.

Management consists of regular transfusion, splenectomy when indicated, and treatment with iron chelating agents to control iron overload. Multiple transfusions carry the risk of infection, and it is advisable to immunise the patient against hepatitis B. The current practice is to maintain the haemoglobin at a high level of 12 g/dl. The advantage is to suppress hypertrophy of the bone marrow, which in turn reduces excessive gastro-intestinal absorption of iron, and also the stimulus to hypersplenism because immature erythrocytes are no longer entering the blood stream. The result is that iron overloading is reduced as well as blood requirement by preventing hypersplenism.

Thrombocytopenia and an increasing need for blood transfusion are indicators for splenectomy. The procedure increases the risk of life threatening infections, and immunisation with vaccines against *H. influenzae* B and *S. pneumoniae* is indicated, as is also the prophylactic administration of oral penicillin 250 mg daily,

Figure 26.1 The hair-on-end appearance in the skull X-ray in thalassaemia

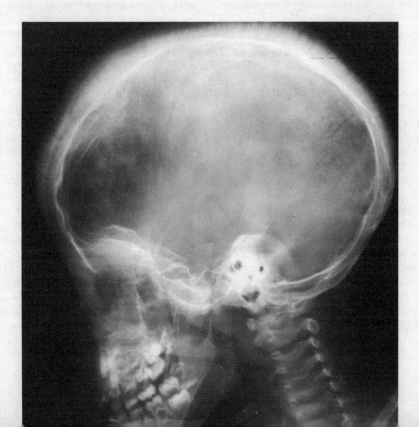

and antimalarials in areas of known endemicity.

Iron chelation treatment is required sooner or later in all patients. Regular intramuscular injections of desferrioxamine (20 mg/kg), at least five times weekly stabilises body iron at 16 g. Subcutaneous infusion (20–40 mg/kg over 12 hours) during the night daily or on alternate days is more effective, and stabilises body iron at 3 g. Iron excretion is helped by vitamin C (200 mg daily) given orally. At the time of transfusion 6 g of desferrioxamine given intravenously helps the excretion of large amounts of iron.

A bone marrow transplant from a sibling is likely to become a definitive form of treatment in the near future.

Prevention Marital and prenatal counselling, antenatal diagnosis with termination of pregnancy in cases of homozygosity, and greater popular awareness of the condition has led to a marked fall in new cases of thalassaemia being diagnosed in a number of Mediterranean countries.

β-thalassaemia minor

In this disease the anaemia is usually mild. But severe symptoms similar to the major disease have been described. Haematological features show minor morphological changes but in others a picture similar to major disease is seen.

Heterozygous thalassaemia with other haemoglobinopathies gives rise to a mild disease.

Heterozygous state is thought to confer advantage through protection against malaria. In some malarious areas as many as 20 per cent of the population may be heterozygotes.

α-thalassaemia

There is defective synthesis of α-chain. In foetal life when haemoglobin F ($\alpha_2\gamma_2$) should be forming, only γ chains are synthesised. These aggregate to form four γ chains. This situation gives rise to haemoglobin Bart's. This condition is incompatible with foetal life. It gives rise to hydrops foetalis and still-births.

In adult life, β-chains are synthesised forming β_4. This situation gives rise to haemoglobin H disease, a milder form of thalassaemia. It is commonly encountered in China, the Mediterranean countries, India, Indonesia, Burma and Thailand.

Abnormal haemoglobin in H disease ranges from 5–30 per cent, the rest is either A or A_2. Clinically, haemoglobin H disease gives rise to chronic recurrent anaemia with attacks of jaundice, fever, joint and abdominal pains. On haemoglobin electrophoresis, H moves ahead of Bart's, hence the two can be differentiated.

Glucose–6-phospate dehydrogenase (G-6-PD) deficiency

Glucose-6-phosphate dehydrogenase is an enzyme occurring in red cells of normal individuals. Certain individuals inherit a deficiency of this enzyme. In the presence of such a defect, the red cells are haemolysed on exposure to various agents and foods.

G-6-PD deficiency has been demonstrated in many parts of the world, particularly in the Mediterranean region, the Middle and Far East and Africa. The incidence is variable, being 10–19 per cent in East Africa.

Available evidence shows that G-6-PD deficiency offers selective advantage to the carriers against effects of falciparum malaria infection in a manner similar to that in the case of the sickle-cell trait. In such malarial areas the gene has survived because of the advantage conferred on the heterozygote. Thus the incidence of G-6-PD deficiency can be greater than 20 per cent in some populations. A high incidence of G-6-PD deficiency in patients with sickle-cell anaemia has been noted by several authors.

The enzyme is inherited as sex linked recessive and has many variants. The two clinically important are: the negro type and the caucasian type. In the negro type, the deficient individuals have 15 per cent of normal enzyme activity while in the caucasians the enzyme activity is as low as one per cent. The caucasian type therefore causes a much more severe disease than the negro type. In the negro type the younger red cells have more enzyme activity than the older cells.

Patients with this enzyme defect have abnormal glutathione metabolism when their red cells are exposed to oxidising substances. Glutathione which is normally in reduced form maintains the integrity of the erythrocyte. In the oxidised form the cell wall of the erythrocyte becomes abnormal and the cell is destroyed, leading to a variable degree of haemolytic anaemia. The first drug to be associated with G-6-PD in the etiology of a haemolytic anaemia was primaquine. Since then many common drugs and substances have been implicated. They include 8-aminoquinolenes and other antimalarials, sulphonamides, sulphones, acetylsalicyclic acid, phenacetin, para-animosalicyclic acid, chloramphenicol, vitamin K, ascorbic acid, broad beans (fava beans), naphthalene (moth balls), derivatives of nitrofurans, dimercaprol, methylene blue, phenylhydralazine, trinitrotoluene, niridazole, neosalvarsan, male fern and even bacterial, parasitic and viral infections.

The enzyme defect is otherwise harmless until the red cells are exposed to oxidising substances. The severity of haemolysis depends upon the variant of the enzyme defect, the dose of the offending agent and the duration of exposure. The haemolysis begins around the third day after administration of the precipitating agent. Rarely does it begin immediately. The anaemia is variable and is usually self-limiting taking about three to ten days after exposure. The haemolysis may be sufficiently severe to cause haemoglobinuria which can simulate black water fever.

G-6-PD deficiency can cause neonatal jaundice and even kernicterus. It is a common cause of neonatal jaundice in the Chinese.

The diagnosis is suspected from history. Deficient enzyme is detected by brilliant cresyl blue dye test or methaemoglobin reduction test. Enzyme assay is more specific.

Management consists of removal of the precipitating agent, estimating the degree of anaemia and giving blood transfusions where there is severe anaemia.

Anaemia due to malaria

Red cells which are parasitised by the malaria parasite haemolyse easily when the parasites burst out at maturity. Parasitised cells are also trapped and destroyed in the reticulo-endothelial tissue, mainly in the spleen, bone marrow and the liver.

Plasmodium falciparum attacks both young and old red cells while the other species of malaria tend to parasitise the older cells only. The resulting anaemia is therefore much more severe in falciparum infection than in the others.

Peripheral blood shows many red cells with parasites. Polychromasia, anisocytosis, poikilocytosis and target cells are common. The red cells are usually normal in size and colour.

Clinically the patient has anaemia and the features of malaria such as fever, diarrhoea and vomiting, weakness, enlarged spleen, anorexia and failure to thrive. The anorexia may lead to dietary deficiency. Haemolysis may also depress the bone marrow thus complicating the anaemia. There is usually temporary bone marrow depression in severe malarial parasitaemia.

Anaemia of malaria is one of the three commonest causes of anaemia at Mulago Hospital in Kampala.

The management consists of treating both the anaemia and malaria. Nivaquin is given for malaria. When anaemia is severe, blood transfusion is life-saving. Many patients need a course of oral iron on recovery from the acute episode.

Anaemia due to lack of haemopoietic tissue
Marrow depression

Bone marrow activity is commonly depressed by chemical, toxic, and physical agents. The marrow depression may affect all the blood-forming precursors or selectively depress the erythroid precursors. Table 26.2 shows the agents that are capable of depressing the marrow.

Table 26.2   Agents that can depress bone marrow

Drugs:	Chloramphenicol, barbiturates, aminopyrin, santonin, tridione, sulphanomides, nitrogen mustard, 6-mercaptopurine.
Toxic agents:	Infections, uraemia, herbs.
Chemical:	DDT, Lead.
Physical agents:	Radiation.
Miscellaneous:	Haemolytic disorders, sickle cell disease, hereditary spherocytosis, multiple transfusions and malnutrition.

In some instances, the offending agent cannot be easily traced. Such cases are classified as idiopathic. Very rarely congenital or primary erythroid hypoplasia is seen.

The clinical features are dependent on the severity of the anaemia and the co-existing causative factors. There is history of weakness, prostration and easy fatigue. The presence of neutropenia may be associated with repeated infective episodes.

Haematological investigations show low haemoglobin with little or no reticulocyte factors. There is low cell count and platelet count. Diagnosis is confirmed by bone marrow examination which shows maturation arrest and generalised cellular depression.

The patients do not respond to haematenics. Blood transfusion with packed and sedimented red cells is the main treatment. Some authors advocate steroids, and testosterone. The primary cause of the marrow depression should be identified and removed or treated where possible. Some authorities prefer to give routine antibiotics for prophylaxis against intercurrent infection.

Infiltration of bone marrow

The marrow may be infiltrated by neoplastic and infective deposits thus rendering it inefficient in the formation of red blood cells or all the blood elements.

The neoplastic deposit and infiltrations are seen in lymphomas, neuroblastoma, leukaemia, Hodgkin's disease. In leishmaniasis, the bone marrow is heavily infiltrated by *Leishmania donovani* bodies. Bone marrow infiltration also occurs in lipid and glycogen storage diseases. The patient will show both the features of the original disease and of anaemia. Treatment is directed to both the offending disease and the anaemia. Blood transfusion is mandatory if the anaemia is severe.

Anaemia of protein-calorie malnutrition

Anaemia of varying degrees occurs in children with malnutrition. In some cases the haemoglobin on admission falls to its lowest value in the second week of treatment. The anaemia is usually mild and is thought to result from a combination of protein deficiency, iron deficiency, intercurrent infections and parasitic infestations. Protein deficiency has been shown experimentally to cause anaemia.

The blood picture varies according to the deficient nutrient. It can be of any morphological type: normocytic, normochromic macrocytic, hypochromic or even dimorphic. The clinical picture is that of pallor together with the features of the co-existing malnutrition.

Biochemical changes include low serum levels of vitamin B_{12} and folic acid. There is also depression of specific iron binding beta-globulin in the serum causing a reduced iron binding capacity in about a third of the patients. Low serum iron levels of 73.7 μg/100 ml with a range of 25–155 μg/100 ml have been reported by several workers. In some instances low plasma levels of vitamin E associated with severely shortened life span of red cells has also been reported. On the other hand, there is no basic defect involving production of erythropoietin.

The bone marrow also shows variable findings ranging from no abnormalities to cases with severe depression of erythropoiesis. The significant bone marrow changes are: depresed cellularity of red cell precursors with a high myeloid erythroid ratio, low number of reticulocytes and pathological megakaryocytes. True megaloblasts and giant stab cells can be usually seen in the marrow. In the author's experience in East Africa, three of every 20 patients with protein calorie malnutrition had megaloblasts in their bone marrow.

This anaemia responds slowly to treatment, due to its multiple etiology. Mild anaemia responds to correction of protein deficiency. Patients with megaloblastic anaemia respond well to folic acid and also to B_{12}. Administration of vitamin E helps to correct shortened life span in some cases. Some workers have found that eight per cent of the cases had refractory anaemia which responded only to administration of pyridoxine. In different situations there may be different factors acting singly or in combination to cause the anaemia. A careful analysis of the dietary history and a knowledge of common deficiencies in the local foods, together with laboratory investigation will help to identify the main deficiency in the individual patient. Treatment of the protein-energy malnutrition on a mixed diet will help to correct the broad deficiency of nutrients. Intercurrent infections should be looked for and treated simultaneously with the malnutrition in order to get a satisfactory haemoglobin response.

Megaloblastic anaemia

Megaloblastic anaemia in the tropics is largely due to nutritional deficiencies rather than Addison's pernicious anaemia which is comparatively rare.

Megaloblastic anaemia is not as common as other types of anaemia and constitutes about two per cent of all anaemias seen in hospital cases in Uganda. In Kenya megaloblastic anaemia has been described mainly on the coast where it occurs on a seasonal basis in both children and adults.

The majority of the cases are due to either folic acid or vitamin B_{12} deficiency or are associated with kwashiorkor. Rarely, it is seen in association with sickle-cell anaemia, during treatment with folic acid antagonists in leukaemia, after prolonged treatment with anticonvulsant drugs, particularly sodium hydantoin, in premature infants, and in infestations with the fish tapeworm.

Folic acid is available in green vegetables, plantains, liver and kidney. Vitamin B_{12} on the other hand is more commonly available in foods of animal origin. Dietary intake and body stores are not as critical for B_{12} as for folic acid hence megaloblastic anaemia of B_{12} deficiency is rare compared to that caused by deficiency of folic acid. B_{12} and folic acid deficiencies are difficult to differentiate without good laboratory facilities. But since folic acid deficiency is commoner, treatment should be started with folic acid. Physiological doses of 0.4 mg daily for 10 days usually induce haematological response in folate deficiency but not in B_{12} deficiency.

A special form of megaloblastic anaemia has been described in the tropics which is associated with hyperpigmentation of hands and feet. Sporadic cases have been reported from Sri Lanka, Nigeria, Indonesia and India. This anaemia, which is also associated with ataxic tremors, responds well to treatment with B_{12}. Other forms of megaloblastic anaemia are seen in the tropics which do not respond to either folic acid or B_{12}, but to pyridoxine.

The diagnosis is suspected on peripheral smear which shows macrocytes in association with raised reticulocyte count. Mean corpuscular volume of the erythrocytes is increased. The diagnosis is confirmed by bone marrow biopsy which shows the presence of megaloblasts. Management consists of removing the underlying cause and supplying the missing nutrient.

Leukaemia

The incidence of childhood leukaemia in most of the indigenous people of the tropics is said to be less than that seen in the temperate countries. It is lowest in the Chinese, while in Western Nigeria and Jamaica the incidence is reported to be similar to that found in Western countries. The low incidence is therefore doubted. Calculations of the incidence from hospital data using the expected number of patients do not reveal true low incidence. The reason for the reported low incidence has variously been thought to be mis-diagnosis, lack of facilities and the pressure on beds so that all severe anaemic children are transfused and discharged home before the investigations are completed. Other authorities think that in the tropics where lymphomas are common, these solid tumours may be variants of leukaemia, thus representing a different host reaction. By comparison with the reported incidence in the past, the incidence is rising. This rise may be real or due to improving laboratory facilities. Under-diagnosis is unlikely in centres like Ibadan and Kampala which have been well staffed for many years with paediatricians and pathologists who are familiar with the presentation of leukaemia. Besides the low incidence of leukaemia in the tropics there are two other peculiarities, namely the high incidence of chloromatous leukaemia and of myeloid leukaemia.

The clinical features are the same as those seen in temperate countries but the age group is older. In the temperate countries leukaemia is commonest in the age group of two to five years. In the tropics most reports describe older children affected.

The main clinical features are: fever, pallor, haemorrhages with purpuras, hepatosplenomegaly and lymphodenopathy. Leukaemia should be suspected in children presenting with PUO and unexplained anaemia. The other peculiar presentation seen in the tropics is proptosis.

The diagnosis depends upon finding abnormal cells in the peripheral smear. A bone marrow biopsy gives a definitive diagnosis. All patients with pallor and leucopenia should have a bone marrow examined to rule out leukaemia. Management is based on supportive as well as definitive treatment. For supportive therapy haemoglobin should be checked and blood transfusion given for anaemia. Sedatives and analgesics may be required for pain. Infection is common in these children because of diminished immunological response. This should be looked for and treated by appropriate antibiotics. The parents should be told the nature of the disease and the prognosis.

The outlook in leukaemia is much improved with increased understanding of the natural history of the disease. In particular irradiation of the CNS together with intrathecal methotrexate at an early stage in the disease helps to avoid relapse and has greatly changed the prognosis. The aim of treatment is to induce remission on diagnosis by means of prednisone and vincristine and maintain the state of remission with methotrexate. If relapse occurs, remission is induced again with prednisone and vincristine and maintained with 6-mercaptopurine. Many of the above chemo-therapeutic agents are not easily available in small district hospitals. On the other hand, the careful supervision necessary and the range of complications both because of the disease and the treatment require that such patients should be referred for management to the larger centres.

Bone marrow transplantation is increasingly used in the management of leukaemia. Long term prospective studies will provide a true measure of its usefulness.

Burkitt's lymphoma

Burkitt's lymphoma is common in the tropics particularly in Africa where it is endemic in Uganda and Nigeria. Cases have been reported in other tropical areas including India and South America. Isolated cases have also been reported in North America and Europe. Outside Africa, the tumour is endemic in Brazil and New Guinea.

Burkitt's lymphoma is a malignant neoplasm seen in children. Boys are affected twice as frequently as girls. It is most frequently seen in the five to nine year age group and rarely under the age of two years or in adults. About ten per cent of cases occur in children over 15 years. Geographically its distribution is similar to malaria. It is largely limited to the lowlands where malaria commonly occurs and is rare in the mountainous areas. Climatically it is limited to warm and humid areas with temperatures not less than 16°C and rainfull not less than 30 inches. Because of this geographical and climatical distribution, it has been suggested that it is induced by a virus like the herpes virus or the Epstein–Barr virus acting on a host in whom the immune response has been altered because of malaria. Other viruses have been isolated from patients but their significance is not clear. It has been further suggested that the majority of the children exposed to the virus develop immunity to it and only a few develop the tumour. This view is supported by finding antibodies in the serum of the patients and the observation that when serum of cured patients is injected in patients with the tumour, the mass regresses.

Burkitt's lymphoma represents 50–70 per cent of childhood malignancies in Uganda and in Ibadan, being several times more common than leukaemia. Because of this high prevalence it was thought in the past to be a biological variant of lymphatic leukaemia.

Seventy per cent of the patients present with facial swelling involving the mandible or maxilla. The facial swelling is painless and grows rapidly destroying the eye and displacing the teeth. The second common presentation is abdominal swelling due to glands or abdominal organs such as kidneys, the ovaries or the liver. It may present with sudden flaccid paralysis of the lower limbs due to cord pressure by the tumour. Superficial glands are rarely involved. Infiltrations may involve the pericardium, meninges, endocrine glands, pituitary, thyroid and adrenals. The disease may present as a solitary swelling of the salivary gland, the neck gland, the testes, the thyroid or the shaft of femur. It is considered to be multicentric in origin whereby multiple sites are involved either at the same time or at different stages.

For purposes of classification and for monitoring response to treatment the clinical features are staged as follows: Stage I a single facial tumour; Stage II two facial tumours; Stage III consists of Stage II plus intra-abdominal, intrathoracic or osseous involvement while Stage IV consists of features of Stage III plus CNS involvement whereby tumour cells are found in cerebrospinal fluid.

Diagnosis is made on histology. Touch preparation is helpful at surgery when the imprint preparations of sections of the tumour are stained with Giemsa stain which makes the identification of abnormal cells easy. Histological appearance consists of sheets of Burkitt's lymphoma cells interspersed with normal histiocytes giving the 'starry sky' appearance. The tumour should be differentiated from retinoblastoma, neuroblastoma and nephroblastoma, all of which it resembles both clinically and histologically.

The prognosis is poor. Those in stages I and II have slightly better prognosis. Those in stage IV have the worst prognosis even with intensive treatment. The tumour usually proves fatal within four to six months if left untreated. However, in some isolated instances spontaneous remission has been observed.

The tumour responds favourably to cyclophosphamide (Endoxan) and methotrexate. The dose of cyclophosphamide is 30–40 mg/kg body weight given as a single dose intravenously. A marked regression of the tumour is observed in patients with stage I and II disease. Myelosuppression with leucopenia occurs between 5–10 days after treatment and recovery from white cell count is seen 10–16 days after treatment. If necessary a second or third dose of cyclophosphamide may be administered when leucopoiesis is normal. Patients should be followed regularly and at the first sign of relapse the above treatment should be repeated.

With the above treatment survival rates are good if the disease is localised. Those with visceral involvement (stage III) may die soon after treatment and surgery. If they survive the initial period, long term remission can be expected in about 67 per cent of cases. Patients in stage IV have a poor prognosis.

Further reading

Newborn

Boon W H. Vacuum extraction in obstetrics. *Lancet* 1961; il: 662.

Ebrahim G J. *Care of the newborn in developing countries.* London and Basingstoke: Macmillan, 1978.

Kagwa J A, Alpidousky V K. Subaponeurotic haemorrhage in newborn infants. An analysis of nine instances in African infants. *Clin Pediat* 1972; 11: 224–227.

Ogunlesi T O. Idiopathic thrombocytopaenic purpura in Nigerians with special reference to Onyalai. *E A fr med J* 1962; 39: 227–231.

Van der Horst R L. Exsanguinating cephalhematomata in African newborn infants. *Archs Dis Childh* 1963; 38: 280.

Nutritional anaemia

Baker S J. Nutritional anaemia – a major controllable public health problem. *Bull Wld Hlth Org* 1978; 56: 659–675.

Biggam Sir A, Wright F J. Tropical diseases and helminthic infections. *In:* McLeod J, (ed). *Davidson's principles and practice of medicine*. Edinburgh: Churchill Livingstone, 1991.

Bwibo N O. Haemoglobin response following intramuscular iron dextran (imferon) in children with iron deficiency anaemia. *E Afr med J* 1970; 47: 254–257.

Finch C A. Iron nutrition. *Ann N Y Acad Sci* 1977; 300: 221–227.

Jelliffe D B, Blackman V. Bahima disease – Possible milk anaemia in late childhood. *J Pediat* 1962; 61: 774–779.

Johnson A A, Latham M C, Roe D A. Nutritional anaemias in the English speaking Caribbean: a review of the literature. *Am J Pub Hlth* 1982; 72: 285–289.

Khan A A. Red cells haemorrhagic disorders and white cells. *Under:* Disorders of the haemopoietic system. *In:* Jelliffe D B, Stanfield P J, (eds). *Diseases of children in the tropics and subtropics*. London: Edward Arnold, 1978.

Layrisse M, Roche M, Baker S J. Nutritional anaemias. *Monograph Ser* WHO 1976; 62: 55–82.

Rao B S N. Physiology of iron absorption and supplementation. *Brit Med Bull*. 1981; 37: 25–30.

Woodruff A W. Recent work on anaemias in the tropics. *Br med Bull* 1972; 28: 92–95.

Haemoglobinopathy

Evans J P M. Practical management of sickle cell disease. *Arch dis childh* 1989; 64: 1748–1751.

Model B, Petrou M. Management of thalassaemia major. *Arch dis childh* 1983; 58: 1026–1030.

Leukaemia

Allinson A. Do viruses cause cancer in man? *Lancet* 1968; i: 1141.

Aur R J A, Simone J, Hutsu H O et al. A comparative study of central nervous system irradiation and intensive chemotherapy early in remission of childhood acute lymphocytic leukaemia. *Cancer* 1972; 29: 381.

Brown R E, Wright B J. Malignancies in African children. How do these differ from malignancies in the U.S.? *Clin Pediat* 1967; 6: 106.

Burkitt D. Determining the climatic limitations of a children's cancer common in Africa. *Br med J* 1962; 2: 1019.

Burkitt D, Hutt M S R, Wright D H. The African lymphoma. Preliminary observations on response to therapy. *Cancer* 1965; 18: 399.

Burkitt D, Wright D H. Geographical and tribal distribution of the African lymphoma in Uganda. *Br med J* 1966; 1: 569.

Davies J N P, Owor R. Chloromatous tumours in African children in Uganda. *Br med J* 1965; 2: 405.

Edington G M, McLean C M U. Incidence of the Burkitt tumour in Ibadan, West Nigeria. *Br med J* 1964; 1: 264.

Goldstein J A, Bernstein R L. Burkitt's lymphoma and the role of Ebstein-Barr virus. *J Trop Ped* 1990; 36: 114–120.

O'Cobor G T, Davies J N P. Malignant tumours in African children with special reference to malignant lymphoma. *J Pediat* 1960; 56: 526.

Wright D H. Cytology and histochemistry of the Burkitt lymphoma. *Br J Cancer* 1963; 17: 50.

Wright D H. Burkitt's tumour and childhood lymphosarcoma. *Clin Paediat* 1967; 6: 116.

Ziegler J L, Morrow R H, Fass L, Kyalwazi S K, Carbone P P. Treatment of Burkitt's lymphoma with cyclophosphamide. *E Afr med J* 1970; 47: 189.

27 *Diseases of the digestive system**

The tropical intestine

In tropical countries where protein–energy malnutrition is widely prevalent, the small intestine undergoes characteristic changes in its function and structure which are further aggravated by associated parasitic and microbial infections. Moreover, anaemia of multi-factorial etiology may further complicate the picture. Genetic variability may add a further dimension to the problem. This subject is discussed under the headings: structural mucosal changes; functional mucosal changes; and problem of enteral infestations and infections.

Structural mucosal changes

The intestinal mucosa is one of the sites of a high rate of protein synthesis and cell turnover. Not surprisingly, it shows changes of atrophy in protein-energy malnutrition. The atrophic changes consist of shortening and broadening of the villi, and formation of convolutions and ridges in place of finger shaped villi; the enterocytes become cuboidal and the brush border shows atrophic changes. In addition there is marked round cell infiltration of the lamina propria. The changes are seen throughout the small intestine and there is some evidence that the jejunum may undergo more extensive changes than the ileum. These mucosal changes are rather non-specific and may be seen in several other conditions like giardiasis, gluten-sensitive enteropathy and tropical sprue.

In healthy individuals among the indigenous population of tropical countries, muscosal changes have been described which are less marked than in patients with kwashiorkor but quite distinct from the normal mucosal pattern of Western countries. These changes may be due to environmental, diet-

* By S P. Lamabadusuriya, Professor of Pediatrics, University of Colombo, and G J. Ebrahim.

ary or other ill-defined causes, and may be an adaptive mechanism in response to a different intestinal environment.

There is evidence to suggest that mucosal recovery is slow despite adequate nutritional rehabilitation, and may take up to three or four years. Other workers, however, have shown reversion to the normal appearances within six months. These diverse findings may be due to the multifactorial etiology of such mucosal changes in states of protein–energy malnutrition.

Furthermore, atrophy of the gastric mucosa and hypochlorhydria have been described in children with protein–energy malnutrition. These alterations are partly responsible for the reduced gastric bactericidal barrier and for the associated overgrowth of bacteria in the gastric and duodenal aspirates of such children. Production of intrinsic factor does not seem to be impaired, although the absorption of vitamin B_{12} may be suboptimal.

Functional mucosal changes
Digestive enzymes

There is overwhelming evidence that undernutrition produces a depletion of intestinal enzyme activity; this includes the different types of disaccharidases, dipeptidases and alkaline phosphatase. Most workers have concentrated on lactase activity. This situation is further complicated by the fact that there are many genetic variations for lactase activity in different ethnic groups. In some races like the Bantu, low levels of lactase activity are found after the weaning period in normal individuals. Since protein–energy malnutrition is common at this age, these ethnic variations in lactase activity may further complicate the picture and in a few cases may even contribute to the nutritional state. Moreover, assessment of recovery of brush border enzyme activity after nutritional rehabilitation is rendered difficult because of the above reasons.

Pancreatic structure and function appear to be markedly affected in the severely malnourished child. Lipase, trypsin, chymotrypsin and amylase all decrease in activity and contribute to malabsorption.

Malabsorption

Intestinal malabsorption has been documented in children with protein–energy malnutrition. Malabsorption of diverse substances such as fat, nitrogen, triolein, oleic acid, vitamin A palmitate, glucose, d-xylose and vitamin B_{12} has been demonstrated. As the children recovered, malabsorption of such substances also gradually reversed. It seems as if protein depletion per se causes malabsorption by affecting mucosal function throughout the gut.

Intestinal motility

Decreased intestinal motility has been shown in malnourished children. This may lead to stagnation of intestinal contents and promote bacterial overgrowth of the upper small intestine with all the resultant effects which will be described later.

Problem of enteral infestations and infections

It is well known that most malnourished children suffer from helminthiasis and other associated parasitic infestations like giardiasis. Heavy giardial infection by itself leads to malabsorption of various nutrients and mucosal abnormalities are usually associated with such infestations. Hook worm infestation not only produces an iron deficiency anaemia with its effects, but also causes a protein-losing enteropathy. Iron deficiency anaemia produces mucosal abnormalities which may lead to malabsorption. Furthermore, steatorrhoea has been noted in patients with hook worm infestation. Ascariasis can provoke malabsorption in a variety of ways, one of which is due to production of the anti-enzyme ascarase in excessive amounts.

Bacterial overgrowth of the upper small intestine in protein–energy malnutrition has been well documented in many studies. These anaerobic bacteria metabolise the physiological bile salts found in the duodenum and jejunum and produce unconjugated monohydroxy and dihydroxy bile salts such as deoxycholate. Thus the concentration of physiological bile salts is lowered together with the production of toxic bile salts. These toxic bile salts like the deoxycholate cause malabsorption of glucose, amino acids, and secretion of water and electrolytes in the

Table 27.1 Disaccharidase deficiency (a) and monosaccharide malabsorption (b)

(a)	Primary	Sucrose–isomaltase deficiency	Rare
		Lactase deficiency	Very rare
	Secondary	Lactase deficiency	Very common
		Multiple deficiency	May accompany secondary lactase deficiency
(b)	Primary	Glucose–galactose malabsorption	Rare
	Secondary	Temporary monosaccharide malabsorption	Not uncommon

jejunal mucosa. These mechanisms contribute to the diarrhoea and malabsorption in patients with various grades and types of protein–energy malnutrition.

Gastric microflora In healthy individuals fluid aspirated from the stomach is usually sterile, except during meals which introduce organisms from the mouth and food. The stomach's defences against bacterial invasion comprise low pH, mucus, lysozyme and immunoglobulins. Changes in pH affect resistance to bacteria. In hypochlorhydria, for example, the number of bacteria found in the stomach increases, and so also is the susceptibility to infectious agents like cholera and salmonella. In children with persistent diarrhoea and malnutrition there is bacterial overgrowth in the stomach. More recently *Helicobacter pylori* have been identified as occasionally infecting the gastric mucosa. These spiral bacteria lie in gastric crypts protected from the acid juice by the mucus layer. Their presence is often associated with gastritis and ulceration.

Sugar-induced diarrhoea in children

Over 50 years ago it was first reported that intolerance in dietary carbohydrate can lead to profuse and protracted diarrhoea in children. Since then much work has been done in this field and presently several types of sugar malabsorption in children are identified. These are classified in table 27.1. The secondary types of sugar-induced diarrhoea are far more frequent than the primary forms.

Clinical features

The predominant symptom of sugar intolerance, regardless of the underlying type of intolerance, is diarrhoea which may be very profuse in infants and young children. The undigested or malabsorbed sugar within the small intestinal lumen attracts large volumes of water by osmosis which results in a profuse, watery diarrhoea. Faecal organisms in the large bowel metabolise these sugars to produce short chain organic acids which increase the osmolarity further and lower the pH, thereby impairing the absorption of water by the colon. Further, bacterial activity in the large bowel produces carbon dioxide, so that these patients pass frequent stools with large amounts of flatus. The stools are very watery and hardly contain any solid material and therefore may be mistaken for urine. If in doubt, a rectal examination will provoke the passage of watery stools with flatus. Often there is reddening, excoriation and even ulceration of buttocks in such infants. In older children the symptoms are less marked, severe diarrhoea is rare but abdominal distension, cramps and flatulence are more marked, especially after the ingestion of the offending sugar.

Diagnosis

The diagnosis is relatively easy in cases of sugar intolerance. An accurate clinical history and assessment of the symptoms should alert the clinician to such a diagnosis, which can then be established by a variety of tests and procedures.

The pH of the stool in a breast fed baby is usually acidic whilst in an artificially fed baby it is alkaline. A stool pH of below 5 in an artificially fed baby should alert the clinician regarding the possibility of sugar intolerance. The amount of reducing substances in the stool can be estimated using Clinitest tablets or Benedict's solution, using a modification of the method described for detection of glycosuria.

It is essential that the watery component of the stool should be examined promptly soon after passage. If there is a delay, the specimen should be frozen immediately after collection. Normal infants and children have only traces of sugar in their stools and a concentration of greater than 0.5 per cent is abnormal. Sucrose is not a reducing substance and will not be detected by this method; prior hydrolysis of the specimen with hydrochloric acid is necessary if sucrose malabsorption is suspected. The total amount of reducing substances in the stools can be estimated and the individual sugars passed in the stool can be identified by paper chromatography, but this information is not essential for adequate diagnosis and management.

Other tests of intestinal sugar absorption are available. These are more useful in older children and are generally not needed in younger patients.

Sugar tolerance tests may be useful in older patients when sugar intolerance is suspected, but diarrhoea is not present at the time. A loading dose of the suspected sugar is given in a dose of 1–2 g/kg, in a fasting state, and serial blood glucose levels are estimated half hourly for the next two hours. Normally a rise of 20–30 mg/100 ml occurs within two hours. Abdominal symptoms usually followed by passage of fluid stools containing sugar are noted in patients with clinically significant sugar malabsorption. The response to different sugars may help distinguish different forms of sugar intolerance, for example a normal response to fructose but impaired responses to glucose and galactose in the rare syndrome of glucose–galactose malabsorption.

The barium–lactose meal has been adapted for use in children. A 50 ml dose of barium is administered together with 2.2 g/kg of lactose followed one hour later by a single plain film of the abdomen. The rapid passage of dye through abnormally dilated loops of small bowels correlates with other evidence of sugar intolerance.

Direct estimation of mucosal enzyme activity is rarely indicated in the diagnosis of sugar intolerance in children. Secondary lactase deficiency is by far the commonest type seen, and its clinical and pathological features are now firmly established. Consequently, direct estimation of small intestinal disaccharidase activity is no longer needed for the satisfactory diagnosis and management of the secondary type. Mucosal disaccharidase assays should be reserved for cases in which diagnosis is doubtful or where a life-long hereditary disorder such as sucrose–isomaltase deficiency is suspected.

In vitro tests of sugar uptake by small intestinal biopsy specimens are at present used for research rather than routine diagnostic purposes. This procedure has been useful in demonstrating impaired uptake of glucose and galactose in glucose–galactose malabsorption.

The conclusive test for the diagnosis of sugar intolerance is the clinical response to removal of the suspected sugar from the diet. If the diagnosis is correct there should be a prompt improvement in symptoms and the stool pattern, followed by a rapid weight gain; a suboptimal response should raise doubts about the diagnosis.

Treatment

The mainstay of therapy is the removal of the offending sugar from the diet. In secondary sugar intolerance, exclusion of the sugar for a temporary but variable time is indicated, whilst long-term dietary restriction is needed in the congenital forms of sugar intolerance. For the management of transient lactose intolerance following gastroenteritis, substitution of soya-protein milk for a lactose-containing milk is often helpful. It must be emphasised that in the breast fed infant secondary lactose intolerance following a bout of diarrhoea is very rare. Breast feeding should be continued throughout the episode of diarrhoea.

Secondary disaccharidase deficiency

The disaccharidases occur in the brush border lining the luminal surface of the intestinal epithelial cells and are susceptible to injury in any disease where damage to the small intestinal mucosa occurs. Examples of such diseases include gastroenteritis, parasitic infestations, protein–energy malnutrition, iron deficiency anaemia and coeliac disease. It is also common in infants after gastro-intestinal surgery, particularly after the relief of large bowel obstruction in the neonatal period. Secondary lactase deficiency is the commonest form of sugar intolerance in infants and children and is often secondary to an episode of infectious gastroenteritis. Since protein–energy malnutrition is a precipitating factor for secondary disaccharidase deficiency, undernourished children are more prone to secondary sugar intolerance following bouts of diarrhoea. Moreover, since lactase is the last brush border enzyme to reach maturity during foetal development, prematurity predisposes to lactose intolerance during outbreaks of diarrhoea in special care units. Furthermore, lactase is present in lower concentrations than other brush border enzymes and is the last disaccharidase to regenerate after mucosal damage. Therefore, the most important type of secondary disaccharidase deficiency is lactase deficiency. Other disaccharidase deficiencies like sucrase may co-exist but do not occur by themselves.

The clinical features of secondary disaccharidase deficiency are similar to those of the primary deficiency states, but follow soon after the predisposing factor, for example, acute gastroenteritis. When a lactose-free milk formula is substituted there is a rapid improvement within the next 48 hours but complete recovery of lactase activity and the ability to digest lactose may take a few weeks or months. During this recovery period, gradual re-introduction of lactose-containing milk should be attempted and if a relapse occurs, lactose should be withheld again for a further period.

It must be emphasised that cow's milk protein allergy can mimic lactose intolerance very closely and the patients may respond in a similar way to the omission of cow's milk since it contains both lactose and protein fractions. Further tests are required to differentiate between these two conditions, which involves the tolerance to separate milk protein fractions and lactose.

Transient monosaccharide malabsorption

This has been observed in the following conditions: (1) post infantile gastoenteritis; (2) after upper small bowel surgery in infants and (3) in malnourished babies.

The clinical features are similar to those of secondary disaccharidase deficiency but the patient will not respond to the substitution of a lactose-free milk containing glucose, galactose or fructose. Metabolic acidosis and hypoglycaemia may complicate the disease. Initially intravenous feeding is required followed by carbohydrate-free oral feeds. Recovery may take a few weeks or several months. The pathophysiology of this condition is not fully understood and it may be related to bacterial overgrowth of the upper small bowel leading to the dehydroxylation and deconjugation of physiological bile salts, which in turn may interfere with the absorption of these monosaccharides.

Tropical sprue

Tropical sprue is an enteropathy of unknown origin occurring in residents or long stay visitors in certain parts of the tropics. It is characterised by chronic diarrhoea, malabsorption and signs of multiple nutritional deficiencies like glossitis, angular stomatitis, anaemia and hypoproteinaemia. Laboratory investigations reveal steatorrhoea and other defects of absorption, as well as altered jejunal morphology on biopsy. There is a spectrum of clinical signs and symptoms varying from the mild to the very severe forms. Some patients present with only isolated complications of malabsorption such as megaloblastic anaemia without any gastro-intestinal symptoms.

In many areas of the tropics chronic and recurrent diarrhoea as well as malnutrition are common problems. The environmental contamination leads to the ingestion of a variety of pathogens. Moreover, parasitic infestations with *Giardia, Strongyloides, Capillaria* and others cause persistent diarrhoea, malabsorption and eventually histologic changes in the gut mucosa. Dietary protein deficiency can also cause enteropathy and investigation of apparently healthy subjects often reveals a high prevalence of minor abnormalities of intestinal structure and function. Intestinal tuberculosis is common in many undernourished communities. Other known causes of malabsorption such as coeliac disease or regional enteritis also occur in the tropics. In such a situation it is difficult to decide whether the clinical signs and symptoms of tropical sprue represent a disease with a single etiology or a syndrome caused by a mixture of conditions.

Clinical features

Tropical sprue (also called postinfective tropical malabsorption) usually begins with an acute intestinal infection which may be bacterial, viral or parasitic. The most commonly isolated bacteria are *Klebsiella*, *E. coli*, and *Enterobacter*. Varying degrees of damage to the enterocyte have been reported in different studies, and the changes become more severe as the disease progresses, though a 'flat' mucosa is extremely unusual. Serum folate levels fall progressively and by four months or so the levels are very low. Folate deficiency aggravates the damage caused by bacterial colonisation. Small intestinal transit time is prolonged in most established cases of tropical sprue due to increased secretion of the hormone enteroglucagon.

Tetracycline reduces the symptoms by eliminating bacterial overgrowth, and leads to cure. Folic acid helps in the recovery of enterocyte function.

The most common and characteristic sympton is diarrhoea. Fever and general malaise may be present in about a quarter of the patients either at the same time as the diarrhoea or preceding its onset by two or three days. Initially the stools contain mucus and blood. Later they become large and bulky. There is a feeling of distension and anorexia together with abdominal pain.

In some cases the diarrhoea lasts for only a few days. In others it may persist for weeks or months. Clinical signs of malnutrition begin to appear as the diarrhoea continues. There is a failure to gain weight. Loss of subcutaneous fat, anaemia, glossitis, and other signs of nutritional deficiencies appear as the disease progresses. The type and severity of the deficiency state will depend upon the local diet and the body stores of the individual patient prior to illness. This would explain the differences in the clinical picture in cases described from different countries.

In one series of 11 children reported from Puerto Rico the common signs and symptoms were as shown in Table 27.2.

Natural history of tropical sprue

Spontaneous remission and 'cure' has been reported in more than half the number affected with sprue. However, in about ten per cent of the cases presenting with symptoms the disease persists causing bouts of intermittent diarrhoea. The longer the symptoms persist, the less likely is spontaneous remission. Without treatment, the mortality rate in such cases can be as high as 30 per cent.

Pathophysiology

Changes in jejunal morphology are seen as early as one week after the onset of symptoms. The histological changes are non-specific and resemble those described in other enteropathies.

A characteristic feature of the enteropathy of sprue is the inability of the small intestine to absorb folate. There is some evidence to show that folate metabolism may be disturbed resulting in a folate-losing enteropathy. Folate requirements may be also high in tropical sprue. It is known that folic acid deficiency by itself can affect gut function and cause malabsorption of other nutrients. The malabsorption and enteropathy of tropical sprue may thus be related to the disturbance of folate absorption and the resulting deficiency.

Extensive bacterial overgrowth in the small intestine with a variety of microflora has been documented in sprue. The bacterial overgrowth interferes with absorption of vitamin B_{12} in the same way as in the 'blind loop' syndrome. Treatment with oral broad spectrum antibiotics causes rapid improvement in some cases again suggesting the role of the microflora in disturbed B_{12} metabolism.

Hypoalbuminaemia, diminished absorption of fat and decreased water and electrolyte transport have also been recorded and contribute to the high mortality from sprue.

Table 27.2 Signs and symptoms of tropical sprue

Signs and symptoms	No.
Weight loss or failure to gain weight	11
Anorexia	10
Weakness	10
Pallor	10
Chronic diarrhoea	10
Glossitis	8
Abdominal pain	4
Burning tongue	2
Vomiting	1

Treatment

Many patients respond to bed rest and a nutritious diet. Several authors have reported improvement with hospitalisation and an adequate food intake alone.

All patients show a rapid response to folic acid with or without vitamin B_{12}. But abnormal gut function persists so that more than half the cases need to take these vitamins on a long term basis.

In various series from different parts of the world a good response to broad spectrum oral antibiotics has been noted. Return to normal function is rapid when antibiotics have been added to folic acid and B_{12}. In particular, antibiotics are useful in those patients who do not respond to the vitamin therapy alone. Tetracycline is the antibiotic commonly recommended.

Preventive programmes

The etiology of tropical sprue is not known but an infectious agent, most probably a virus, has been suggested. This hypothesis is based on the observation that there is usually evidence of transmission within a household, clustering of cases around the index case and the occasional epidemic outbreaks. The occurrence of tropical sprue in servicemen and other expatriates who are long term residents in the tropics also favours the hypothesis of an infective etiologic agent instead of toxic substances, such as rancid fat, or dietary deficiencies.

The widespread presence of the so-called 'tropical intestine' in both the indigenous as well as expatriate residents in the tropics, and the heavy contamination of the upper small intestine in tropical sprue, which is analogous to the situation in malnourished children, strongly suggest that inadequate nutrition and environmental contamination are important contributory factors. Recurrent injury to the bowel mucosa by helminthic and protozoal infestation may further predispose to enteropathies in the tropics. Improved nutrition and safe water, together with facilities for early diagnosis and treatment, will greatly influence the incidence of many tropical enteropathies.

Necrotising enteritis (pig bel)

This condition has been described from New Guinea where it occurs in small outbreaks following ritual feasting on undercooked pork. Hence the name pig bel in Pidgin English. Following the reports from New Guinea, cases have been also reported from Uganda and Ghana.

Most of the pathological changes are found in the third part of the duodenum and the upper jejunum which become inflamed and oedematous. Thrombosis of the mesenteric vessels leads to necrosis and perforation of the bowel. *Clostridium perfringens* type C can be grown from the gut and from the mesenteric nodes. The condition is thought to be a gangrenous arteritis due to the ingestion of clostridial toxin in the festive meat.

Most patients are below five years of age. They present with shock, coma and a toxic state of acute onset, or as surgical emergencies with paralytic ileus, perforation and peritonitis. In some the acute stage would have passed before reaching the hospital and the presentation then is with surgical problems like adhesion and fistulae formation.

In the acute state, which is a common mode of presentation, the abdominal signs may be vague and indefinite in the early stages. Fever, coma and jaundice are often the main symptoms so that a provisional diagnosis of enteric fever, hepatitis or acute gastroenteritis is commonly made.

The treatment is supportive with intravenous fluids to treat shock, gastric aspiration and administration of gas-gangrene antiserum or specific antiserum against *Cl. perfringens* type C if available. Broad spectrum antibiotics are given by mouth. Surgery is indicated if the intestinal obstruction is not relieved by conservative means or if signs of peritonitis or tender abdominal masses develop. The mortality in necrotising enteritis is high. Those recovering may go on to formation of strictures or fistulae leading to malabsorption. More recently a vaccine has been developed using the toxoid of *Cl. perfringens* type C.

Veno-occlusive disease

Hepatic veno-occlusive disease is a progressive form of portal hypertension. Histology of the liver shows central vein dilatation and fibrosis. It is a potentially fatal cause of ascites and hepatic failure. The commonest cause is exposure to herbal teas and brews containing hepatotoxic pyrollizidine alkaloids. Epidemics have been reported from Jamaica, India, Afghanistan and several other countries after contamination of grain stores with the alkaloids, or after consumption of alkaloid containing plants or bush teas. The plants are ingested as food (ackee), or infused in water.

The pyrallozidine alkaloids comprise over 180 compounds which occur in at least eight plant families (for example ragwort and comfrey), which have a wide geographical distribution. Hepatotoxicity is also related to host susceptibility, ingested dose, and the route to exposure. Infants are particularly susceptible, and can be affected by an exposure of less than one week. Older children and adults develop symptoms after an exposure lasting over several months.

The treatment is mainly supportive and symptomatic with adequate rest during the acute illness, nutritious diet and vitamin supplements. High protein diet with raised energy content is recommended except in liver failure or if fats are not tolerated. Salt and water restriction may be necessary to control ascites and oedema. Frequent paracenteses may be necessary to relieve the abdominal distension and to make the patient comfortable.

Indian childhood cirrhosis

This disease is peculiar to the Indian subcontinent though some case reports have come from Sri Lanka, Burma and Bangladesh. Even though a large number of Indians have now lived for many generations in other countries, both tropical and temperate, the disease has not been reported from them, indicating the strong influence of an environmental factor.

The maximum incidence is between the first and the third years of life and up to three-quarters of the cases occur in this age group. There is a high familial incidence, and amongst the cases investigated, 20–40 per cent have occurred within the same family.

The history is of gradual and progressive abdominal enlargement. The liver has a characteristically hard consistency and a sharp edge on palpation. Jaundice is often the symptom leading to admission, and indicates a terminal stage. Death occurs within weeks or months of onset of jaundice, and is due to liver failure, bleeding, anaemia or secondary infection.

In the early stages clinical diagnosis is not easy, especially since liver function tests are not very discriminatory. Liver biopsy is the best way of making a diagnosis. In the advanced case histology of the liver shows widespread damage of cells with presence of hyaline inclusion material, vacuoles, inflammatory infiltrate and pericellular fibrosis. In the advanced stage almost every cell contains orcein staining granules representing copper deposition.

Most affected children give a history of being fed on cow's milk. In traditional Indian homes brass vessels are used for storage and cooking of food. Most such vessels have an inner lining of tin, and it has been shown that when this inner lining is not renewed regularly milk stored in the vessel absorbs copper especially when boiled in the vessel.

Inj. penicillamine 20mg/kg/day helps in the early stages of the disease, but is ineffective once jaundice has set in. Health education concerning avoidance of brass vessels for cooking and storing food has been shown to lower the incidence of the disease amongst affected communities.

Chronic inflammatory bowel disease

Crohn's disease and ulcerative colitis are the two major forms of presentation. Over the last decade new forms of inflammatory bowel disease have been described, and major changes have taken place in the investigation and management of Crohn's disease and ulcerative colitis. It is significant that lack of breast feeding and episodes of diarrhoea during infancy have come to be identified as predisposing to the development of Crohn's disease.

Early symptoms of *Crohn's disease* are non specific, and consist of lethargy, abdominal pain, and chronic diarrhoea. In the fully established disease, which may be months or years later, loss of weight and growth retardation, abdominal pain and diarrhoea, variable bowel habits, and psychological problems are most common. On clinical examination, growth faltering, anaemia, perianal abnormalities (anal fissures, skin tags or anal fistula), and abdominal tenderness are found.

By contrast early symptoms of *ulcerative colitis* are more specific. Diarrhoea, bleeding per rectum, abdominal pain, tenesmus and loss of weight are common findings.

After excluding infection with parasites (amoebiasis, giardiasis, and helminthic infection), and bacteria (shigella, salmonella, campylobacter, yersinia and tuberculosis) the diagnosis is confirmed by means of contrast studies of the bowel, colonic endoscopy and biopsy.

Crohn's disease responds well to an elemental diet in which all intact protein is replaced by amino acids. Success rates for remission are about 80 per cent, and linear growth is much better compared to children treated with steroids.

Sulphasalazine is valuable in the management of

ulcerative colitis (40–60 mg/kg in the acute attack; 20–30 mg/kg as maintenance dose). Topical corticosteroids (prednisolone enema or suppositories) are effective during acute attacks. Surgery may be needed in those who do not respond to medication.

Further reading

Booth I W. Chronic inflammatory bowel disease. *Arch dis childh* 1991; 66: 742–744.

Cook G C. Aetiology and pathogenesis of postinfective malabsorption (Tropical Sprue). *Lancet* 1984; i: 721–723.

Rollins B J. Hepatic veno-occlusive disease. *Am J Med* 1986; 81: 297–306.

Tanner M S, Portmann B. Indian childhood cirrhosis. *Arch dis childh* 1981; 56: 4–6.

28 Diseases of the nervous system*

Paediatric neurology is concerned not only with acute diseases of the central nervous system but also with the study of the disorders that affect the maturation and function of the nervous system during its critical period of development in the early years of life, that is, developmental paediatrics. It differs in this important respect from adult neurology because of the profound effects intercurrent illness has on the further development of the nervous system. In Western countries paediatric neurology is becoming increasingly concerned with developmental assessment and the early detection of deviations from the normal pattern of neurological and intellectual development from birth through to the early years of school life.

The developing central nervous system (CNS) is

* By P. Barnes, Consultant Paediatrician, Bedford General Hospital, Bedford, and G. J. Ebrahim.

particularly vulnerable to a host of insults operating from the time of conception through infancy to late childhood. The brain is the most rapidly growing organ after birth and cell replication is nearly complete by the age of six months, although cell hypertrophy continues until about three years of age. By then the brain has reached 80 per cent of its adult weight although body weight is only 20 per cent of the final adult weight. Maturation of the brain proceeds as myelination takes place with the development of new behaviour patterns and loss of primitive reflexes. These proceed in an orderly sequence and damage to the brain may result in interference with functions that have already developed or in the failure of future patterns of behaviour to develop, or in persistence of primitive patterns of function and behaviour, or regression to these. The maintenance of adequate nutritional and

Table 28.1 Major causes of insult to the CNS

Pre-natal	
Intrauterine infection	Cytomegalovirus, rubella, herpes, toxoplasmosis, syphilis, HIV
Developmental malformations	Hydrocephalus, microcephaly, cortical atrophy
Maternal exposure to X-rays	
Disorders of pregnancy	Maternal illness, premature labour, placental disease
Perinatal (often multiple)	
Bad obstetric history	Infertility, previous abortions, stillbirths or neonatal deaths, antepartum haemorrhage, pre-eclampsia, premature labour
Difficult labour	Disordered uterine action, cephalopelvic disproportion, malpresentation, intrapartum asphyxia
Post-natal	Apnoea or asphyxia, intracranial haemorrhage, hypoglycaemia (especially light-for-dates infant), neonatal jaundice, prematurity or post-maturity, neonatal tetanus
Post-natal	
Catastrophic febrile illness with convulsions or altered consciousness	
Malaria	
Meningitis – pyogenic or tuberculous	
Dehydration	Cerebral thrombosis
	Gastroenteritis
Encephalopathy of 'encephalitis', acute infections, diseases or immunisation	
Sickle cell anaemia	
Trauma	
Metabolic	Hypoglycaemia, hypernatraemia, lead, inborn errors of metabolism

metabolic needs of the developing brain is reflected in its blood supply – the infant brain receives 60 per cent of cardiac output compared with 15 per cent in adults. The CNS has no stores of energy, it derives this mostly from carbohydrates and utilises particularly vitamins of the B group. Protein – calorie malnutrition interferes with brain cell growth and replication, the protein content, DNA content and lipid content are all reduced and myelination is halted. These changes are more marked in the cerebellum than the cerebrum. Some of these effects of malnutrition are discussed on page 311. These are a matter of great concern in developing countries since the period of maximal brain growth and maturation coincides with the peak time of malnutrition.

In particular, the present trend of bottle feeding and the use of over-dilute formulae for economic reasons has led to an increased incidence of malnutrition and diarrhoea in very young infants. The stresses imposed by fever and infection on the developing central nervous system and its metabolism, together with its low epileptic threshold is reflected in the high incidence of febrile convulsions and disastrous sequelae. The major insults experienced by the CNS in infancy are listed in table 28.1 and the sequalae are summarised in table 28.2.

Neurological problems of children in developing countries

Neurology clinics are now established in children's departments in several teaching hospitals in Africa and India, and data from some of these have enabled

Table 28.2   Effects of damage to the CNS

Intellectual deficit – Mental retardation

Neurological deficit
  Epilepsy
  Hyperkinesis
  Behaviour problems
  Cerebral palsy – Hemiplegia, diplegia, dyskinesia
  Specific defects – Vision, hearing, learning, speech

NB Defects are often multiple – for example, mental
  retardation and epilepsy; epilepsy and behaviour
  problems are often associated.

Table 28.3   Major neurological problems of children as reported from four centres

Centre	Kampala	Ibadan	India	Lagos
Type of clinic	All neurological problems	All neurological problems	Cerebral palsy only	Cerebral palsy only
Mental sub-normality	68 (50%) (Neurological deficit in 2/3 of these)	249 (28%)	272 (71%)	†
Neurological deficit but mentally normal	33 (25%)	–	108 (29%)	NS
Behaviour disorders	41 (30%)	37 (4%)	NS	NS
Epilepsy	59 (43%)	NS	53 (13%)	†
Poliomyelitis	*	160	*	NS
Total No. Patients	138	865	380	361

Notes:
* Separate clinics existed – not included in the study.
NS Not stated
† Major associated defect
Multiple handicaps common and some patients are included in more than one category.

Sources: Kampala – Egdell H G, Stanfield J P. Paediatric neurology in Africa: a Ugandan report. *Br med J* 1972; 1: 548.
Ibadan – Elam H P. A panoramic view of the children's neurology service in Ibadan, Nigeria. *Develop Med & Child Neurol* 1967; 9: 784.
India – Basu B. Cerebral palsy in childhood. *J Indian med Ass* 1967; 49: 477.
Lagos – Animashaun A. Cerebral palsy in African children. *First International Conference on Paediatrics in the Tropics.* Ibadan, 1969.

the content of paediatric neurology and its common problems to be defined. A direct comparison between these clinics is difficult because of differing presentation of data and classifications but the overall picture from each is very similar.

Major problems common to all (table 28.3)

These are mental retardation, 'cerebral palsy' which includes a variety of neurological disorders mainly with motor dysfunction, epilepsy, behaviour disorders and the effects of poliomyelitis. Special poliomyelitis rehabilitation clinics exist in some hospitals.

Presenting symptoms fall broadly into four groups (table 28.4). Although these referrals were selected there seems no reason to suppose that they would be significantly different in the other clinics in view of the similarity of their problems. About one-third of the children were referred to the clinic because of anxiety/concern by parents of their failure to achieve the expected levels of development. The remainder were about equally divided between those who had delayed development plus fits, those with fits alone and a miscellaneous group. Behaviour problems were the presenting complaint in only a small number. Conspicuous by their absence are psychosomatic disorders and behaviour which trouble the child but not society. These might well be assumed to be unresponsive to Western type medicine and are therefore not brought to clinics. Indeed the community may set its own limitations to referral by its attitudes to Western medicine as a whole and to certain conditions such as epilepsy.

The clinical findings in the different studies were very similar (table 28.5). The most common neurological deficits found were tetraplegia and hemiplegia, less often paraplegia and rarely monoplegia. Patients are more likely to seek attention for more serious disabilities, hence the prevalence of tetraplegia in all series. Spasticity was the commonest disorder followed by athetosis and hypotonia.

The remarkable absence of ataxia is partly due to the tendency of African mothers to carry their children for longer periods when they have disability and partly due to its tendency to improve with time thereby causing less concern to parents. Less common findings include deafness, blindness, speech disorders, hyperkinesis and physical violence. A considerable number of children were found to have multiple handicaps. The Uganda data showed that two-thirds of the mentally subnormal children also had neurological deficits and the Indian data revealed that 13 per cent of children with cerebral palsy had epilepsy.

Table 28.4 Presenting neurological symptoms in Kampala

Not achieving expected level of development	40
Fits only	30
Fits + delayed development	29
Behaviour problems	9
Miscellaneous*	30
Total	138

* Including not walking or talking; deaf; school refusal; headaches; 'confusion'; fainting attacks; terrors; stutter etc.

Source: Egdell H G, Stanfield J P. Paediatric neurology in Africa: a Ugandan report. *Br med J* 1972; 1: 548.

Table 28.5 Findings in cerebral palsy

	India	Nigeria	Uganda
Anatomical			
Hemiplegia	14.5%	NS	7%
Diplegia (tetraplegia)	61.5%	NS	26%
Paraplegia	22.5%	NS	4%
Monoplegia	0.3%	NS	0.7%
Triplegia	0.3%	NS	–
No. of Cases	275*		138†
Neurological Findings			
Spasticity	72%	57%	26%
Athetosis	5.5%	33%‡	5%
Hypotonia	7%		7.5%
Ataxia	nil	2.5%	2%
Others	5.5%	5.5%	
Associated			
Mental Retardation	71%	NS	50%
Epilepsy	13%	NS	42% (approx)
Total No. of Cases	380	365	138†

NS not stated.
* with spasticity only.
† not all had neurological deficit. This figure is total in the series.
‡ Includes pure athetosis and mixed cases with pyramidal and extrapyramidal spasticity.

Sources: India – Basu B. Cerebral palsy in childhood. *J Indian med Ass* 1967; 49: 477.
Nigeria – Elam H P. A panoramic view of the children's neurology service in Ibadan, Nigeria. *Develop Med & Child Neurol* 1967; 9: 784.
Uganda – Egdell H G, Stanfield J P. Paediatric neurology in Africa: a Ugandan report. *Br med J* 1972; 1: 548.

Etiology

History taking is often limited by the absence of any previous medical records, children may be accompanied by other members of an extended family group. Memory of a past event is not always accurate, and in some cases the history has to be taken through an interpreter. In spite of these limitations symptoms can be clearly related in many cases to the time of birth or some significant post-natal event. Whilst in other cases symptoms appear to have evolved gradually over a variable period of time.

The experience from Africa and India shows clearly that acquired post-natal events are even more important than the formidable hazards of birth and the peri-natal period and can be identified in all the 60 per cent of cases. From the Ugandan data it was shown that most of the post-natal cases had a normal birth and that the commonest mode of post-natal onset (in 50 per cent of cases) was a catastrophic acute febrile illness often with fits – often inadequately treated in the early stages. These post-natal events emphasise the effects of the many environmental hazards to which young children in developing countries are exposed and the devastating effects of such illness as acute bacterial meningitis, encephalitis, the common infectious diseases, malaria, convulsions associated with any acute febrile illness, malnutrition and dehydration. Inadequate or late treatment is responsible for the survival of brain damaged children who would otherwise have died.

The hazards of birth are often multiple and include abnormalities of pregnancy, dystocia and difficult labour, peri-natal asphyxia, birth trauma, prematurity, postmaturity, hyperbilirubinaemia, neonatal tetanus and other infections. However, data from Uganda showed that only one-third of patients gave either a history of abnormal birth or symptoms dating from birth. In the Ibadan study slightly more than half of the cases of cerebral palsy, however, were considered to be congenital (53 per cent) although a cause was only recognised in half of these. In the Indian study of cerebral palsy a peri-natal cause was identified in 40 per cent of cases. This contrasts with the experience in developed countries where the events of birth are the largest single cause of neurological handicap and acquired post-natal causes accounted for only 6.4 per cent of 400 mentally retarded children. These studies emphasise only the grosser aspects of chronic neurological disease and must surely be 'the tip of the iceberg' with many lesser degrees of handicap existing undetected and untreated within the community.

It is clear therefore that many of the disabilities seen in paediatric neurology clinics are preventable and could be reduced by better obstetric care, the early diagnosis and treatment of acute infections, maintenance of a high immunisation rate and malaria prophylaxis, and prevention of malnutrition. Much can be done by health workers to educate the community and especially teachers, about the nature of mental retardation, epilepsy and physical handicaps so that children need not be further handicapped by social and educational ostracism. Finally some modification in the training and attitudes of doctors and medical assistants, nurses and health visitors is essential if they are to diagnose and treat more effectively the chronic neurological and behavioural problems which are being increasingly recognised. The success of polio rehabilitation clinics demonstrates what can be done when existing resources are fully utilised.

Neonatal convulsions

Fits are not always easy to recognise in the newborn. Many babies make momentary jerky movements when asleep and also when awake. A normal startle or Moro response is often misinterpreted by both inexperienced nurses and mothers as a convulsion. Tonic–clonic convulsions are rare and fits in the newborn consist mainly of tonic generalised muscle contractions with extension of the limbs and neck and a fluttering or deviation of the eyes and sometimes apnoea and cyanosis. Focal or multifocal jerking at about three per second may also occur. The three main causes of convulsions in the newborn are brain damage, metabolic disturbances and infections of the CNS (table 28.6). Fits occurring in the first three days of life are usually the result of a perinatal cerebral insult or occasionally a cerebral malformation. Intrapartum asphyxia is particularly dangerous. Convulsions as a result of asphyxia are usually tonic and there is a considerable risk of permanent brain damage particularly in those cases with poor muscle tone. There is a significant mortality and as many as 20 per cent of survivors may be handicapped. In addition, studies in Edinburgh have shown that significant metabolic disturbances may also be present in this group of infants presenting with convulsions and brain damage associated with asphyxia at birth. In the study about one-third had hypocalcaemia and one-third hypoglycaemia. In addition there were other clinical disturbances such

Table 28.6   Etiology of neonatal convulsions

Age	Cause	Associated factors
Birth → 3 days	Brain injury – from asphyxia or haemorrhage Hypoglycaemia – small-for-dates infants Malformations of the brain Associated biochemical factors: Hypoglycaemia Hypocalcaemia	Placental insufficiency
From 5th day onwards	Biochemical disturbances: Hypocalcaemia and hyperphosphataemia Hypomagnesaemia and hyperphosphataemia Hypoglycaemia Neonatal tetanus Kernicterus	Artificial feeding
Any age	Bacterial meningitis and septicaemia Uncommon causes: Congenital infections Inborn errors of metabolism	

as apnoea, the need for tube feeding, apathy, hypotonia, diminished reflexes and cranial nerve palsies as well as permanent neurological and intellectual deficits. Conditions associated with 'placental insufficiency' such as severe pre-eclampsia, small-for-dates infants and possibly twins appear to cause a significant lowering of both calcium and glucose in infants during the first three or four days of life.

Fits occurring from the fifth day onwards are more likely to be associated with a biochemical disturbance, particularly hypocalcaemia and less often hypomagnesaemia with an associated hyperphosphataemia. A smaller number are due to hypoglycaemia. There is a significant association with artificial feeds and some may be related to maternal deficiency of vitamin D. The fits are focal and clonic in type and may occur whilst feeding. Cyanosis and loss of consciousness is not common. Hypertonia especially in the extensor muscles may be noted. Many infants appear 'hyper alert'. In the absence of any associated brain damage, neurological and intellectual sequelae are rare. Treatment consists of adding 1 ml of ten per cent calcium gluconate or calcium lactate to each feed for about a week.

Meningitis and septicaemia are other important causes of fits and of course may occur at any age from birth onwards. Rarer causes are congenital infections for example, cytomegalovirus and toxoplasmosis and the rarer inborn errors of metabolism.

Convulsions must be differentiated from apnoeic attacks or choking attacks or neonatal tetanus. This should not be too difficult although occasionally mild cases of tetanus may not be easy to differentiate. Bizarre irregular movements of the limbs and a history of neonatal jaundice should distinguish convulsions from kernicterus. A lumbar puncture and blood culture are essential to exclude meningitis and septicaemia. The differentiation between brain damage and a biochemical disturbance is to be made on clinical grounds. The use of the Dextrostix reagent strip (Ames Laboratories Limited) is valuable in diagnosing hypoglycaemia. In the absence of laboratory facilities for estimating serum calcium, the addition of calcium gluconate to feeds may produce a therapeutic response.

Convulsions and epilepsy in childhood (table 28.7)

Convulsions are one of the commonest emergencies seen in out-patient departments. Whilst they are an every day occurrence to medical and nursing staff, they are extremely frightening to parents who may have their own beliefs about causation and eventual outcome. Their anxieties may be fully justified for many may have seen their own or others' children die or suffer brain damage on account of a convulsive illness.

Table 28.7 Etiology of fits (after neonatal period)

Infections	Intra-uterine infections, meningitis, encephalitis, cerebral abscess, malaria, parasitic infections
Febrile convulsions	Acute infections outside the CNS
Encephalopathy	Acute infectious diseases Post immunisation Acute 'toxic' encephalopathy

Metabolic	'Spontaneous' hypoglycaemia; hypocalcaemia; hypomagnesaemia
	Water and electrolyte disturbances
	Toxins: lead, tetanus
	Inherited disorders: phenylketonuria
	                    : Hunter–Hurler
	                       mucopolysaccharidoses

Space-occupying lesions	Abscess, tumour, subdural haematoma
Congenital malformations of CNS	Tuberose sclerosis; hydrocephalus; Sturge–Weber
Cerebral palsy Mental retardation Epilepsy Post traumatic Progressive degenerative disorders of the CNS Hypertensive encephalopathy Photosensitive	

Convulsions with fever

Convulsions in children may be associated with an acute febrile illness from any cause, especially malaria, measles, otitis media and viral upper respiratory infections. They may occur at any time from soon after birth until about the age of five, with a peak incidence between six months and two years. Boys are more commonly affected than girls. It is estimated that between five and seven per cent of all children in Britain experience one or more febrile fits and this figure may be as high as 10 per cent in the tropics. There is some evidence of a genetic predisposition with a higher than expected incidence amongst close relatives. A child who has had one febrile convulsion has an increased risk of between 12 and 40 per cent of having another with a subsequent febrile illness. Recurrence of febrile fits is more common in females; in those children with a family history of febrile convulsions, and if the first febrile convulsion occurred at a young age.

Convulsions were the presenting complaint in 20 per cent of almost 4000 admissions to the children's emergency room in Ibadan in 1968. Fifteen per cent were 'febrile' with illnesses not directly involving the central nervous system. Hypoglycaemia was present in many, probably related to the earlier administration of indigenous therapeutic agents. In Lagos febrile convulsions had the highest mortality of all diseases in childhood. One third were due to malaria. In the non-malarial group, the chief pathological findings were oedema of the brain, a large thymus and a generalised increase in lymphoid tissue suggesting recurrent stimulation of the reticulo-endothelial system. High morbidity and morality was also found in a study in Kampala. In 109 children with febrile convulsions and altered consciousness there were 29 deaths and neurological deficits occurred in 17 of the survivors. The clinical course was related to the CSF findings, those who had a pleocytosis had a longer stay in hospital, longer period of fever and greater incidence of residual neurological signs. The relative infrequency with which viruses are isolated is emphasised by several authors.

Catastrophic infections associated with severe

febrile convulsions are very important as a common cause of permanent neurological and intellectual damage. This is often aggravated by delays in presentation which may be due to a variety of reasons but often because of the long distances involved in travelling to medical centres. It was found that fever in the early stages was not always treated promptly or vigorously enough, antimalarials were given too late, water and electrolyte disturbances were not corrected adequately or early enough, and fever was allowed to continue too long unchecked. The ultimate deficits, especially in infancy, are thought to be directly proportional to the degree and duration of both the fever and the acute disturbance of the brain. There is now convincing evidence that prolonged or severe or repeated episodes of febrile convulsions cause mesial temporal sclerosis. The scar so produced becomes an epileptic focus with the development of chronic temporal lobe epilepsy in adult life. Surgery may be of benefit in selected cases.

The mechanisms producing febrile convulsions are uncertain but are probably related to the immaturity of the rapidly developing brain, its inherently low threshold to fits at this age and to the metabolic disturbances following the onset of fever. It may be significant that convulsions are commonest at the onset of an illness when the temperature is rapidly rising and are much less common after a few days of established fever. In some instances convulsions may be the earliest sign of a fever.

A febrile convulsion is a seizure associated with fever in infancy or childhood, usually between three months and five years, without evidence of intracranial infection or a defined cause. Seizures in children who have suffered a previous non-febrile convulsion are excluded in this definition.

In children who have a prolonged seizure lasting more than twenty minutes, or those who have not completely recovered within one hour it is reasonable to suspect meningitis, encephalitis, metabolic or a neurodegenerative disorder with a seizure precipitated by fever, or cerebral palsy with intercurrent infection.

Admission to hospital is usually governed by the following considerations

(1) Complex convulsion, lasting for more than 20 minutes with focal features, repeated in the same episode of illness; or incomplete recovery after one hour.
(2) The child is less than 18 months old.

Blood glucose should be estimated if the child is still convulsing or is unrousable when seen. A lumbar puncture is not necessary in every case, but the decision not to do a lumbar tap should always be reviewed a few hours later. A lumbar puncture is indicated if there are clinical signs of meningitis, in the case of a complex seizure, if the child is unduly drowsy or irritable, if there are signs of systemic illness, or if the child is less than 18 months old. In a comatose child a thorough clinical examination should be carried out before doing a lumbar puncture.

The management of febrile convulsion consists of bringing the fever down with paracetamol (120–250 mg/kg every four to six hours depending on age). Rectal diazepam (500 micrograms/kg) or inj.paraldehyde 2 to 4ml) may be used to control any further seizures. Prophylactic anti-convulsant treatment is indicated only if there is a clear neurological abnormality (for example microcephaly, hydrocephalus or cerebral palsy), or if there are frequent recurrences of febrile seizures (for example two or more in a spate of six months).

The risk of recurrence during the two years after the first seizure is 30 to 40 per cent. Almost half the second seizures occur within six months of the first, and three quarters within a year. Recurrence is determined largely by age, being more common in those less than 18 months old. A family history is also a significant factor.

There is no evidence that prolonged therapy with anticonvulsant prevents the development of epilepsy later. In one of the largest series on febrile convulsions it was shown that three factors are associated with an increased risk of epilepsy by the age of seven years. These are: (1) presence of epilepsy in a parent or a sibling; (2) a developmental abnormality noted before the first seizure, and (3) occurrence of a complex first seizure (defined as lasting more than 15 minutes; focal; more than one seizure in 24 hours). The risk of epilepsy by age seven years is two per cent with the presence of one risk factor and 10 per cent if there are two.

From the practical point of view children with febrile seizures can be classified into three groups.

(1) Those who are *neurologically normal*. In them the prognosis is good with only one to five per cent risk of epilepsy.
(2) Those who are *neurologically abnormal*. The prognosis depends on the degree and type of abnormality, and is particularly poor in very young children.
(3) The third group are those with a *family history of epilepsy* in first degree relatives. In them the risk of epilepsy irrespective of febrile convulsions,is two to five per cent.

Some common causes of acute fever with convulsions

Some common causes of acute fever with convulsions but without other physical signs are

(1) Pyogenic meningitis – lumbar puncture is essential.

(2) Ear and throat infections often cause high fever with convulsions and delirium. It is negligence not to examine the ears and throat of every febrile child, bearing in mind that the febrile state itself may cause slight congestion.

(3) Malaria – if there is no response to adequate antimalarial treatment in 48 hours the diagnosis should be reconsidered, or malarial infection resistant to the common anti-malarials should be looked for.

(4) Measles. It may be the prodromal stage before the rash appears. Presence of Koplik's spots may help to establish the diagnosis.

(5) Typhoid. Fever and abdominal pain are often the only symptoms of typhoid. The child is toxic and looks ill.

(6) Miliary tuberculosis. Fever and a toxic child may be the only symptoms. Cough may not be significant.

(7) Urinary tract infection. For diagnosis a *fresh* specimen of urine must be examined microscopically and obtained by suprapubic bladder puncture if necessary.

(8) Gastroenteritis – if uncomplicated it is seldom accompanied by significant fever. If the child is febrile, consider infection due to a specific pathogen, for example, *Salmonella* or *Shigella* or malaria.

(9) Non-specific fevers, often due to viruses. It may also be the prodromal stage of specific viral infections such as adenovirus infection or infective hepatitis, measles, poliomyelitis.

In addition to lumbar puncture, examination of a thick blood film for malaria parasites and a fresh specimen of urine are essential. More detailed investigations will depend upon the suspected diagnosis and available laboratory facilities.

Most children have outgrown the tendency by the age of five or six years and parents can be reassured that their children will not be epileptic. However, if the first febrile fit was prolonged, lasting 30 minutes or more, or the convulsions focal, or if abnormal neurological signs were diagnosed at the time of the first seizure, the risks of recurrent afebrile convulsions are much higher. In some series when these indicators were present the risk was reported to be as high as 58 per cent. Most recurrent afebrile convulsions occur within 10 years of the first febrile fit and 47 per cent within one year.

Traditional remedies for convulsions

It is hardly surprising that such a frightening and potentially fatal condition has attracted a wide range of therapeutic 'remedies' and traditional medicines from indigenous practitioners. Some are based on traditional beliefs of the cause of fits, often strongly interwoven with witchcraft, magic and taboo. Unfortunately many are almost as harmful or even more harmful than the fits themselves and produce additional complications. In Western Nigeria the application of heat to the soles of the feet and the palms of the hands is part of the traditional treatment to drive out evil spirits and the resulting burns may cause severe deformities as well as secondary infection including tetanus. Also in parts of Western Nigeria a preparation made by fermenting tobacco leaves in cow's urine is given to children with convulsions. This preparation contains a potent hypoglycaemic agent which causes further brain damage. In some parts of India and West Africa severe conjunctivitis and permanent damage to the eye may be caused by rubbing irritants such as pepper into the eyes and mouth of unconscious patients in an attempt to resuscitate them. Finally status epilepticus may result from the inadvertent injection of drugs such as nikethamide (Coramine) in rural dispensaries by medical assistants and nurses in mistaken attempts to rouse and resuscitate children. Simple health education in clinics and dispensaries can do much to prevent these tragic sequelae.

Pyogenic meningitis

In pyogenic infections of the meninges the critical first step is the acquisition by the host of the infecting organism through nasopharyngeal colonisation. A variety of microbial virulence factors help the infecting organisms to establish mucosal attachment, for example presence of a capsule (as in the case of *H. influenzae* and *S. pneumoniae*); an outer membrane protein; fimbriae (as in the case of *N. meningitidis*), and so on. Once the mucosal barrier is crossed and access to blood stream achieved, the infecting organisms are able to avoid host defences by a variety of mechanisms.

Fever, convulsions, neck stiffness and increasing drowsiness are the classical symptoms and signs of meningitis. In the very young infant the clinical picture can be atypical. For example, fever may be absent in overwhelming sepsis. Neck rigidity is difficult to elicit in the very young. Instead a full fontanelle is a useful sign to look for.

Since the outcome depends on early diagnosis and institution of specific treatment, it is essential that a lumbar puncture is performed early, and the fluid sent for culture. Whilst awaiting the results treatment can be commenced empirically, as shown in table 28.8, and later modified according to the sensitivity tests. The causative organisms vary according to age, and their sensitivity to antibiotics may vary from one geographical region to another.

The penetration of the antibiotics into the cerebrospinal fluid is important. All beta lactam antibiotics penetrate poorly, except when the meninges are inflamed. The acid pH of purulent cerebro-spinal fluid inhibits bactericidal activity of the aminoglycosides. There is also the problem of antagonism between antibiotics.

There is now emerging resistance to penicillin in the pneumococci. In such instances a third generation cephalosporin (cefotaxime or ceftriaxone) should be used. Similarly, penicillin resistant meningococci are being increasingly reported. In the case of *H. influenzae* resistance to chloramphenicol

Table 28.8 Common organisms and the starting treatment

Age	Common organisms	Starting treatment
0–4 weeks	E. coli Gp.B strepto. L. monocytogenes	Ampicillin + aminoglycoside or Ampicillin + 3rd generation cephalosporin
1 month- 3 months	E. coli Gp.B strepto. L. monocytogenes H. influenzae S. pneumoniae	Ampicillin + 3rd generation cephalosporin or Ampicillin + aminoglycoside
3 months- 18 years	H. influenzae N. meningitidis S. pneumoniae	Ampicillin + chloramphenicol or 3rd generation cephalosporin

Table 28.9 Dosage schedule of antibiotics for treating pyogenic meningitis

Antibiotic	Daily dose
Penicillin G	10–20 mg/kg
Ampicillin	250 mg 4 to 6 hourly
Chloramphenicol	50–100 mg/kg
Gentamicin	2–3 mg/kg every 8 hours
Cefotaxime	100–150 mg/kg
Cefuroxine	60 mg/kg

is rare, but if found the antibiotic should be changed to cefotaxime or cefuroxine.

The outcome is much improved in the case of meningitis due to gram negative organisms. Cure rates of 78 to 94 per cent are reported in some series, in contrast to mortality rates of 40 to 90 per cent previously.

The dosage schedule for the different antibiotics is in table 28.9.

Prophylactic treatment may have to be considered in the case of *H. influenzae* and *N. meningitidis* for all individuals sleeping and eating in the same household, for all preschool children in day nurseries, and for room mates in dormitories. Rifampicin is the preferred drug, together with the administration of the appropriate vaccine where possible.

Epilepsy

The distinguishing feature of epilepsy is recurrent seizures which are brief and usually unprovoked stereotyped disturbances of consciousness, behaviour, emotion, motor function or sensation resulting from cortical neuronal discharge.

The diagnosis of epilepsy is largely on clinical grounds. It is based on a detailed description of events experienced by the patient, or observed by an eye-witness. Hence the basic rule about diagnosing epilepsy is never to make the diagnosis without good clinical evidence. Febrile convulsions, breath holding attacks, pseudoseizures, syncope and metabolic disturbances need to be excluded. Once the diagnosis of epilepsy is accepted, an adequate classification of the seizures, and of the syndrome must be attempted.

Specific investigations like the EEG can sometimes help, provided one bears in mind that between 10 and 15 per cent of the population may have an abnormal EEG. Using a more rigid definition for abnormality, only one per cent of a non-epileptic population will have an EEG which can be called abnormal. Amongst those with seizure disorders a single routine EEG is likely to show an abnormal pattern in about 50 per cent. The EEG is particularly helpful in distinguishing absence seizures from complex partial ones, and generalised seizures from focal ones.

Based on the characteristics of the seizures, four specific seizure types are described as follows

(1) Myoclonic seizures or 'spasms'
– the typical pattern is one of brief jerks in arms and legs, often occurring in series.
(2) Absence seizures
– the pattern is one of sudden loss of consciousness with staring and blinking. Immediate recovery of consciousness follows.
(3) Partial seizures
– consciousness is unaffected in simple ones, but impaired in complex ones. Symptoms are according to focal localisation.
(4) Generalised tonic-clonic seizures (GTCS)
– typically there is a fall, followed by tonic–clonic convulsions, followed by deep sleep.

Taking these specific seizure types as starting points, the various childhood epileptic syndromes are classified according to age of onset as shown in table 28.10.

Neonatal onset

Early myoclonic encephalopathy. The seizures can be fragmentary or massive myoclonia, and usually tonic or particularly motor. Characteristically there is severe neurologic abnormality and early death.

Onset in infancy

Spasms. The characteristic form is the West syndrome. Repetitive flexor, extensor or mixed spasms are associated with developmental delay or regression. Response to treatment is poor, and neurological or intellectual deficits invariably occur.
Myoclonus. In the *benign* form repetitive myoclonic jerking occurs in otherwise normal infants. The seizures respond to treatment, and the long term outlook is good.
In the *severe* form clonic seizures start usually after a febrile episode. Later generalised myoclonic attacks supervene. EEG abnormalities in the form of spike and wave patterns, photosensitivity, and focal abnormality appear later. Response to anticonvulsants is poor, and developmental arrest is the usual outcome.

Table 28.10 Epileptic syndromes associated with specific seizure types

Myoclonic seizures or 'spasms'
Neonatal onset
   Early myoclonic encephalopathy

Onset in infancy
  'spasms'
  Myoclonus
    Benign myoclonic epilepsy
    Severe myoclonic epilepsy

Onset first 5 years
   Myoclonic – astatic epilepsy
   Lennox – Gastaut sundrome

Onset 2–12 years
   Epilepsy with myoclonic absences

Onset in adolescence
   Juvenile myoclonic epilepsy
   Other syndromes

Absence seizures
Typical
   childhood onset
   adolescent onset
  with bilateral myoclonic jerking

Atypical with slow spike-wave
   astatic epilepsy
   and other syndromes

Partial seizures
  Neurological findings normal, specific EEG changes
   Benign partial epilepsies of childhood and adolescence

  Progressive neurological and intellectual deficit

Generalised tonic-clonic seizures (GTCS)
  With typical absences
   Childhood absence epilepsy
   Juvenile absence epilepsy

  With myoclonia
   Juvenile myoclonic epilepsy

  Occurring on awakening
   Epilepsy with GTCS on awakening

Onset in childhood

Myoclonic, or myoclonic-astatic seizures accompanied by absences are the modes of presentation in myoclonic astatic epilepsy. The response to treatment is variable and so is the prognosis.

Resistance to anticonvulsants and slow mental development are also seen in the Lennox–Gestaut syndrome, which presents with tonic seizures or at times with atypical absences.

Childhood absence epilepsy is characterised by sudden onset of loss of consciousness with mild clonic, tonic or atonic features or automatisms. The seizures are frequent and in 40 per cent of cases are associated with generalised convulsions. A characteristic spike and wave pattern is seen on EEG. There is good response to treatment, and the disorder remits by the time of puberty.

In epilepsy with myoclonic absences bilateral rhythmic myoclonus accompanies loss of consciousness. The spike and wave pattern is seen on EEG. There is resistance to anticonvulsants, and mental deterioration is common.

Benign partial epilepsies have a strong family history. They usually remit at puberty. Patients present with tonic–clonic contractions involving the face, lips, tongue. Drooling is common because of involvement of the pharyngeal muscles. Unilateral parasthesia is commonly complained of. In some forms there are visual symptoms, because of the involvement of the occipital cortex. Severe headache may be complained of after the seizure.

Onset in adolescence

The seizure disorder of adolescent onset may have absences, myoclonus, or generalised convulsions as their predominant features. In most cases attacks occur on awakening in the morning.

Treatment

No drug is without risk, and the treatment of epilepsy has to be weighed on a risk versus benefit basis. With modern drugs there are strong reasons for early commencement of treatment, but probably not until two seizures have occurred. On the other hand when a second attack has followed quickly after the first one (less than one month) early institution of treatment is necessary, since there is a close association between the number of attacks before starting treatment and the ultimate prognosis.

The principles of treatment can be outlined as follows

(1) Single drug therapy should be the aim. Remission can be expected in 75 per cent of the cases with monotherapy.
(2) Once drug treatment has been started the aim should be to withdraw it as early as feasible. High remission rates have been reported consistently in those who have been seizure free for two years.

(3) Carbamazepine or sodium valproate are appropriate for most seizure disorders. Only in status epilepticus or childhood absence seizures is there a good reason for considering other drugs.
(4) If the drug chosen initially proves ineffective at the highest tolerated dose, a second drug may be tried; but alone.
(5) The chosen drug should be introduced at low dose and built up gradually.

The commonly used anticonvulsants are listed in table 28.11.

Stopping treatment

About 75 per cent will remain in remission on withdrawal of treatment after a seizure free period of two to four years. The period of withdrawal varies between six weeks and one year.

The unconscious child

Disturbance of consciousness complicates many childhood illnesses in the tropics and the admission of an unconscious child is a daily event in many clinics and emergency rooms. Unconsciousness may result from diffuse disorders, either intracranial or extrinsic, or from localised brain disease (table 28.12).

Diffuse disorders

Intracranial

Infections of the central nervous system
Bacterial and tuberculous meningitis. Both may have reached an advanced stage when the child is brought to hospital, unconscious and convulsing or both. Meningitis ranks high in the list of 'top ten' disorders of children and is an important cause of mental retardation. Early lumbar puncture in all suspected cases is essential.
Viral meningo-encephalitis. Although a large number of viruses have now been identified as causal agents of encephalitis, confirmation of a specific viral agent in many cases is still difficult because of the laboratory techniques involved. Encephalitis is an occasional complication of the common infectious diseases – measles, mumps and less often varicella, as well as whooping cough. In varicella cerebellar involvement may be a prominent feature. Occasionally encephalitis complicates immunisation procedures (see page 312).

Table 28.11 Commonly used drugs in epilepsy

Drug	Seizure disorder	Starting dose mg/kg/ day	Target dose mg/kg/ day	Frequency of dose times/ day
Carba-mazepine	Tonic-clonic seizures	5	12.5	2 or 3
Clonazepam	Myoclonus other spasms	0.025	0.05	2 or 3
Diazepam	Status epilepticus	–	–	–
Ethosuxi-mide	Absences	10	15	1
Phenobar-bitone	Tonic-clonic Newborn	4	6	1
Phenytoin	Tonic-clonic Partial seizures	5	7	1 or 2
Sodium valproate	Tonic-clonic Myoclonus Absences	10	20	1 or 2

Table 28.12 Common causes of loss of consciousness

Diffuse disorders

Intracranial
Infections – meningitis, encephalitis, encephalopathies
Epilepsy
Vascular disorders
Head injury

Extrinsic
Anoxia
Metabolic – gastroenteritis (water and electrolytes)
  hypoglycaemia
  diabetic (hyperglycaemic) coma
  uraemia
  hepatic failure
  hypomagnesaemia
Hypertensive encephalopathy
Accidental poisoning

Localised brain disease
Supratentorial
Infratentorial – tumours, abscess, granuloma, (vascular)

Cerebral malaria. This diagnostic label is frequently attached to all children in areas where *Plasmodium falciparum* malaria is endemic and who present with a short febrile illness, convulsions, malarial parasites in the blood and unconsciousness. Cerebral malaria requires energetic treatment for it has a high mortality and those who recover are often left with significant neurological deficits. However by no means all children with fever, fits and malarial parasites in their blood have cerebral malaria and uncritical use of this diagnosis may result in other serious conditions such as meningitis being missed.

Trypanosomiasis. CNS signs are prominent because of early involvement of the nervous system. Unsteadiness of gait and tremors are followed by the gradual onset of lethargy and somnolence from which in the early stages the patient is readily roused. With increasing involvement of the CNS the child acquires a dull, stupid look. The diagnosis should be suspected in any child with a prolonged history of these symptoms if he is known to come from an endemic area. Examination of a thick blood film, gland puncture, or CSF should confirm this.

Parasitic infections. Certain parasitic infections may be complicated by a diffuse encephalitis. These include

(1) Cysticercosis. Diffuse cysticercosis occurs after eating raw meat containing the larvae of *Taenia solium* (pork tape worm). Convulsions are the commonest presentation, although occasionally acute raised intracranial pressure is the earliest sign. Calcification of cysticerci in tissues including the brain, takes place slowly and is rarely seen in childhood.

(2) Schistosomiasis. Ova of *Schistosoma japonicum* are disseminated throughout the body in many organs. Deposits in the brain produce convulsions, coma, and a variety of focal signs. Subsequent granulomatous development around the ovum may produce signs suggestive of a space-occupying lesion or neoplasm. Ova of *S. mansoni* and *S. haematobium* seem to disseminate more to the spinal cord and produce a transverse myelitis.

(3) *Paragonimus westermani* (paragonimiasis). Cerebral paragonimiasis is a common extrapulmonary manifestation of infection with this fluke and may present with a wide range of neurological disorders, including epilepsy, encephalitis, meningitis, cerebral tumour, hemiplegia or a progressive encephalopathy, as well as ophthalmological signs. Granulomata and subsequent calcification occur round the ova.

Epilepsy

Post ictal unconsciousness rarely lasts more than half an hour, although many children recover consciousness and go to sleep for another hour or two. A bitten tongue or incontinence are supportive evidence. The presence of a co-existent head injury should always be excluded by carefully palpating the scalp and, if necessary, X-raying the skull. Pupil and eye movements are usually normal, although the plantar reflexes are usually extensor and a transient Todd's paralysis may be seen. Prolonged coma suggests encephalitis.

Subarachnoid haemorrhage and other vascular accidents (see page 319).

Head injury

This is suggested by the circumstances in which the patient is found and by careful examination of the scalp for signs of trauma.

Extrinsic or systemic causes

Anoxia

Anoxia may follow acute respiratory obstruction, for example, in croup, convulsions, tetanus, whooping cough, inhalation of vomit or in drowning. Severe anoxia accompanies respiratory and cardiac arrest. Maintenance of normal pupillary responses and reflex eye movements suggests a better prognosis. The persistence of dilated pupils, the occurrence of clonic fits and an extensor plantar reflex indicate the likelihood of permanent neurological damage.

Metabolic disorders

Gastroenteritis. Some degree of CNS disturbance, fretfulness and irritability is common in severe gastroenteritis. Febrile convulsions may complicate the illness if fever is prominent. The most serious complication of dehydration is cerebral thrombosis in either the larger venous sinuses or as multiple disseminated thrombi in the smaller veins. Both are common autopsy findings in the tropics. Local or diffuse cerebral infarction, hemiplegia and intellectual retardation may also follow. Hyperosmolar (hypertonic or hypernatraemic) dehydration is fortunately much less common in the tropics than in temperate climates. Infants under three months are more vulnerable because of their immature renal function and the fever which increases insensible fluid loss. Evidence from Britain suggests that artificial feeding is a significant factor since the salt content of cow's milk is about three to four times that of breast milk. Hyperosmolarity and the associated electrolyte imbalance causes a severe disturbance of cerebral function. The clinical features are irritability proceeding to apathy, delirium and coma. Convulsions are common and one third of cases may exhibit neurological disturbances during the illness. Rehydration should be slow as too rapid a correction of the fluid and electrolyte imbalance may result in further fits and possibly cerebral haemorrhage. The mortality rate is about 10 per cent and up to 15 per cent of survivors are left with some neurological or intellectual handicap.

Hypoglycaemia. Severe symptomatic hypoglycaemia alone is not a common cause of coma or convulsions but it may complicate a number of other disorders and demands treatment in its own right. Spontaneous hypoglycaemia should always be considered in the differential diagnosis of epilepsy and readily excluded by the Dextrostix estimation of the blood sugar. The accidental ingestion or therapeutic use of a number of toxic substances in different parts of the world is associated with profound hypoglycaemia, often resulting in permanent brain damage or even death. Children seem particularly vulnerable to the hypoglycaemic effects of alcohol and all children admitted with a history of ingestion of alcohol or spirits should be given an intravenous glucose infusion (5 or 10 per cent) until they have fully recovered consciousness. Other examples include the vomiting sickness of Jamaica caused by eating unripe ackee fruit, and the use of a cow's urine – tobacco mixture in Western Nigeria for the traditional treatment of convulsions. The mixture is prepared by fermenting raw tobacco leaves in cow's urine and is given either by mouth or rubbed onto the skin. Significant amounts of nicotine may be absorbed from the skin. Children treated with this mixture are deeply unconscious and many die in hypoglycaemia. The symptoms are severe and very low CSF glucose levels were observed leading to the demonstration of profound hypoglycaemia, which far from relieving the symptoms of convulsions, aggravated them. The mixture was later shown to contain a powerful hypoglycaemic agent. Hypoglycaemia is known to complicate severe kwashiorkor; it is also a diagnostic feature of Reye's Syndrome.

Diabetic (hyperglycaemic) coma – ketoacidosis and deep acidotic breathing will be present. Routine urine testing suggests the diagnosis.

Uraemia – confusion, stupor or coma may be present. A metabolic acidosis and hyperventilation will also be present.

Hepatic failure – confusion and apathy proceed to coma. A flapping tremor and foetor hepaticus are late signs. Coma may occur in severe fulminating hepatitis, or as a terminal event in chronic liver disease and cirrhosis, for example, Indian childhood cirrhosis. In veno-occlusive disease liver failure may be either acute or chronic.

Hypocalcaemia (tetany). Neonatal convulsions are considered on page 297. In the older child, tetany may follow prolonged vitamin D deficiency and malabsorption states, especially with steatorrhoea and occasionally following too rapid fluid replacement after acidosis and dehydration.

Magnesium deficiency. This too may cause neonatal tetany. It has been shown that convulsions due to magnesium deficiency in severe kwashiorkor are associated with a poor prognosis and are aften a preterminal event.

Hypertensive encephalopathy
This is likely to occur in children whenever the blood pressure exceeds 160/90 and is followed by headache, fits, focal deficits, for example, aphasia, cortical blindness or hemiplegia, and coma. The most common cause is renal disease, acute glomerulonephritis, renal failure or haemolytic-uraemic syndrome, but occasional causes are coarctation of the aorta, steroid overdose and, rarely, a neuroblastoma. The blood pressure and femoral pulses of every unconscious child should always be examined.

Accidental poisoning
Accidental poisoning is an important and not uncommon cause of sudden unconsciousness and sometimes convulsions in a young child who has been quite well some hours earlier. Children are naturally curious and will put almost anything and everything into their mouth, the range of poisonous substances to which they have access is probably infinite. Certain groups of substances, however, predominate and are classified below. Doctors, nurses and paramedical staff should familiarise themselves with the specific local poisons and their clinical effects.

(1) Drugs may be accidentally ingested by the child or administered by the mother in ignorance of the correct dose. Instructions may not have been given clearly, she may have completely misunderstood the instructions or may have believed that a larger dose would result in quicker recover. Particularly dangerous are aspirin, linctus codeine and chlorpromazine. Other common drugs accidentally ingested include ferrous sulphate, barbiturates, drugs used in the treatment of psychiatric disorders (tri-cyclic antidepressants and diazepam) and sometimes digoxin. The neurological complications of some other drugs are considered in table 28.13.

(2) Indigenous and traditional therapy, native medicines and herbal preparations – many of these contain potent alkaloids (for example, the common tropical weed *Datura* contains hyoscyamine and hyoscine (scopolamine)) or other substances producing a bewildering number of side effects. Some may be used in the traditional treatment of convulsions.

(3) Household preparations – kerosene, universally available, is by far the commonest. Alcohol, domestic cleaning agents and disinfectants are also common.

(4) Environmental hazards – these may be acute, for example pesticides such as DDT, organophosphorus compounds and paraquat, or chronic, like exposure to lead.

(5) Accidental poisoning can also be due to the following

(a) Toxic fruits and plants – well-known examples are the ackee fruit of Jamaica and bitter cassava in West Africa.

(b) The bites and stings of insects, snakes and other animals. The Elapidae (cobras and krait) produce a potent neurotoxin which produces increasing paralysis and inco-ordination, terminating in respiratory paralysis though without loss of consciousness. Toxin

Table 28.13   Drugs causing coma and convulsions

Drugs causing drowsiness and coma
  Barbiturates
  Opiates including codeine and pethidine
  Ethyl alcohol and methyl alcohol
  Salicylates
  Antihistamines – Phenergan (promethazine), Largactil (chlorpromazine)
  Lead and mercury
  Digitalis
  Carbon tetrachloride
  Boric acid
  Tricyclic antidepressants

Drugs causing convulsions
  Aminophylline – overdose given intravenously
  Kerosine and other petroleum distillates
  Organophosphates and other insecticides, DDT
  Atropine
  Phenol and related disinfectants
  Lead and iron
  Amphetamine
  Salicylates
  Plant poisons
  Camphor
  Respiratory stimulants – nalorphine, nikethamide lobeline and leptazol.

of vipers produces widespread haemorrhages and interference with blood coagulation, vasomotor failure, cardiac failure and convulsions.

(c) Many species of both sea and river fish in the tropics are poisonous, particularly the larger carnivorous fish. If consumed they cause a variety of neurotoxic symptoms including paraesthesia and sensory symptoms as well as abdominal pains, muscle weakness and sometimes convulsions and even death from respiratory paralysis. The condition, ciguatera, is well known in the Pacific, Japan and the Caribbean areas.

A diagnosis of accidental poisoning may be suggested by the sudden onset, circumstances in which the child is found and access to a drug or toxin, normal findings on physical examination and the absence of localised brain disease. Some poisons produce a characteristic clinical picture and symptoms, others generalised depression of the CNS with coma whilst still others may excite the CNS causing convulsions. In general, the pupillary reflexes are preserved except with derivatives of the opiates, tricyclic antidepressants and organophosphorus compounds, and there is preservation of eye reflex movements, that is the eyes remain central at rest. Symmetrical conjugate eye movements occur with head rolling or flexing or extending the neck (except in deep coma).

Localised brain disease

Unilateral lesions of the cerebral hemispheres rarely cause unconsciousness until their size is such as to cause a rise in intracranial pressure with displacement or herniation through the tentorium. The clinical features depend upon the site (see space-occupying lesions page 320).

Hysteria

This is rarely prolonged. It may be suggested by increasing resistance to attempts to open the eye or limb movements. Pupil responses, the respiratory pattern and muscle tone are all normal. A useful test is the cold water caloric stimulation of the ears which produce a normal response of nystagmus.

Investigations

Only after an adequate airway has been secured and effective respiratory support provided are examination and investigations carried out. A full history of the circumstances in which the child has been found is obtained together with as much of his previous history as is possible. A full general examination including a careful search for trauma of the head, limbs, abdomen and spine, is followed by a full neurological examination paying particular attention to general responses, neck stiffness, pupil reactions and eye movements, muscle tone in the limbs and movements in response to stimuli especially to any asymmetry of response. The pattern of respiration is noted.

Urine should be examined routinely for protein, glucose, reducing substances and ketones, and the Phenistix reagent strip test will be positive in the presence of salicylates. Where facilities exist blood urea, electrolytes, glucose and calcium should be measured. In certain circumstances it might be possible to send away serum or urine to regional laboratories if drugs or toxins are suspected. X-ray of the skull may reveal a fracture or separation of the sutures. Lumbar puncture, important to exclude meningitis, should not be done if there is papilloedema or other evidence of raised intracranial pressure. The need for other investigations will be determined by the clinical picture and provisional diagnosis and availability of facilities.

Nursing care of the unconscious child

The unconscious child should be nursed semiprone so that the tongue does not fall back and obstruct the airway and secretions do not accumulate in the mouth and pharynx. The position should be changed from side to side every two hours. Unless the child is easily roused, an oral airway should be inserted, or in a deeply unconscious child an endotracheal tube may be necessary. Secretions should be sucked away gently with aseptic precautions, to avoid trauma to the mouth.

Head injury or neurological observations chart should be used to record, (1) the level of unconsciousness, (2) pupil size and reaction, (3) pulse rate, (4) respiratory rate, and (5) blood pressure. The frequency of observations depends on the state of the child, but in a seriously ill patient it should be quarter hourly. Observations should be carried out and recorded preferably by trained and experienced staff (or at least supervised by them) who must understand the significance of what they are doing and report immediately any signs indicating raised intracranial pressure or cerebral displacements. These are dilatation of the pupils, increase in pulse pressure, slowing of the pulse rate, an increase or decrease in the respiratory rate and any alteration in its pattern particularly causing periodic breathing (Cheyne–Stokes) and the development of paresis in any limb. The level of consciousness should be recorded using statements such as 'drowsy but answers rationally' or 'responds to loud commands'. The onset and site of any fits should be reported immediately.

Nutrition and hydration

If a child does not recover consciousness rapidly or remains deeply unconscious a nasogastric tube should be passed. The stomach can then be emptied and feeds can also be given this way indefinitely. An intravenous drip may be established for infusion of blood, or hypertonic solutions and may replace a nasogastric tube if there is ileus but in general it is only a short-term measure.

General care

General care includes attention to the eyes and mouth, pressure points as in adults, avoidance of overheating or chilling and where appropriate nursing within a mosquito net. Catheters should be avoided because of the risk of introducing infection.

Physiotherapy is important and should be started in the acute phase with breathing exercises and postural drainage and tracheobronchial toilet. Passive movements are carried out at all joints to avoid contractures. Physiotherapy may also play an important part in rehabilitation if there are neurological sequelae, especially in learning to walk again and to use the hands.

Management

The state of consciousness of the patient and response to specific stimuli is carefully recorded. The terms commonly used to record consciousness are clouding of consciousness, stupor and coma. Clouding of consciousness implies reduced wakefulness or drowsiness. The patient is easily distracted, cannot think rapidly and has a short attention span. Unless he is distracted his eyes will close and his attention is lost. Stupor is a degree of unresponsiveness from which the patient can only be roused by vigorous stimulation. In coma, he is unrousable and unresponsive. However, the most important single factor in management is the accurate serial documentation of the level of coma. Neurological examination is used to provide evidence of either diffuse

brain disease or brain stem dysfunction. Hence the importance of recording accurately and serially pupil responses, eye movements and the respiratory pattern.

If brain stem pathways are intact, the cause of coma will usually be found in either diffuse brain disease (for example infection or trauma) or toxic or metabolic depression of neuronal function. Primary intrinsic brain stem lesions are uncommon in children but secondary damage from mechanical shifts can occur because of pressure from an expanding supratentorial mass. In these circumstances neurosurgery may be life-saving.

Coma will also occur if the normal metabolic requirements of the brain are not met. These include a reduction in cerebral blood flow by 50 per cent or more, a fall in arterial oxygen tension to below 40 mm mercury and a fall in blood sugar level to below 40 mg/100 ml.

Specific treatment of unconsciousness consists of diagnosing the cause and treatment or removal of the cause.

Nutritional disorders of the CNS

Infantile beri-beri

Infantile beri-beri is due to thiamine deficiency occurring in breast fed infants whose mothers themselves are thiamine deficient. It can also occur in artificially fed infants if the feed is deficient in thiamine. It is fairly widespread in South-east Asia and the Philippines especially where polished rice is the staple diet, but is uncommon where unpolished or undermilled rice is eaten, for example, India and Sri Lanka. Recognition of the cause and the introduction of unpolished rice has caused a steady decline in the incidence in recent years. Thiamine is necessary for the complete oxydation of carbohydrates and during its absence intermediate breakdown products accumulate, for example, pyruvate and other bisulphate binding substances. Clinical symptoms usually appear about the age of two or three months and are described on page 263. Meningeal and gastro-intestinal symptoms tend to be more chronic and less dramatic, particularly in older infants. The meningeal symptoms may simulate meningitis with head retraction, bulging fontanelle, muscle rigidity in the limbs and staring eyes with dilated pupils. Without treatment these symptoms progress to convulsions, coma and death. Occasionally muscle paralysis occurs. CSF examination is normal. Associated gastro-intestinal symptoms include abdominal distension and tenderness, most likely due to muscular tenderness, and constipation. Some of the cerebral symptoms may be due to oedema of the brain and at autopsy petechial haemorrhages are often seen in the grey matter around the third ventricle. In chronic adult cases there is demyelination in the posterior columns and peripheral nerves. Clinical features in adults are predominantly muscle tenderness, muscle weakness and sensory loss.

Treatment

There is a prompt response to thiamine 25–100 mg intravenously or intramuscularly. Correction of the diet and treatment of the mother is also essential.

Chronic malnutrition in older children

The symptomatology often reflects inadequate intake of energy and protein, mixed vitamin deficiency and other essential dietary factors including minerals. Symptoms may be precipitated by any intercurrent infection or drugs interfering with or blocking metabolic pathways, for example, isoniazid in the treatment of tuberculosis may result in a pellagra-like syndrome which can be prevented by giving pyridoxine 5–10 mg daily.

Beri-beri

In older infants and children the symptoms are predominantly those of a neuritis and encephalopathy.

Pellagra

Pellagra is due to a deficiency of niacin. The precursor of this is tryptophan. Food such as milk and eggs which are deficient in niacin but rich in tryptophan therefore do not cause pellagra. The disease is endemic in the Near East, Africa and in south-east Europe in areas where maize is the staple carbohydrate but it is also seen from time to time in non-maize eating countries such as India and parts of Latin America. Isolated niacin deficiency is uncommon in children. It produces a peripheral neuritis of the glove and stocking type and an encephalopathy with confusion and disorientation.

Riboflavin

This is widely distributed in plant and animal foods. Minor degrees of deficiency are probably fairly widespread throughout the whole of South-east Asia, Africa and Latin America. Symptoms tend to appear with protein calorie malnutrition. There are no specific CNS signs.

A syndrome of unknown etiology with rhythmic coarse tremors involving especially the face and limbs, hypotonia, mental regression (apathy and indifference) and an anaemia, macrocytic in the majority, has been described from India. Most patients were underweight, breast fed and from poor homes. They improved after vitamin B_{12} injections, but this and other treatment had no effect on the tremor which gradually subsided.

Tropical myelopathies

Tropical myelopathies are of two types viz. ataxic and spastic. In the ataxic type there is sensory ataxia with loss of proprioceptive functions. Spastic paresis, on the other hand, is characterised by spastic lower limb palsy with minimal sensory deficit.

Tropical ataxic neuropathy is usually of nutritional origin. There are often other clinical signs of nutritional deficiency, like stomatitis, angular cheilitis, glossitis and dermatitis, associated with the neurological syndrome. In many instances the condition is precipitated by infection, like malaria or chronic diarrhoea. Post infective malabsorption is a common cause. Women who are pregnant or lactating are specially vulnerable. Visual impairment and nerve deafness has been described in a significant number of cases. Parenteral administration of vitamins of the B group brings about rapid improvement in two-thirds of the cases.

Another etiological factor of nutritional origin is chronic cyanide poisoning in communities whose staple food is cassava. This type of myelopathy also occurs in epidemic form, especially in times of drought (for example 'mantakassa' in Mozambique, and 'konzo' in Zaire). The cyanogenic glycosides of cassava get normally detoxified during the traditional processing sequence of soaking, drying, and storage. After ingestion further detoxification occurs by metabolic pathways requiring sulphur containing amino acids. Deficiency of such amino acids in the diet can make cassava dependent communities specially vulnerable.

In tropical spastic paraparesis the main lesion occurs in the pyramidal tract, especially in the lumbar region. Two clinical types have been described viz. acute and chronic, or slow.

The acute type is associated with malnutrition and post infective malabsorption. Another etiological factor is a neurotoxin, as in the case of lathyrism which has been reported from India, Bangladesh and Ethiopia. In these countries agricultural workers are customarily paid in seeds of the plant lathyrus sativus. It contains the neurotoxic amino acid, beta-oxalyl-amino-alanine (BOAA). The flour made from the seed is often used to adulterate gram flour.

Soaking the seed in warm water for several hours prior to consumption leaches out the toxin and makes the seed safe.

The slow type of myelopathy is usually seen in adults, and is of infective origin. In the Jamaican myelopathy 60 per cent of the patients tested positive to syphilis. In other series described from Central and South America, the Caribbean and Africa 85 per cent of the patients had antibodies against HTLV-I virus on Elisa. The course of the disease is chronic and relentlessly progressive.

Neurological changes in protein – energy malnutrition (PEM, kwashiorkor)

The neurological changes in the acute stage are well-known. Misery, listlessness and apathy combined with inertia are commonly present and the child responds with irritability when disturbed. A smaller number may show muscle tremors or oculogyric crises. In severe cases drowsiness develops, occasionally progressing to coma and ending fatally. Convulsions may be a preterminal event in a small number and resemble tetany with a normal serum calcium. There is also a decline in performance in locomotion, expression, comprehension and in social spheres which recovers fully with treatment. Such recovery is more quick when the mother remains in close contact with the child.

The symptoms in PEM are dependent on multiple factors. It has been pointed out that PEM and magnesium deficiency share many common features and that magnesium supplements are an essential part of the comprehensive management of PEM as they facilitate recovery and reduce mortality. Magnesium is essential to normal activity and stability of the brain and many magnesium-dependent enzymes are involved in normal brain metabolism at cellular level. Magnesium and pyridoxine are inter-related through biochemical pathways, and convulsions may result from a deficiency of both. Magnesium is also an activator for all enzymes requiring thiamine pyrophosphate as a co-factor. It is likely that the encephalopathy of PEM is the result of an interaction between deficiency and imbalance of essential and non-essential amino acids, together with a deficiency of enzyme functions particularly those relating to the vitamin B group, and further exaggerated by the deficiency of mag-

nesium and potassium. However, this is almost certainly a simplified view.

Peripheral nerve involvement has been demonstrated. Motor nerve conduction and velocity were found to be significantly reduced in PEM as compared with controls but were reversible in survivors. Abnormal EEG tracings in the acute stages improve with treatment and recovery. A syndrome of coarse tremors has also been noted in African children recovering from PEM, with cogwheel rigidity and increased tendon jerks. The cause is unknown but recovery is spontaneous.

The vexed question of the longterm effects of PEM on subsequent brain function and intellectual performance remains as yet unanswered and will have to await the outcome of careful longterm studies, some of which have already begun. A fundamental problem in interpreting all such studies lies in the selection of standards of normality and controls which are used and these must be critically examined before interpreting any results. The situation at present can be summed up as follows

(1) The critical period of postnatal brain growth coincides with the age at which malnutrition is most prevalent throughout the world. The most critical period is in the first six months or so and it is possible that prolonged breast feeding is protective, particularly in the first year. A decline in breast feeding and early infantile marasmus may therefore have very serious significance.

(2) Experimental studies on malnutrition in young animals clearly show that the ultimate effects on the CNS are dependent on species, age of insult, its severity and duration. Different tissues respond in different ways and the timing of the period of malnutrition is critical. The evidence in animal experiments suggests that when malnutrition occurs at the critical phase it does cause permanent sequelae. Nevertheless their relevance to the human situation is still far from clear.

(3) So far no clear evidence has emerged from long term studies to indicate that subsequent physical growth and development of children treated for severe PEM in early childhood is in any way different from that of siblings or controls from the same economic and social background.

(4) Evidence on brain size and mental development is less conclusive but there are some pointers from a few studies from Central and South America which suggest that children who have been malnourished or who live in poor surroundings, or who had suffered a serious period

of semi-starvation very early in life, were not the equal of their peers when faced with IQ tests at the ages of three to six years. Children who had had malnutrition before the age of six months had the greatest deficit compared with those who had been affected between 6 and 30 months. It does seem that in assessing subsequent intellectual performance the age at which malnutrition occurs, its severity and duration and the influence of other adverse environmental factors may be critical.

Neurological complications of immunisation procedures

All immunisation procedures carry a small but definite risk of serious neurological sequelae. The low incidence of these complications however must be measured against the undoubted benefits that mass immunisation brings in terms of reduction of morbidity and mortality in many communities.

Pertussis

Although controversy still exists in Britain about both the efficacy and risk of complications following pertussis immunisation, the importance of whooping cough as a major killer in infancy in many parts of the world leaves no doubt as to the need for continuing immunisation. Present evidence suggests that reactions are most likely to occur after the first or second immunisation, and in children with a past history of fits, a reaction to a previous immunisation, those with pre-existing brain damage and those with an intercurrent infection. The most common reactions are fretfulness, screaming and irritability and fever usually within 24 hours of immunisation. More serious is the onset of persistent screaming, convulsions and encephalopathy within the first week after immunisation and commonly within 24 hours. One-third of these patients may die, and another third may be left with residual and often severe brain damage.

The majority are mentally retarded with or without epilepsy or infantile spasms and may have other lesions such as a hemiparesis etc. The risk of these reactions has been estimated as being between 1 in 100 000 and 1 in a million and could be reduced by avoiding immunisation of children with intercurrent infections and neurological abnormalities.

Measles

The incidence of encephalitis in natural measles has been estimated as 1 in every 1000 cases. The onset is usually about four or five days after the rash appears and the mortality rate is about 20 per cent. Less severe neurological changes, convulsions and abnormalities of behaviour, occur in about 4 per 1000 cases. The successful production of effective attenuated live vaccines has enabled large scale mass vaccinations to be carried out in many parts of the world and the incidence of side effects reported has been remarkably low. With attenuated live vaccines only five to ten per cent of children develop fever of 39.4°C (103 °F) or over and the risk of convulsions is slight, compared to natural measles. Convulsions were reported in several trials usually six to nine days after vaccination, coinciding with the height of the febrile reaction. It has been estimated that these occurred in about 1 per 1000 as compared with 4–8 per 1000 in natural measles in the USA and Europe and 10 per 1000 in natural measles in the tropics. Some are undoubtedly febrile fits triggered off by the fever of a reaction to a vaccination although some may possibly be specifically caused by the live vaccine. EEG tracings have been found to be abnormal in over 50 per cent of children with natural measles but in less than five per cent after measles vaccination. The overall incidence of encephalitis following vaccination has been remarkably low and in some series the incidence of deaths has not been greater than amongst the controls. The estimated rate in the USA in 0.9 cases per million doses of vaccine.

Post vaccinial encephalomyelitis

This is rare under the age of three. It may follow either primary vaccination or re-vaccination after a long interval. The onset is acute, between 8 and 15 days after vaccination with some disturbance of consciousness, fits, involuntary movements of the extra-pyramidal type and dysarthria. Fever and meningism are often present. Involvement of the spinal cord with a transverse myelitis and paraplegia may also be present. CSF protein is increased (up to 120 mg/100 ml) and there is lymphocytic pleocytosis with up to about 100 cells per cubic millimetre. The mortality is nearly as high as 20 per cent but in those who recover neurological sequelae may be less severe than after vaccinial encephalopathy. There is evidence of a perivenous encephalitis with widespread foci of perivascular demyelination and perivenous microglial proliferation. The lesions are predominantly in the subcortical white matter of the brain. It is believed to be an allergic reaction with an auto-immune basis, the target organ being the white matter of the CNS. On this basis treatment with steroids has been suggested but the results are of doubtful value.

Other much less common reactions include meningism about five or six days after primary vaccination, and a polyneuritis. A local brachial neuritis or circumflex nerve mononeuritis simplex may complicate vaccination. Epilepsy and polio may be aggravated by vaccination.

The overall incidence of CNS complications is very small. In primary vaccination it is highest in the first year of life and lowest between the ages of one and four years, rising again after the age of 15 years.

Neuropathy
Bacterial exotoxins

Diphtheria exotoxin is elaborated at the site of infection and has a predilection for cardiac muscle, the nervous system and kidneys. Histologically there is a toxic peripheral neuritis involving particularly the nerves to the heart, palate, eyes and larynx. Three forms of paralysis are seen. (1) Palatal and pharyngeal is much the commonest appearing about the third week and causing regurgitation of fluids through the nose and nasal speech. The pharynx is involved and there is also cough and dysphagia. (2) Ocular paralysis appears about the fifth week with strabismus and paralysis of accommodation. (3) Peripheral neuritis appears late, is often transient and there is full recovery. The commonest feature is ataxia and absence of deep reflexes. The most serious is diaphragmatic (respiratory) paralysis.

Clostridium botulinum (botulism) causes weakness and paralysis including bulbar palsy in many cases which proceeds to respiratory paralysis and death. Symptoms appear 12–48 hours after eating contaminated food.

Acute infectious polyneuritis (Guillain–Barré Syndrome)

The cause is uncertain but is believed to be viral. There is often a history of a preceding mild upper respiratory infection or febrile illness some days or some weeks earlier, and occasionally follows a recognisable illness such as infectious mononucleosis,

Demyelinisation in the peripheral nerves and nerve roots and sometimes degenerative changes in the anterior horn cells may be found. It may be analogous to parainfectious encephalomyelitis but occurring in the peripheral nerves.

Clinical features

There is a sudden onset of weakness, usually symmetrical and most severe in the lower limbs and distal muscles which become hypotonic with diminshed reflexes. Meningeal irritation, rare in adults is quite common in children. Except for the facial nerve, cranial nerves are rarely involved. Respiratory paralysis requiring mechanical ventilation is the most serious complication and may affect up to ten per cent of cases. Muscle tenderness and paraesthesiae may occur but sensory symptoms are uncommon. Symptoms progress for a week or ten days before recovery begins. Recovery may be slow, over many months and at times never complete. There is no treatment. Steroids have little effect on the course of the disease. Landry's paralysis is a severe form with rapidly progressing ascending paralysis and respiratory paralysis. The disease must be differentiated from acute poliomyelitis in which the meningitic illness is usually more severe and the onset of paralysis slower, less symmetrical and more patchy.

Other diseases in which neuropathy occurs
Leprosy

This is the commonest neurological disorder in the tropics affecting peripheral nerves (see also chapter 15).

Acute infectious diseases

These include typhoid, typhus, mumps, scarlet fever. The clinical picture is similar to infectious polyneuritis.

Tick paralysis

Hard (ixodid) ticks are normal parasites of domestic and wild animals but may become attached to the skin of humans for several days. They are commoner in girls than boys as they are able to hide in the longer hair. Sudden paralysis may follow the bite of a single gravid female tick, probably from a toxin injected from the salivary glands. There is an acute ascending usually bilateral flaccid paralysis which may be complete within 12–24 hours with death from respiratory paralysis. If however the tick can be removed whole, including the mouth parts, before bulbar paralysis sets in, then recovery is possible.

Drugs and chemicals

Vincristine may cause a mixed motor and sensory neuropathy after prolonged use. Lead neuropathy is uncommon in children. The insecticides parathion and malathion are slowly absorbed through the skin and may cause a neuropathy after prolonged contact.

Triorthocresylphosphate (a constituent of lubricating oil) has caused disastrous outbreaks of paralysis after contaminating food or, as in Morocco, following the adulteration of cooking oil. In survivors recovery may be incomplete.

Ammoniated mercury ointment is still quite popular because it is cheap and effective in the management of septic skin rashes in infants, but sufficient mercury may be absorbed to give acrodynia (pink disease) and neuropathy. Mercury is also an ingredient of many 'whitening' creams used for cosmetic purposes. The classical symptoms of mercury poisoning are anorexia, photophobia and irritability together with cold red extremities and refusal to walk or stand. There is hypotonia and absence of reflexes.

Acute toxic encephalopathy

This is an ill-understood disorder occurring mainly in infancy and early childhood in which convulsions followed by delirium and coma with fever and vomiting develop acutely during the course of many common illnesses. These include gastroenteritis, clinically insignificant upper respiratory infections, dysentery and cholera, pneumonia, most of the common exanthemata and infectious diseases and smallpox vaccination. It is often fulminant and there is a high mortality, survivors are frequently left with a severe neurological deficit. The etiology and pathogenesis is obscure but suggests vulnerability of the developing brain to some factor, possibly toxic, infectious or metabolic or an abnormal immune response. The main pathological finding is cerebral oedema, together with some degeneration of neurones. There is a marked absence of inflammatory reaction.

Localised neurological signs are unusual apart from extensor plantar responses. Papilloedema may be absent but abnormal pupillary responses if present indicate brain stem compression. Assymmetrical pupillary responses falsely suggest a mass. Decereb-

ate posture may develop as a preterminal event. Lumbar puncture is contra-indicated because of the high intracranial pressure.

There are no specific laboratory signs to help in the diagnosis which may mimic the encephalopathy of a number of metabolic disorders although the characteristic findings in these should help to distinguish them. Conditions which may have to be considered in the diagnosis include acute bacterial meningitis, viral encephalitis, post-infectious encephalomyelitis, Reye's syndrome, cerebrovascular accident and trauma, subdural haematoma, lead encephalopathy, hypertonic dehydration, and space-occupying lesions.

Management consists essentially of supportive measures and control of convulsions and fever, with close monitoring of the vital signs. Control of cerebral oedema may be attempted by the use of (1) dexamethosone 1 or 2 mg four or six hourly, or (2) hypertonic intravenous infusions such as mannitol – given slowly by intravenous drip over about 30 minutes, dose 2g/kg in 20 per cent solution, or 15 per cent urea in invert sugar 0.5–1 g/kg over about 20–30 minutes.

Reye's syndrome

This syndrome of acute encephalopathy and fatty degeneration of the viscera especially the liver, has now been reported from many different parts of the world. It is a severe and often fatal disorder of unknown etiology and pathogenesis, commonly observed following a mild prodromal illness such as gastroenteritis, respiratory viral infection, chicken-pox and influenza B. The pathological findings in the brain are those of marked cerebral oedema accompanied by some neuronal degeneration, but there is no cellular infiltrate or demyelination. The liver shows often intense fatty degeneration, liver cells being heavily infiltrated with fat and depleted of glycogen. There is no hepatocellular necrosis. The clinical features suggest either a viral infection or some form of intoxication but intensive screening has failed to reveal any toxins except in Thailand where aflotoxin ingestion has been linked with the syndrome. In Canada exposure to insecticide has been suggested but remains unproven. In spite of the relationship to outbreaks of influenza B, chicken-pox and other viral infections, no virus has ever been isolated from the liver or brain. More recently an enzyme deficiency has been suggested but remains unproven. Aspirin ingestion has also been suggested.

Clinical features

The onset is acute often following a mild prodomal illness with convulsions and gross disturbance of consciousness rapidly proceeding to coma and often death within a day or two. Vomiting is variable but may be severe and protracted. Focal neurological signs are conspicuously absent, there is no meningism and papilloedema appears late. Mild or moderate liver enlargement appears in only about half the cases and jaundice is rare. The presence of irregular respiration or acidotic breathing may arouse suspicion. The diagnosis is difficult in life though may be suggested by biochemical abnormalities. The most striking finding is hypoglycaemia which is reflected in a low CSF sugar as well as raised serum transaminases, and a prothrombin activity of less than 60 per cent of normal. Serum bilirubin may be normal or slightly elevated. Plasma bicarbonate is low as the metabolic acidosis develops. Blood ammonia and serum amino acids are also raised but the detection of these is outside the scope of most laboratories. Needle biopsy of the liver which may be so helpful in confirming the diagnosis is often precluded by prolonged prothrombin time. CSF is normal.

The differential diagnosis includes all conditions considered in acute toxic encephalopathy but the visceral findings distinguish Reye's syndrome from all other encephalopathies.

There is no specific treatment. Supportive measures are aimed at correcting hypoglycaemia (by high carbohydrate intake) and the acidosis. The fluid intake may need to be restricted to reduce the risk of cerebral oedema. Fresh frozen plasma or fresh whole blood may be required if a bleeding diathesis develops. Mannitol or dexamethasone may be used to control cerebral oedema.

Para-infectious encephalomyelitis

This appears to be an allergic type of reaction following many acute infectious illnesses, measles, rubella, varicella, mumps, whooping cough and sometimes after immunisations and injections of antiserum. Pathological findings in the brain are vascular congestion and haemorrhage from small vessels, perivascular infiltration and perivenous demyelination.

Clinical features

The onset is usually acute with headaches, fever drowsiness and malaise followed by convulsions stupor and coma. Ataxia and cerebellar involvement

is a feature in varicella. Varying degrees of paralysis follow including an involvement of the cranial nerves. Lower motor neurone paralysis indicates spinal cord involvement. There is no specific treatment, steroids appear to be of no value. The presence of coma, convulsions or a hemiparesis are adverse signs, the mortality may be as high as 10 per cent in varicella and up to 20 per cent in measles.

A localised brachial neuritis may follow immunisation procedures. It has been suggested that it could be a localised form of the Guillain–Barre syndrome.

Slow virus infections

Subacute sclerosing panencephalitis (SSPE)

This and kuru are only two of a number of chronic and subacute degenerative disorders of the CNS in which there is evidence of infection by a slow virus or other transmissible agent. The term 'slow virus infections' is applied because of the slow progression of the disease. The reasons for this unusual behaviour are unknown and pose many interesting problems as yet unanswered regarding the nature and properties of the viruses which cause these peculiar effects on the brain and their effects on the patient's immune response to the infection. In tissue cultures the measles virus of SSPE remains tightly bound to the cells and can only be detected with difficulty, the patterns of intracellular growth too are quite difficult. The measles virus can be cultured from both biopsy and post mortem specimen. Although the virus can be isolated, very high measles antibody titres are found in both the CSF and serum and circulating immune complexes of viral antigen combined with antibody can be demonstrated. The disease may represent qualitative variation in the patient's response to measles infection and may be genetically determined. In most cases there is a history of clinical infection with measles before the age of two but the onset of symptoms in SSPE is between 6 and 11 years with an average interval of 6½ years. Symptoms are those of a progressive loss of cerebral function (dementia) with a slow onset over many months. There are associated personality changes, lethargy, regression of speech and myoclonic jerks may appear. There is inco-ordination with both extra-pyramidal signs. The EEG pattern is characteristic. The pathological findings in the brain are those of perivascular inflammation and neuronal degeneration. There is also glial proliferation. The neurones may show nuclear and cytoplasmic inclusions. Demyelination is usually only slight. There is no treatment and the disease is progressive.

Kuru

Although this disease is confined to New Guinea it has attracted considerable attention because of its clinical features. It occurs mainly in children over the age of four and in adult women. The earliest symptoms are tremor and ataxia accompanied by a change in personality. These rapidly progress with the development of coarse tremors, choreiform movements and inability to walk, followed by inability to sit or even swallow. Most patients are dead within a year. A transmittable agent has been recovered from the brain of patients with kuru but clustering within families suggests possible genetic factors as well. The prevalance of the disease is related to ritual feasting after the death of a relative in which children and women participate. The rites involve ingestion of small portions of the brains of the dead relative.

Neurological complications of commonly used drugs

A number of drugs are widely used and often indiscriminately prescribed for the symptomatic and therapeutic treatment of common symptoms and conditions in young children in paediatric outpatient departments and clinics. Their side effects are often ill understood by those who prescribe them, often medical assistants and nurses, and may appear after only a modest overdose or even the normal dosage. Drug action may be especially potentiated by factors such as dehydration from vomiting, diarrhoea, fever or inadequate fluid intake or by interaction with the second drug sometimes given to treat symptoms produced by the first drug. Mothers themselves may mistakenly continue to administer medicines rather than fluids to an ill child and thus increase the dehydration, continue to give drugs after symptoms have subsided, or increase the dose believing that the child will recover more quickly. Overdosage with many drugs produces drowsiness or even coma and respiratory depression. The phenothiazines (for example, Largactil) and metochlopromide (Maxalon) may produce bizarre and alarming extrapyramidal symptoms without loss of consciousness. Acute dystonic reactions are probably the commonest with painless spasmodic contractions and rigidity of various muscle groups producing trismus, torticollis, opisthotonus, oculogyric crisis and bizarre postures. Other effects may include restlessness and jitteriness or pseudo-Parkinsonism with muscle weak-

ness and lack of movement but without tremor. The clinical picture may suggest hysteria, encephalitis, chorea or tetanus but the complete relaxation of affected muscles between spasms and during sleep and the normal movement of muscles other than those subject to spasms differentiates it. No treatment other than total withdrawal of the drug is necessary in most cases. Severe acute dystonic reactions can be controlled by giving intravenous promethazine (Phenergan) 6–12 mg or by intramuscular diphenhydramine (Benadryl) 10–20 mg.

Chlorpromazine (Largactil)

This drug is widely used as anti-emetic. It causes central and autonomic depression and potentiates reaction of other sedatives and narcotics. High dosage produces 'chlorpromazine intoxication', a state of dazed bewilderment. Acute dystonic reactions may occur as described above. Other side effects include drowsiness, hypotension, a lowering of body temperature and a dry mouth.

Prochlorperazine (Stemetil)

Phenothiazines with a piperazine side chain such as prochlorperazine can produce quite marked restlessness and are more likely to cause extra-pyramidal signs and acute dystonic reactions.

Metochlorpromide (Maxalon, Primperan)

This anti-emetic may produce restlessness and the more severe types of dystonic extra-pyramidal reactions. Its action is potentiated by phenothiazines and *the manufacturers specifically advise against using the two drugs together*.

Diphenoxylate (Lomotil)

The manufacturers recommend that this drug widely used in the treatment of diarrhoea, *should not be given to children under the age of two years*. It is structurally related to pethidine and may produce drowsiness, coma, respiratory depression and apnoea. In addition constricted pupils, muscular hypotonia and abdominal distension, nystagmus and convulsions may occur. Atropine present in the preparation may produce fever, flushing and tachypnoea. Several reports draw attention to the appearance of symptoms many hours after the drug has been taken and the need for observation to be continued for as long as 72 hours since the onset of respiratory depression may not appear until at least 24 hours after ingestion of the drug. The pethidine antagonist nalorphine is a specific antidote, in a dose 1 or 2 mg intramuscularly or intravenously repeated after 15–30 minutes according to the clinical response.

Chloroquine

Intramuscular injections of chloroquine may be followed by convulsions and sudden death. Parenteral adminstration should be reserved for emergency use only, as in cerebral malaria, and never in a dose exceeding 5 mg/kg. Intravenous injections should never be given.

The tricyclic antidepressants (amitriptyline and imipramine)

These produce drowsiness, ataxia, coma and convulsions. In addition restlessness, hallucinations, nystagmus and increased reflexes may be observed. Dilatation of pupils may occur particularly with imipramine. Even more important are the cardiac arrhythmias which develop including ventricular premature systoles, hypotension and cardio-respiratory arrest.

Piperazine

Neurotoxic symptoms may appear several days after the first dose. The syndrome is popularly known as 'worm wobble'. Symptoms include dizziness, drowsiness, disorientation, muscle weakness and hypotonia, ataxia and inco-ordination. In severe cases myclonic jerks or even status epilepticus may occur. EEG changes have been reported after normal doses. Neurotoxic symptoms are most likely to occur in the presence of established neurological disorders, chronic renal insufficiency and concurrent administration with phenothiazines such as chlorpromazine. Piperazine is an acetyl choline antagonist and prevents its replacement at neuromuscular junctions causing temporary paralysis.

Aspirin

Because of its widespread use in the management of fever, accidental overdosage of aspirin is now one of the commonest causes of poisoning. It is most likely to happen when adult doses are given in the presence of high fever and restricted fluid intake or excessive loss. Hyperventilation is an early sign, accompanied by irritability and excitement which is then followed by coma.

Kerosene (paraffin)

Its universal presence in most homes makes it another common cause of accidental poisoning. The usual complication is a severe lipid pneumonia but absorption of sufficiently large amounts from the intestine causes drowsiness, convulsions and coma.

Lead

Lead poisoning is important because the diagnosis is often missed and it has a high mortality and morbidity. In children poisoning is usually a chronic process, lead being accumulated slowly in the body but because of the vulnerability of the central nervous system symptoms may appear after only relatively short exposure and the clinical presentation is usually acute. In mild cases weakness, irritability, pallor and anaemia, headache and anorexia may be the presenting symptoms. More severe cases may present acutely with symptoms suggesting meningitis with raised intracranial pressure, papilloedema, convulsions and neck stiffness or as an acute encephalopathy with severe convulsions often difficult to control and raised intracranial pressure from cerebral oedema. The diagnosis should always be considered in any case of 'status epilepticus' which is difficult to control in spite of adequate doses of anticonvulsant drugs. Less common presentations in children include peripheral neuropathy, ataxia and optic atrophy. Encephalopathy may be precipitated by any acute intercurrent infection or metabolic disturbance such as acute gastroenteritis. It is seldom possible to estimate blood lead levels but the diagnosis may be suggested by the presence of papilloedema and increased protein and pressure in the CSF, glycosuria and proteinuria and anaemia resembling that of iron deficiency. Evidence of lead ingestion may be seen on plain X-rays of the abdomen. Basophilic stippling of the neutrophils and 'lead lines' of increased radiological density in the epiphyses are late signs. Common sources of lead include lead paint either in the house or on toys, lead pipes in areas of soft water, or old car batteries which may be used as a source of fuel, for storage purposes, or for play. Another source is 'surma' a lead containing eye shadow and cosmetic used in many parts of India and Pakistan on both mothers and their children. The powder may contain as much as 70 per cent lead. Outbreaks of lead poisoning from surma have recently been reported amongst immigrant children in England. Pica is common in mentally defective children but may also occur in normal children as part of a behaviour problem and is also said to be a sign of iron deficiency. Lead poisoning is said to be commoner amongst children who eat earth or nibble and chew paint or furniture.

Cerebral oedema may be reduced temporarily by an intravenous infusion of a 20 per cent solution of mannitol, 2.5 g/kg over about 20–30 minutes. The gut should then be purged of lead before starting treatment with calcium disodium versenate (calcium EDTA). This is given as a daily intravenous infusion as a 0.2–0.4 per cent solution in a dose of up to 70 mg/kg per day for five days. The course can then be repeated after two or three weeks. An alternative treatment is oral d-penicillamine 20 mg/kg per day for seven days.

Symptomatic lead poisoning has a high mortality and a significant number of survivors are left with mental retardation or other neurological deficits.

Ferrous sulphate

Restlessness, collapse, convulsions and coma are later manifestations of iron poisoning appearing after the initial haematemesis and circulatory collapse. In children who eventually recover neurological sequelae are uncommon.

Vascular disorders
Cerebral thrombosis

Thrombosis of the large venous sinuses and thrombophlebitis of the cortical vessels is a complication of many acute illnesses. The two most important pathological processes involved are, (1) extension of an inflammatory lesion to include the affected vessel, and (2) dehydration in which the viscosity of the blood is increased. Children with cyanotic congenital heart disease are especially vulnerable. In many illnesses both processes operate together.

Involvement of the affected vessel in an inflammatory lesion

In bacterial meningitis, especially when the onset of treatment has been delayed, and in meningo-encephalitis there may be diffuse involvement of small vessels (and at times large vessels also) with widespread small areas of cerebral oedema or even infarction and cortical atrophy. Coma and convulsions are frequent and are followed by focal signs, hemiplegia or cranial nerve paralysis. The child may recover only to be left with neurological or intellectual deficit.

The commonest local inflammatory lesions are suppurative otitis media and mastoiditis with spread to the surrounding bone such as the petrous temporal resulting in lateral sinus thrombosis. Other inflammatory lesions including osteomyelitis of the skull, cerebral abscess, tuberculoma or sepsis following trauma may all cause thrombosis in an adjacent venous sinus.

Cavernous sinus thrombosis

The anatomical situation and structure of the cavernous sinuses makes them susceptible to septic thrombosis secondary to infection on the head and neck, travelling along the emissary veins which carry extracranial blood to the sinuses. Important routes are via the superior ophthalmic vein communicating with all tributaries of the facial vein, emissary veins from the pharyngeal and pterygoid plexuses, those from the mastoid and auditory veins through the petrosal sinus, and cerebral as well as meningeal veins. The frequency of bilateral thrombosis is due to the interconnections within the sinus. The widespread signs and symptoms of cavernous sinus thrombosis are due to the anatomical relationship with the internal carotid artery and its sympathetic plexus which pass through the sinus, and the closeness of the third, fourth and sixth cranial nerves together with the maxillary branch of the fifth, as well as of the pituitary gland. The source may therefore be any of the common sites of infection on the face especially around the eyes and nose, abscesses and boils, sepsis secondary to trauma of the face or scalp, osteomyelitis, orbital cellulitis, sinusitis, pharyngitis or dental sepsis, otitis media and mastoiditis. Occasionally even remote sepsis like, for example, on the legs, may be responsible.

The child is severely ill and febrile. A characteristic clinical picture develops with the occlusion of the cavernous sinuses. Initially it may resemble orbital cellulitis but the peri-orbital pain and oedema are much more marked, proptosis occurs early and chemosis of the eyelids may be startling. If the eye is not already closed by oedema, there will be marked papilloedema and loss of vision. A progressive ophthalmoplegia occurs and with the involvement of the trigeminal nerve there is loss of the corneal reflex and anaesthesia. Meningeal irritation may be present and convulsions and coma may develop at any time. Involvement of the pituitary may cause sudden collapse due to adrenal insufficiency. The diagnosis is established when eye signs become bilateral. Blood culture is often positive although the CSF is rarely so.

Treatment

A combination of antibiotic therapy should be used, selected so as to be effective against all the likely infective agents, particularly Gram positive organisms. The antibiotics should be given intravenously or intramuscularly for 72 hours. Treatment can then be modified on the basis of subsequent laboratory reports. Special attention should be given to the local care of the proptosed eye to protect the cornea. Hydration must be maintained but sedatives should be avoided.

Effects of dehydration

Superior sagittal sinus thrombosis is a common site of thrombosis in severe dehydration accompanying diarrhoea.

Other vascular disorders
Cerebral embolism

This is uncommon and is seen mainly in children with cyanotic congenital heart disease (Fallot's tetralogy) and occasionally in bacterial endocarditis. Hemiplegia is the most common sequel.

Fat embolism may complicate sickle-cell crises and also fractures of the long bones, particularly the femur. It is often fatal.

Cerebrovascular anomalies

Congenital aneurysms on the circle of Willis and occasionally elsewhere rupture either spontaneously or as a result of trauma causing subarachnoid haemorrhage. The onset is sudden with headache and loss of consciousness, irritability and photophobia. Neck stiffness may be difficult to detect in the early stages and in profound coma. Diagnosis is by lumbar puncture. Treatment is surgical, if facilities are available. A small proportion recover on conservative treatment with bed rest and good nursing care, but the risk of recurrence is high.

Subarachnoid haemorrhage
This is uncommon in children. In a review of 57 patients collected during a period of 11 years in Ibadan, subarachnoid haemorrhage was diagnosed in 10, of whom 9 died. Three had sickle-cell anaemia and the bleeding was presumed to be secondary to sickling. Angiomata rather than aneurysms have been found to be a commoner cause of subarachnoid haemorrhage in children in Thailand and Malaysia.

Other cerebrovascular anomalies include arteriovenous malformations and fistulae. Some of these may be associated with fits and neuro-cutaneous syndrome such as the Sturge–Weber syndrome.

Auscultation of the head may reveal the presence of a bruit.

Other causes of intracranial haemorrhage
These are disorders of the blood, blood dyscrasias, idiopathic thrombocytopenic purpura, sickle-cell anaemia, haemophilia and vitamin K deficiency in the newborn. Mycotic aneurysms may develop after septicaemic or pyemic states and rarely vitamin C deficiency may impair capillary integrity.

Acute infantile hemiplegia
This occurs chiefly in infants and young children complicating a variety of febrile illnesses, often with convulsions and unconsciousness. The pathogenesis is probably similar to that in venous thrombosis, namely inflammation and/or dehydration, or possibly an embolism of a cerebral artery. It has also been suggested that arteritis of the carotid artery secondary to infection of the throat or cervical glands may also be a cause. Cortical atrophy may develop later. After recovery, hemiplegia or a monoplegia, dysarthria, or intellectual retardation and convulsions are likely sequels. The CSF is usually normal, thus differentiating it from subarachnoid haemorrhage. The non-progressive nature of the hemiplegia distinguishes this condition from cerebral tumour, abscess and other lesions.

Neurological complications of sickle-cell anaemia

These are the result of intravascular sickling within cerebral vessels. In a careful study of seven patients with neurological deficits using angiography, partial or complete occlusion of a large vessel and discrete obstruction in the internal carotid artery were demonstrated in six patients. Involvement of the anterior and middle cerebral arteries and also vertebral artery was observed. This suggested that large vessel occlusion was not the result of back stasis from capillaries to major vessels as has been widely believed but may be the result of occlusion by sickling in the vasa vasorum and in the nutrient arteries that supply the walls of larger vessels. The process appeared to be progressive as repeat angiography showed the development of collaterals. This agrees with the impression gained in Kampala that patients who have once experienced intracerebral episodes of sickling seem liable to recurrences. The incidence of neurological complications in sickle-cell anaemia is difficult to assess. Experience in the sickle-cell clinic in Kampala, Uganda, indicates that intracerebral sickling is fortunately not common, but when it does occur the effects are seldom reversible and often devastating, with serious neurological and intellectual deficits. A much higher incidence of complications was found in another study when a quarter of the 89 patients developed neurological symptoms over a period of five years. Complete recovery took place in only half the episodes. The commonest complications are hemiplegia, coma or disorders of consciousness, convulsions and visual disturbances. Hemiplegia contributes a significant number of cases to acquired cerebral palsy in many areas. Alterations in consciousness may occur with or without convulsions. On recovery there is usually a residual hemiplegia. Cerebral infarction and subarachnoid haemorrhage are occasional complications. Several cases have been reported from Nigeria and where it was thought that the bleeding was probably secondary to sickling. Visual defects vary from field defect to total blindness which may be transient or permanent. It can be an isolated incident or precede or follow a major cerebral crisis. In some instances the blindness is cortical. Vitreous haemorrhages are a characteristic finding in HbSC disease although it is rare in homozygous sickle-cell anaemia. It presents in various ways, as a sudden monocular blindness, sometimes with recurrent episodes or as a gradual loss of vision. Some recover completely, others are left with permanent loss of vision of varying degrees. Other changes found in the eye include micro-aneurysms of the retinal vessels, retinitis proliferans as collateral channels develop with obliteration of retinal vessels.

Less common neurological findings include isolated aphasia, isolated cranial nerve palsies, transient ataxia, hypopituitarism and optic atrophy.

There appears to be no close relationship between neurological complications and sickle-cell crises, acute intercurrent infections, surgery and anaesthesia although these are recognised to be risk factors. In most cases neurological symptoms develop spontaneously in patients who are previously well and wake in the morning to find themselves hemiplegic, or blind or aphasic. In others changes of consciousness appear over a period of hours or in association with a recognised crisis or illness.

The most common pathological findings in the brain are multiple small infarcts and haemorrhages. Large infarcts, subarachnoid haemorrhage in the absence of aneurysms, intracerebral haemorrhage and large vessel thrombi are also known to occur. The meningeal vessels are prominent and packed with sickle-cells. Fat embolism with occlusion of the terminal arterioles is a commoner finding in the HbSC disease and sometimes occurs in adults with sickle-cell anaemia.

The incidence of neurological complications in the sickle-cell trait is no greater than in the general negro population with a normal haemoglobin but nevertheless sudden death and strokes have occurred in young patients with the sickle-cell trait associated with widespread cerebral infarction. There is no evidence of any impairment of cerebral function per se in sickle-cell anaemia. One study found the intellectual status of children with sickle-cell anaemia to be no different from those with normal haemoglobin. This accords with our own observations in the sickle-cell clinic in Kampala. The increased risk of children with sickle-cell anaemia to pneumococcal meningitis is now well recognised and is believed to be due to deficient pneumococcal opsonising activity related to splenic immunological unresponsiveness.

Space occupying lesions

These produce symptoms of raised intracranial pressure such as headache, vomiting, papilloedema and visual disturbances, separation of the sutures and a progressive impairment of consciousness or alteration in behaviour, and focal neurological signs depending on the site of the lesion. These are

(1) Uncal herniation – here the infero-medial part of the temporal lobe (uncus) herniates over the edge of the tentorium due to pressure from above. The resulting compression of the third cranial nerve and the brain stem produces a declining level of consciousness and a third nerve palsy on the same side as the lesion. The pupil dilates and becomes fixed whilst eyeball movements like elevation, depression and adduction fail.

(2) Central herniation is the result of midline downward displacement at the tentorial opening. It produces a progressive deterioration in consciousness, early loss of conjugate eye movements and later disordered patterns of respiration and decerebrate posturing. Damage to the pons is suggested by hyperventilation or breathing with a chaotic pattern, whilst terminal gasping is characteristic of medullary compression.

(3) Infratentorial lesions – unconsciousness results from a direct disturbance of the reticular areas which are essential to the maintenace of an alert state in the cerebral hemispheres. More

rarely it is caused by either an upward shift at the tentorial opening or a downward shift through the foramen magnum. The neurological picture may be identical with brain stem displacement from a supratentorial lesion at any given time but there is a difference in the sequence of events. From the onset there are signs of brain stem abnormality like abnormal pupil responses and dysconjugate or absent reflex eye movements. The pupils are widely dilated by anoxic brain stem damage and may be pin point after a pontine haemorrhage. The presence of normal reflex eye movements indicates intact brain stem pathways.

In many instances children are only brought to hospital in the late stages of their illness when they have progressed to coma or convulsions and the diagnosis is far from clear. A careful history from a reliable witness or attendant and followed by a careful clinical examination and a few simple basic investigations will often yield a surprising amount of useful information enabling a tentative diagnosis to be made. Specialised investigations (angiography) are not without risk and should only be carried out in centres where neurosurgical facilities are available to give a diagnosis or follow with surgical treatment.

Diagnoses to be considered include

Cerebral neoplasms

Cerebral abscess

Subdural effusion

This is still a common complication of bacterial meningitis, usually presenting during the second week with irritability, fever, vomiting and sometimes convulsions. Occasionally an effusion may develop following a febrile illness or dehydration, presumably the result of a small cerebral thrombosis. Diagnosis is by subdural tap.

Tuberculoma

Tuberculomata may be single or multiple. The latter are evidence of disseminated tuberculosis. They may present with a bewildering variety of clinical signs, depending on numbers and site although occasionally intracranial tuberculoma can be silent. The commoner sites are the mid brain, cerebellum and frontal lobes. There is always a very high risk of rupture and subsequent tuberculous meningitis. Calcification occurs in the healing stages. Prolonged antituberculous therapy is required and if a lesion is causing focal pressure symptoms surgical removal may be needed. The diagnosis depends on the relationship between the neurological signs and the presence of tuberculosis elsewhere. More detailed investigations may be needed to locate the actual sites of the lesions.

Parasitic infections

A number of parasites may migrate to the CNS at various stages in their cycle of development for example, toxocara, cysticercoid, amoebiasis, schistosomiasis and paragonomiasis. Parasitic infection of the nervous system may cause either acute symptoms or focal signs due to granulomatous lesions. In addition hydatid cysts may occasionally develop in the brain from the dog tapeworm *Echinococcus granulosa*.

Cerebral oedema

Generalised cerebral oedema may cause a considerable increase in brain volume and a marked rise in intracranial pressure together with convulsions and coma. It is an important feature of several encephalopathies such as acute toxic encephalopathy, hypertensive encephalopathy and lead encephalopathy, benign intracranial hypertension or 'pseudotumour cerebri'.

Benign intracranial hypertension

This may present with cranial nerve palsies, especially the sixth, headache and visual disturbances. The marked papilloedema contrasts with the general well being of the child. It is believed to be the result of diffuse cerebral oedema, the ventricles are normal in size. It was originally described following otitis media and was believed to be due to lateral sinus thrombosis but it is now also known to occur after acute viral infections, vitamin D intoxication, tetracycline and nalidixic acid therapy and following a reduction of steroid dosage in children who have been on treatment for long periods. It may also follow endocrine disturbances and occasionally occurs in girls at the menarche. The condition is self-limiting but responds to steroid therapy and in children who have already been on steroids, the dose should be temporarily increased again. All cases should be thoroughly investigated to exclude a tumour.

Cerebral abscess

This is rare in infancy but remains a difficult problem in older children. The diagnosis often presents considerable difficulties which leads to delay in treatment. Mortality is still high at 30–60 per cent which is only slightly better than that of 30 years ago. The high mortality has been attributed to the difficulties in accurately localising the abscess, to the misuse of antibiotics and to failure to tap the abscess daily. In a series of 200 abscesses, including many adults, 50 per cent of the organisms were *Streptococci* (mainly anaerobic or microaerophilic, that is, difficult organisms to culture), 20 per cent were *Staphylococci* and 15 per cent coliforms.

The clinical features are those of infection, intracranial suppuration and raised pressure as well as focal neurological signs.

Cerebral abscess is always secondary to a source of infection elsewhere and a septic focus can nearly always be found. The most common is chronic middle ear infection with mastoiditis, followed by lung disease, and trauma on the head with fracture or penetrating wound. Children with cyanotic congenital heart disease are particularly prone to this complication. Fever and leucocytosis are common but may be absent if the abcess has become walled off. Raised intracranial pressure and suppuration cause headache often of some weeks duration and vomiting with loss of weight, sometimes resembling tuberculous meningitis. There is almost always some alteration in mental state – irritability, fretfulness, lack of concentration, confusion, lethargy or drowsiness. Menginism may be present. Coma is usually of late onset and is often a pre-terminal event. Papilloedema is a variable feature and may be either absent or marked. A combination of leucocytosis and bradycardia is a helpful sign but bradycardia is by no means always present.

Careful examination may be needed to detect focal signs which include ataxia, hemiparesis, cranial nerve palsies and visual field defects. Focal convulsions may be helpful in localising the site. The interval between the onset of infection and the diagnosis is often quite long, several weeks is not uncommon but a cerebral abcess should be suspected in a child who has signs of cerebral dysfunction lasting ten days or more after an acute infection. The differential diagnosis includes encephalitis, cerebral tumour, tuberculous meningitis and trypanosomiasis in endemic areas. The differentiation from cerebral tumour is often difficult and is sometimes only made at operation.

Diagnosis

Lumbar puncture must be avoided, especially if there is evidence of raised intracranial pressure. Even if there are no clinical signs of raised pressure it is still hazardous and may be followed by a rapid deterioration. Whilst it is necessary to exclude meningitis, the presence of papilloedema, convulsions and localising signs are more likely to indicate an abscess. They are contra-indications to lumbar puncture suggesting instead urgent neurosurgical investigations. It is usually difficult to obtain the accurate localisation of an abscess necessary for successful aspiration, especially where multiple abscesses are present. However in one study the sole exception was in relation to ENT sepsis where the abscess was found to be closely related to a site of sepsis. Carotid arteriography has been found to be accurate in only two-thirds of cases and may in fact be misleading because oedema surrounding the abscess displaces blood vessels particularly the middle cerebrals. Ventriculography, although helpful at times, is an undesirable procedure and sometimes dangerous. The recent introduction of brain scanning gives precise and accurate localisation of an abscess and should result in earlier diagnosis and better management, but unfortunately is not likely to be available except in specialised centres for many years. Factors which contribute to the continuing high mortality are inability to prove the diagnosis especially when early symptoms are ill defined, the presence of multiple abscesses, coma on admission and a ruptured abscess with positive CSF culture. In one study it was found that an abscess in survivors was more often associated with a cranial injury or surgery or with adjacent ENT infection. The following suspicious pointers were also noted

(1) An abscess may present with fever, lethargy and headache without any definite neurological signs.
(2) Bilateral abscesses may be present in spite of unilateral neurological signs.
(3) Multiple unilateral abscesses may be present.
(4) Meningitis not due to *Haemophilus, Pneumococcus* or *Meningococcus* may be secondary to a ruptured brain abscess.
(5) Any neurosurgical procedure may be complicated by the development of a brain abscess.
(6) Arteriography may give negative results but should always be done on both sides, whenever it is undertaken.
(7) Brain abscesses may recur.

Treatment

Investigation and treatment should be carried out in a neurosurgical unit. A lumbar puncture should not be done if a cerebral abscess is suspected. If antibiotic treatment is to be given, penicillin is the drug of choice, the dose being one or two mega units six hourly. A primary septic focus elsewhere should be sought and treated appropriately. A full ENT examination is essential. If the patient is in coma, intravenous mannitol may bring about temporary improvement.

Paraplegia

All grades of severity may be seen in children presenting in out-patient clinics. The commonest cause is tuberculosis of the spine (Pott's disease). The history is usually one of slow and increasing progression of symptoms with obvious deformity of the spine and a variable degree of spasticity, weakness and sensory loss in the legs together with sphincter involvement. X-rays confirm destruction of bone in one or two vertebrae. A tuberculous focus can usually be found elsewhere although occasionally a primary focus in the pedicle itself can cause paraplegia. A paravertebral abscess may also be present.

Burkitt's lymphoma is the second commonest cause of paraplegia in Uganda and West Africa (see page 283). In some instances it may be the earliest clinical manifestation whilst in others it may be the presenting symptom in spite of generalised disease. The distinction from tuberculosis is easy because the history is much shorter, as symptoms may have been present from a few days to a few weeks before referral, the paraplegia is usually flaccid at the outset and there is no spinal deformity. Sensory changes vary from mild to complete loss with sphincter involvement. Radiological changes may be present in the vertebrae and a paravertebral mass may also be demonstrated. Myelography and laminectomy reveal single or multiple extradural deposits.

Trauma can result in paraplegia – road accidents and falls especially from trees are the common injuries in children. In countries where schistosomiasis is endemic, a *Schistoma* granuloma in the spine is an occasional cause of paraplegia.

Epidural and paravertebral *abscess*, usually secondary to a septicaemic spread from a focus elsewhere, can at times cause paraplegia.

Spastic paraplegia has been described in association with *vitamin deficiencies* in Jamaica.

Lathyrism is one of the oldest known forms of paraplegia. It is especially prevalent in central India but is also seen in other parts of the world from time to time, for example, south-east Europe. The toxic agent is in the seeds of *Lathyrus sativus*, a hardy winter crop grown extensively in India for human and animal use, particularly when other crops have failed. The human disease occurs when the diet containing more than one-third of *Lathyrus* seeds is eaten for a period of three to six months or more. Symptoms begin with the acute or subacute onset of muscle cramps, weakness and stiffness in the lower limbs with progression to paraplegia in some. The toxic agent is believed to be ß-N-oxalyl-L ß-diamino-proprionic acid which is known to be an amino acid antagonist in microorganisms. Histology of the spinal cord shows microglyosis in the anterior and lateral horns, partial degeneration of motor tracts and anterolateral sclerosis in the dorso-lumbar area.

Subluxation of the atlanto-axial joint due to tonsillar or retropharyngeal abscess is an unusual cause but can result in progressive paraplegia.

Cerebral palsy – the diagnosis is usually evident from the history and clinical findings.

Tumours

Tumours which may cause spinal cord compression include neuromas which may be isolated or multiple as in Von Recklinghausen's disease, secondary deposits from a medullo blastoma or malignant astrocytoma or extension through an intervertebral foramen by a neuroblastoma.

Symptoms of spinal cord compression

An intraspinal mass above the level of L1 will compress the cord causing spasticity, weakness and increased reflexes in the limbs and trunk below the compressed segment with extensor plantar responses. Sensory loss involves all segments below the level of the mass but to some extent depends upon the site, thus an anteriorly placed mass will affect predominantly pain and temperature sensation whilst posterior compression of the cord will mainly affect joint and discriminatory sense. A lateral tumour may cause a Brown–Séquard syndrome with spastic weakness on one side and loss of pain and temperature sensation on the opposite side. Symptoms and signs of segmental root involvement such as root or girdle pains, hyperaesthesiae, muscle weakness and wasting, and diminished reflexes in root distribution may also help to determine the site of compression.

Compression of the corda equina roots below the level of L1 causes weakness, muscle wasting and diminished reflexes, and progressive sensory loss in the distribution of the lower lumbar and sacral nerves. There is early impairment of bladder function.

The early symptoms of paraplegia, abnormal gait, a limp, weakness, abnormal reflexes, the presence of root pain and sensory changes and disturbances of micturition demand investigation. X-rays of the spine may reveal changes in the vertebral bodies or pedicles, or a para-vertebral mass. In the presence of the block in the spinal canal, CSF protein is raised and Queckenstedt's test is negative, that is, there is no rise in CSF pressure on compressing the jugular veins. (This test is dangerous in the presence of raised intracranial pressure.) Malignant cells may be seen in the CSF. Contrast myelography using Myodil will outline the position and extent of a mass but is not without some risk and the procedure is best done by a neurosurgeon.

Treatment

Treatment is that of the underlying cause. Laminectomy and surgical treatment are best avoided except in the case of a pyogenic abscess, since they often make the paraplegia worse. Urinary infection can be avoided by training children to keep dry by correlating the intake and output of fluids and expressing the bladder manually every two or four hours. Parents or attendants can be shown how to do this. Avoidance of constipation is also important. Equally important is the early rehabilitation with active and passive movements to keep the legs and especially the feet in their normal attitudes to enable children to stand and walk later. The avoidance of contractures and deformities is particulary important when there is some muscle power which can otherwise be utilised in standing or walking.

Cerebral palsy

Cerebral palsy is the name given to a number of non-progressive disorders of the brain in which impaired motor function is the main symptom. Although the cerebral lesion is non-progressive some of the peripheral effects, in particular contractures, may become progressively worse if untreated.

Table 28.14   Classification of cerebral palsy

Neurological diagnosis	Distribution
Hemiplegia	Right
	Left
Bilateral hemiplegia	–
Diplegia	
Hypotonic	Paraplegic
Dystonic	Triplegic
Spastic or rigid	Tetraplegic
Ataxic diplegia	
Hypotonic	Paraplegic
Spastic	Triplegic
	Tetraplegic
Ataxia	Mainly unilateral
	Bilateral
Dyskinesia	
Dystonic	Monoplegic
Choreoid	Hemiplegic
Athetoid	Triplegic
Tension	Tetraplegic
Tremor	
Mixed forms	

Source: Ingram T T S. Cerebral palsy. In: Disorders of the central nervous system. In: Forfar J O and Arneil G C, eds. *Textbook of paediatrics*. Edinburgh: Churchill Livingstone, 1973.

As the term includes several disorders, there are a number of widely different causes. About half are probably genetically determined, some are due to perinatal injury and the remainder are acquired postnatally. The classification used here is based upon the neurological diagnosis and its distribution and is shown in table 28.14.

Hemiplegia

This implies unilateral limb paralysis usually associated with spasticity. Commonly the upper limb is affected to a greater extent than the lower limb. Boys are affected more often than girls in a ratio of two to one. About half of the cases are congenital. A few are a result of a developmental malformation but the most important cause in the majority is perinatal injury. There are often multiple factors involved, such as, for example, a bad obstetric history together with difficulties in delivery followed by postnatal asphyxia. There is also a high incidence of both prematurity and postmaturity in all published series. Hemiplegia is also the commonest type of acquired cerebral palsy – the majority following an acute and often castastrophic febrile illness in the first year or two of life. Acute infantile hemiplegia is also the end result of many of the other common insults to the central nervous system at this stage.

Clinical features

Lack of movement of varying severity in the limbs and face of the affected side is the main symptom. In congenital cases the affected side is floppy and hypotonic after birth and spasticity only appears after some months. As it does so the mother notices stiffening and flexing of the fingers and thumbs so that there is difficulty in opening the palm of the hand. The baby tends to turn to the normal side. As spasticity increases the tendon jerks become brisker. Acquired hemiplegia usually develops during a recognisable illness often in association with a fit and is most severe immediately following the seizure with a gradual improvement in function. Spasticity appears some two or three weeks later, and increases over the next two months or so. The patient now develops the characteristic posture of hemiplegia – adduction, flexion and internal rotation at the shoulder, semiflexion at the wrist and elbow, pronation of the forearm and flexed fingers over an adducted thumb. In the lower limb the hip is adducted, internally rotated and semi-flexed, the knee is semi-flexed and the foot plantar flexed, sometimes with varus or valgus deformities. The findings in established hemiplegia depend on the degree of involvement. Mildly affected cases are able to use the hand whilst moderately affected cases can use the hand as an assistant to the normal hand. There is loss of voluntary movement patterns which have been acquired late, for example, abduction of the thumb and full supination of the forearm and the ability to extend the fingers. In severely affected cases the limb is of little or no use. In the lower limb muscle imbalance will cause impairment of gait.

There may be some sensory loss in a small number of patients, usually loss of position sense and two point discrimination. Visual field defects may also be present. Vasomotor involvement (loss of vasomotor tone) is common in the affected limbs which are colder, particularly when exposed to low temperatures, often cyanosed and oedematous. They also tend to grow more slowly and may be slightly shorter. Epilepsy is also a common complication.

Bilateral hemiplegia

Hemiplegia on both sides is uncommon (about five per cent of cases of cerebral palsy). The majority are due to developmental malformations of the brain and there are often abnormalities in cardiac, skeletal and other systems. Acquired cases may follow trauma or at resuscitation after cardio-respiratory arrest. Spasticity is generally severe and there is also involvement of the bulbar muscles which are spared in unilateral hemiplegia. In addition the majority are severely mentally retarded and have epilepsy. Because of bulbar involvement there will be early feeding difficulties with regurgitation, inhalation and pneumonia. Most affected children in the tropics will die of intercurrent infection early in life.

Diplegia

In diplegia there is more or less symmetrical paresis of the limbs, but the lower limbs are affected more severely than the upper. Spasticity or rigidity are commonly present and occasionally there may be some bulbar involvement. Almost all cases are congenital due to some development malformation. The pathological findings include cortical atrophy and a microcephaly. The mothers of diplegic infants tend to have a poor obstetric history such as relative infertility and a higher proportion of foetal wastage including neonatal deaths. There is also a higher incidence of diplegia in multiple pregnancy, especially in those with low birth weight.

Clinical features

After birth infants may be either hyperexcitable or lethargic. Symptoms then appear slowly over the following months with delay in motor milestones, especially in locomotion, crawling or walking because of involvement of the lower limbs. If the infant is paraplegic with involvement of the head and upper limbs symptoms will appear early because of poor head control and delay in sitting unsupported. The classical feature is that of scissoring of the legs when the infant is held erect. In the supine position infants develop posture of opisthotonos. Primitive infantile reflexes like grasp, stepping and tonic neck are retained and a tendency for scissoring and spasticity increases as the infant gets older. Reflexes become brisker. With increasing spasticity and flexion, fixed deformities and contractures tend to develop. There is a risk of subluxation of the hip or even dislocation with increasing adduction, internal rotation and semi-flexion. Affected limbs are often cold and cyanosed due to lack of vasomotor tone and growth may be stunted. Sensory loss however is uncommon. If all four limbs are affected, cranial nerve involvement is common with convergent squints, visual field defects, loss of visual acuity or even optic atrophy. Although bulbar involvement is not usually severe, it may be sufficient to cause difficulties in feeding and swallowing, aspiration pneumonia and an early death. This combined with the considerable difficulties in locomotion, increasing spasticity and contractures make the prognosis poor for this form of cerebral palsy in developing countries. The survivors may also have speech problems.

Ataxic cerebral palsy

Uncomplicated ataxic cerebral palsy is characterised by weakness, inco-ordination of movement and intention tremor, generalised hypotonia and unsteadiness. The absence of uncomplicated ataxic cerebral palsy has been noted.

In ataxic diplegia there is more or less symmetrical paresis of the limbs being more marked in the upper than the lower, together with ataxia.

Most cases of ataxic cerebral palsy are congenital due to malformation of the cerebellum or its connecting pathways. Acquired cases may follow any severe insult to the growing brain but also occur after chicken-pox, injury to the posterior fossa from tumour, trauma or surgery and may be a sequel of symptomatic hypoglycaemia. Ataxic diplegia is commonly associated with hydrocephalus complicated by cerebral palsy.

Clinical features

Ataxic type of cerebral palsy is impossible to diagnose during the neonatal period but may be suspected in 'floppy babies' who show few spontaneous movements or if there is associated hydrocephalus. Later there is a lack of voluntary movements and hypotonia, with retardation in motor development, delay in achieving head control, in sitting alone and in walking. There is a characteristic broad-based gait with the arms held out to give extra balance. In uncomplicated ataxic cerebral palsy the intention tremor and hypotonia become less marked in older children.

In ataxic diplegia the findings are those of ataxia with superimposed spasticity which may to some extent depress the intention tremor. The child walks on a broad-based gait but with slightly flexed knees and hips, a tendency to walk on the toes and with a scissor-like motion as in diplegia. Other complications include tendency to develop contractures, epilepsy, speech disorders and mental retardation.

Dyskinesia

This is an impairment of voluntary movements caused by involuntary movements and unwanted changes of tone in bulbar, trunk and limb muscles, rather than paresis or inco-ordination of voluntary movement. The major pathological changes are found in the basal ganglia. Most cases are the result of perinatal brain injury often following difficulties in the perinatal period. There is often a history of intrapartum asphyxia, birth trauma and apnoea after birth. Kernicterus is a particularly important cause.

Clinical types of dyskinesia

(1) Athetosis – slow writhing movements of the distal part of the limb when voluntary movement is attempted. It may complicate hemiplegia but in dyskinesia it is unassociated with paralysis or spasticity.
(2) Choreoid movements – relatively rapid movements mainly in the proximal part of the limbs resembling the movements found in rheumatic chorea.
(3) Dystonic movements – slow involuntary movements in the proximal part of the limbs, often involving the trunk and tending to produce postures resembling opisthotonos.
(4) Tremor – irregular alternating involuntary movements.
(5) Tension – sudden increase in tone when voluntary movements are attempted.

Clinical features

Most cases show involvement of all four limbs, trunk and bulbar muscles. Impairment of function is most likely to be seen in more precise and finer movements, that is, fine manipulation with fingers and produce more intense involuntary activity than grosser movements such as pointing and grasping. Bulbar involvement may cause severe impairment of speech because of the fine muscular movements required.

Abnormal movements may be seen in severe cases of kernicterus in the neonatal period and many infants with dyskinesia have feeding and swallowing difficulties. The neonatal period is followed by latent period lasting from several weeks to several months in which most signs disappear but careful follow-up reveals delay in achieving motor milestones and there is generalised muscular hypotonia. Persistence of the atonic neck reflex beyond the age of six months is an especially important and useful sign. In kernicterus in addition there is a characteristic inability to look upwards from an early age. There is then a gradual onset of unwanted mass movements in the limbs and trunk occurring whenever the baby attempts voluntary movements. For example, attempted movements may cause head retraction on opisthotonos. After a further period of weeks or months these mass movements are replaced by discrete involuntary movements in which any attempt at voluntary movements results in changes of tone and in unwanted involuntary movements.

The major problems

Involuntary movements and alteration in tone cause feeding difficulties and speech problems. It may be three or four years before a child can swallow semi-solids and he may never be able to chew properly. If therefore he survives the hazards of aspiration pneumonia in infancy, he may still fail to thrive and perish from malnutrition. In less seriously affected children involvement of the lip, tongue and palate produces speech problems and difficulties in communication. In children with kernicterus, high tone hearing loss is an additional impairment to language development. In spite of these problems, however, mental retardation and epilepsy is less common than in other forms of cerebral palsy.

Other forms of cerebral palsy

The choreoid syndrome is a form of dyskinesia seen in school children who are described as 'clumsy' or 'fidgety'. They show a mild excess of choreoathetoid movements but more importantly may have learning difficulties. Involuntary movements may be demonstrated by asking the child to stand with his feet together and his hands outstretched. Some children are by nature clumsy, although no involuntary movements may be demonstrated. This may be a mild form of ataxic cerebral palsy.

Associated disabilities in cerebral palsy

These may be of more practical importance than the motor handicap itself and it is often these which make cerebral palsy such a disabling condition. Often multiple handicaps may be present and a high proportion have mental retardation, epilepsy, speech disorders, defects of vision or hearing, as well as educational and behavioural problems. Thus it is

estimated in the UK that only one-third of children with cerebral palsy are of normal intelligence and a quarter have an IQ below 55, that is, are severely educationally subnormal. Children with hemiplegia, dyskinesia or diplegia confined to the lower limbs are more likely to be of normal intelligence. In addition those with normal intelligence may have a specific visuospatial or audiophonic difficulties causing specific learning, reading and writing problems.

Half the children with hemiplegia also have epilepsy, chiefly the grand mal type although focal seizures are also common in hemiplegia, and ataxia. Severely mentally retarded children with all types of cerebral palsy are particularly liable to salaam-type of spasms. Fits are much less common in the simple ataxic and dyskinetic forms. Unfortunately epilepsy makes employment impossible for some children with cerebral palsy who would otherwise be suitable. Behaviour disorders are also commoner amongst children with epilepsy and with mental retardation.

The incidence of cerebral palsy in the UK is about 3 per 1000 live births. There are no statistics from the tropics but reports suggest that it is frequently encountered in neurology clinics and a large proportion of cases are acquired postnatally. One study found that cerebral palsy accounted for over one-third of cases seen in the clinic and just under a half were acquired. In another study about a quarter were of postnatal origin. The most significant finding is that so many of these cases are preventable.

Management of cerebral palsy

This may need to be started before a final diagnosis has been made, particularly with early detection before the classical signs appear. As with all handicapped children management is essentially a team affair with the physiotherapist playing a key role.

Physiotherapy

Both active and passive movement must be encouraged to avoid contractures and deprivation from the lack of voluntary activity. The parents must play a critical role in providing environmental stimulation and experience of movement patterns. The basis of treatment is to inhibit the more primitive reflex patterns and encourage the later developing patterns found in older, normal children. The prevention of deformity is of the greatest importance in hemiplegia and diplegia where there is a tendency for spastic flexion and contractures to develop.

Passive movements are essential if these are to be prevented. Dislocation of the hip, flexion of the knee and plantar flexion deformities may prevent a child who has the potential to walk from eventually doing so. Surgery is to be avoided as a rule since further interference with muscle balance may only aggravate existing deformities.

Occupational therapy

Every effort should be made to stimulate the child as much as possible and to make him as independent as possible. Parents are taught not only passive movements but simple feeding techniques, toilet training and how to make the best use of both of his hands. A simple object such as a ball may be used to help particular movement patterns. Children should be allowed to play with other children as much as possible. The provision of simple nursery facilities with a physiotherapist in attendance should be encouraged as part of the development of paediatric departments. Even in children with multiple handicaps, the successful management of one particular problem such as the satisfactory control of epilepsy or hyperkinesia may lead to an all round improvement, making the child much easier to handle by his parents. Children with lesser disability should be encouraged to do as much as they can but not driven to the point of frustration. It may even be possible for milder cases to attend school and where possible this should be encouraged. Parents should be given every encouragement and support, not only in caring for the child but in helping them to accept his condition. Many severely disabled infants and young children however inevitably succumb to malnutrition from feeding problems, aspiration pneumonia and intercurrent infections, as well as from being abandoned by their parents.

Care and provision of services for handicapped children

The provision of services for handicapped children in most developing countries is virtually non-existent. Such services are expensive and where health budgets are severely limited, priority must understandably be given to other more pressing problems and to preventive services. On the other hand, in the affluent societies of the West reduction in the incidence of infectious diseases and other preventable disorders has resulted in an increasing amount of a paediatrician's time being spent on problems of handicapped children. A modest start in the development of services for handicapped children can be made in many centres by providing out-patient and physiotherapy facilities by interested and motivated staff. It must be realised at the outset that management is a team affair with usually a paediatrician or other interested health professional at the head of the team and a physiotherapist, preferably trained in the problems of the handicapped child, as his key colleague. The facilities will depend very much on what is available locally and how much enthusiasm can be generated in the local community for voluntary help. All religious bodies and international service organisations have a keen interest in services for the handicapped. Though facilities should be closely linked to the hospital, day care centres for the handicapped child need not necessarily be on a hospital site. Day care should be run on an out-patient basis. Distance and cost will prevent many from regular visits, therefore there may be need for temporary hostel accommodation where mothers and children can stay for a short while to be taught the basic techniques of home physiotherapy.

Very severely affected children are unlikely to survive much beyond infancy. The aim should be to select children most likely to benefit from help, that is, mild to moderate cases who can be rehabilitated. Treatment need not necessarily be expensive, a simple piece of equipment can often be made or adapted to suit the special needs of an individual. For the more severely handicapped it may not be possible to do very much. Nevertheless, in children with multiple handicaps attempts to help in one sphere are often rewarding, for a reduction of one disability often helps to reduce the overall burden, making management for the mother much easier and simpler. Later, it may be possible to provide special schooling for educable children although this is not yet available in most developing countries. The aim should be to try and integrate the child back into the normal school and the community.

Medical aspects

The first need is to define the child's problems and then his needs and finally to decide what, if anything, can be done for him. Management should not await a final medical diagnosis which in some instances may only be possible after a period of observation. A full physical and neurological examination, of course, is essential. Intercurrent disease such as anaemia, malnutrition and tuberculosis will require treatment. An attempt should be made to identify the cause of the handicap, for example pre-natal or post-natal. The child may need to be observed on more than one occasion at the centre by the doctor or therapist before a final diagnosis is made. More prolonged observation may be needed if there is only developmental delay since classical signs of cerebral palsy may not appear until later. Diagnosis and assessment are only the first though important step towards management. More exact assessment may involve the services of orthopaedic, ENT, eye and dental specialists whose co-operation and interest should be sought and stimulated at an early stage. Different attitudes and approaches must be developed for the care of handicapped children from those in acute illnesses. It is important for one doctor to be in overall charge on a long term basis co-ordinating the management by other members of the team so that omissions or duplication of services do not occur and parents are not confused by personnel sometimes working at cross purposes.

It is important to draw up a plan of action for each child with as much help as is possible from the parents. Often we underestimate their intelligence, interest and enthusiasm in helping with the child. It is important to explain clearly that 'cure' is not possible and that only a degree of improvement is to be expected. Furthermore, parents must be told exactly how much improvement can be expected and over what period of time. They must be encouraged to do as much as they can for the child and give explicit guidance on every day matters and simple care. They must not be confused by being told too much at once.

All families of handicapped children are under some stress, particularly the mother who may devote time to the child at the expense of her husband and other children. The services of a medical social worker are of special help here.

Special provision will be needed for children who are blind or partially sighted, deaf or partially deaf and who have speech problems. Facilities for many of these children are not yet available and depend to a large extent on the availability of skilled therapists.

Further reading

Bucher B, Poucoard J A, Vernant J C, DeFreitas E C. Tropical neuromyelopathies and retroviruses: a review. *Reviews of Inf Dis* 1990; 12: 890–897.

Gram L. Epileptic seizures and syndromes. *Lancet* 1990; 336:161–163.

O'Donohue N V. Use of antiepileptic drugs in childhood epilepsy. *Arch dis childh* 1991; 66: 1173–1179.

Joint Working Group of the Research Unit of the Royal College of Physicians and the British Paediatric Association. Guidelines for the management of convulsions with fever. *Brit Med J* 1991; 303: 634–636.

Roman G C. Tropical myelopathies and myeloneuropathies. *PAHO Bull* 1987; 21: 293–303.

Tunkel A R, Wispelwey B, Scheld W M. Bacterial meningitis: recent advances in pathophysiology and treatment. *Ann Int Med* 1990; 112: 610–623.

Wallace S J. Childhood epileptic syndromes. *Lancet* 1990; 336: 486–487.

Wright P F. Approaches to prevent acute bacterial meningitis in developing countries. *Bull Wrld Hlth Org* 1989; 67: 479–486.

Section VII

Provision of Care

29 *Provision of care*

It is now common knowledge that a large part of the morbidity and mortality seen in children of the developing countries is preventable. Table 29.1 gives causes of death in children in three different parts of the developing world.

The reasons why these preventable diseases cause a large proportion of illness and mortality are multifactorial. They have been often called the 'diseases of poverty' but their roots also lie in ignorance and tradition. In most rural societies disease is thought to be due to wrong behaviour such as breaking a taboo, or witchcraft, or due to evil spirits. It is also generally believed that for some diseases Western medicine has no cure, like for example obowosi (kwashiorkor) in Uganda. Instead, people put their faith in the indigenous system of health care, of which there may be several (figure 29.1).

Medical services as they have evolved in most countries are largely based on the urban hospital which has 'cure of disease' as its main interest. Such hospitals may serve the needs of the urban elite but do not meet the requirements of the rural societies and have virtually no impact on the determinants of disease in the community. Several studies in different parts of the developing world have demonstrated how the hospital may in fact siphon off scarce resources from the grass roots of the health system instead of being a support to it (figure 29.2).

Table 29.2 compares the capital and running costs of a regional hospital with those of rural health centres in Tanzania as well as the service outputs of the two types of institution. Clearly more is to be gained by developing the rural health centre/sub centre concept than from investing in hospitals.

Table 29.1   Causes of death in children

	Dar-es-Salaam (1969)	Imesi (Nigeria 1959)	Sumatra (Indonesia 1964)
Diarrhoeal disease	9.49%	12%	25%
Respiratory infections	23.7%	12%	11%
Protein–calorie malnutrition	9.0%	12%	26%
Malaria	6.4%	8%	8%
Measles	10.8%	8%	7%
Tuberculosis	1.2%	5%	6%
Anaemia	6.8%		5%
	67.39%	57%	88%

Table 29.2   Costs and service outputs of regional hospitals and health centres in Tanzania

Regional hospital	Rural health centre
Building cost of a 200-bed hospital = £300 000=	15 rural health centres
Recurrent annual expenditure of 1 regional hospital =	Recurrent cost of 15 rural health centres
Annual admissions 9 000	Annual admissions 15 000
Out-patients attended 400 000	Out-patients seen 1 million

The preference of parents in the Punjab for the source of advice
and treatment for some childhood disease (N=60) Kaher et al '72

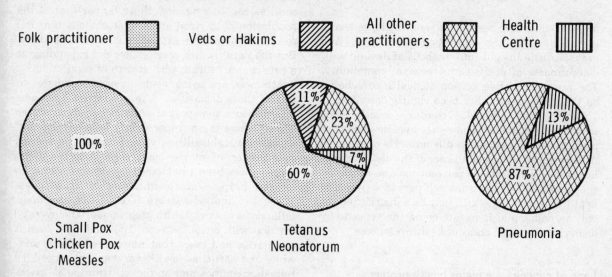

Figure 29.1   Source of health care in rural North India

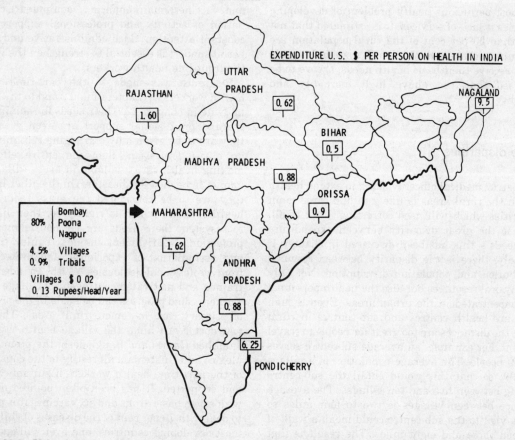

Figure 29.2   Urban rural maldistribution of health expenditure. In Maharashtra, the three main cities consume 80 per cent of health expenditure

The district medical officer's dilemma

Medical education, based as it is on the large teaching hospital, has also evolved on similar lines, and provides little insight into methods of dealing with determinants of disease in a peasant community. The present curative system of health care based on the large hospital has been rightly described as 'importing from abroad yesterday's solutions for tomorrow's problems'. The newly-appointed district medical officer is thus in a dilemma. He is expected to be responsible for health care of the district population of which up to 80 per cent may be rural. On the other hand, he finds himself part of a system of health care delivery which may be a district service only in name, and is in fact doing the opposite by depriving the rural areas of health resources.

Lack of services – a major health problem

The most pernicious health problem of developing countries is lack of services. It is estimated that not more than 20 per cent of the rural population are in regular contact with the health system. If people do not receive their basic health needs, are we to be surprised that they have high morbidity and mortality?

Three disparities

The district medical officer wishing to extend health care in the rural areas is likely to find three main disparities which will need correcting. First of all, there is the great disparity between expenditure and needs – this has been discussed in chapter 1. Secondly, there is the disparity between resource distribution and population distribution. Not only the physical resources but also the health personnel are concentrated in the urban areas. Even though there are health centres and sub-centres in rural areas, the distances are too great for people to travel to them. For example, an average subcentre serves 10 000 people. The average population of a village is 1000, so that this would entail the sub-centre serving between five and ten villages. The average distance between villages is two to four miles so that a visit to the sub-centre could mean a walk of between three and eight miles. The result is that most health centres and sub-centres end up with providing outpatient care for only those villages where they are sited, and large sections of the population go unattended. The third disparity is between the growth of population and the rate at which services can be extended. Since 80 per cent of the population is in rural areas, it is obvious that the so-called population explosion is occurring there. But the rural health services are not expanding at a rate commensurate with growth of population.

Attempts are being made in some countries to correct these disparities. A few countries have now established a new post of a district medical officer (rural) whose main responsibility is to develop and supervise rural health services. Similarly, a district co-ordinator of mother and child health (MCH) services has been established by several countries for the purpose of co-ordinating MCH services. These two individuals are likely to be the main pillars of a district health programme. The average district will have between 100 and 200 health auxiliaries and twice that number of village midwives and part-time health workers. Their need for refresher courses and on-the-job training is great. Moreover, the question of regular supply of drugs and vaccines, maintenance of equipment, co-ordination of activity and professional support needs constant attention. Such administrative and managerial support is essential to strengthen the work of the front-line health workers.

Reference was made to the part-time village health workers in chapters 1 and 2 and to the village midwife in chapter 22. Their needs for administrative and professional support are even greater. If they are to be given only a grudging recognition by an elitist profession, then the entire effort for making health care available in every village and hamlet is headed for disaster. On the other hand, if they are to be considered the grass roots of the health system, which is rightly so, then like any root system their needs are for nourishment and protection. Nourishment implies regular training and assimilation of experience, and protection is from professional jealousies. With an adequately trained and motivated contingent of village health workers rapid progress can be made in the provision of primary care in remote rural areas. The bare-foot doctor of China, the village health worker of Jamkhed (India) and Bangladesh, the promoters in Mexico and Guatemala all testify to the capabilities of the part-time health workers if suitably trained and supported. It has been often pointed out that with seven basic drugs and six vaccines it is possible to deal with 70 per cent of the diseases of children in most developing countries, and even village health workers can become proficient in the use of a handful of medicines.

Identifying the major health problems and their severity

Having put together the various components of a district health team in the form of auxiliaries and village workers, the next step will be to identify the major health problems and their severity. Data on mortality and rates such as infant mortality rate, pre-school mortality, perinatal and maternal mortality are useful. Where national statistics are available it is justifiable to assume that similar rates apply for the district until such time as local data have been gathered. If no national statistics are available, an impression can be obtained by a rapid assessment in one or two villages selected in accordance with their distance from a rural health unit. Exact figures are not absolutely necessary and should not delay health activities. The ideal should not be allowed to become the enemy of the good. Information gathering can continue while services are being provided and health programmes implemented.

Table 29.3 is an example of mortality data gathered by local 'informants' in selected villages in India and provides insight into rural health problems.

The information on mortality is next supplemented with data on morbidity. Hospital admissions and out-patient attendances together with diagnoses made in the health centres and sub-centres can provide valuable information about the common illnesses for which help is sought. Table 29.4 is an example of such information obtained in Tanzania.

Figures like those presented above only mirror the common health needs of the people and are by no means exact. They are useful as a starting point

but the information will need to be supplemented by observations made during 'village rounds' and by talking to the people. The latter provide also a useful tool for estimating the prevalence of chronic disability many of whom may not attend rural health units for treatment. Thus impressions about the prevalence of polio paralysis, blindness and cerebral palsy can be obtained through visits to villages and schools.

Identifying the determinants of disease

Vital statistics and morbidity data are mainly statements of facts and main problems. The determinants of disease are in the homes, the environment and the life styles of the people. Further observations on the knowledge, practices and attitudes, nutritional intake, housing, local belief systems, concepts of disease, and child bearing as well as child rearing practices, are necessary to get to the true etiology of disease. Some of these determinants may be more

Table 29.3   Causes of death in 786 health centre villages in India (1969)

Causes	% Deaths
Violence or injury	3.5
Diarrhoea	9.2
Childbirth complications and pregnancy	1.3
Coughs	24.5
Swellings	8.0
Fevers	20.6
Other infant deaths	11.1
Other clear symptoms	5.0
Miscellaneous, including extreme old age	16.8

Table 29.4   Per cent of outpatients by diagnosis

| | Health centres | | Sub centres (dispensaries) | |
	A	B	A	B
Infections and parasitic diseases	49.4	43.3	33.4	27.3
Nutritional	3.3	0.8	0.3	1.2
Mental disorders and CNS	7.2	5.9	12.1	12.2
Respiratory	10.5	12.9	20.5	17.6
Digestive system	9.1	14.1	26.3	26.6
Genito-urinary	2.5	1.7	–	0.5
Skin	11.7	14.9	4.0	5.9
Accidents, poisoning	1.2	0.5	1.1	2.6
Other diagnoses	5.1	5.9	2.1	5.2

important than the causes described in the conventional text book. The auxiliary who has spent a considerable part of his or her professional life in villages, the part-time health worker, the village school teacher, the agricultural extension worker, the community development officer and above all the villagers themselves can be a mine of information and every opportunity to cultivate their friendship and help should be utilised.

During the training sessions with the auxiliaries and village health workers a considerable amount of information can be gathered about local customs and practices, especially if the training is in the form of discussion groups instead of didactic lectures. The information thus obtained is then used to supplement the vital statistics and other health data to construct a true picture of problems and needs.

Are the services coping?

The mere setting up of the health centres and sub-centres does not create a health programme. In many cases these institutions are nothing more than extensions of the out-patient department of hospitals with virtually no impact on the health situation in the community. It is best to raise in discussions the following questions: How defined needs are met? How adaptable to demand are the services? Are the different health institutions well integrated and mutually supportive or do they work in seclusion? How well are the health services integrated with other community programmes such as education, agriculture and community development?

Coverage of the vulnerable groups

By far the most important question to ask is about coverage. What is the take-up rate by the 'target' population? The vulnerable groups like children, pregnant women and lactating mothers form up to two-thirds of the population of an average rural community. Services for monitoring their health in the form of under-fives' clinics and antenatal services can produce a major impact on mortality and morbidity. The importance and purposes of antenatal care are discussed in chapter 22, and are well known. The importance of the under-fives' clinic, on the other hand, has not been sufficiently appreciated. This clinic integrates an ordinary child welfare clinic with simple out-patient care. Super-

vision of growth and nutrition (chapter 6), immunisation (chapter 7), health and nutrition education (chapter 5), advice on child spacing and early identification of developmental disorder are integrated with diagnosis and management of common illnesses such as malaria (chapter 20), diarrhoea (chapter 11), respiratory illness (chapter 24), anaemia (chapter 5) and skin or eye sepsis. Many other activities can be built around the under-fives' clinics, the objective being to generate competent parenthood, community cohesion and self-reliance. For example, parents' clubs, playgroups, nutrition rehabilitation programmes, adult literacy classes, youth clubs and similar other activities can be generated around the clinic depending upon resources and community response (figure 29.3).

The under-fives' clinic is to be thought of as a basic service for children and not a speciality clinic. Then only can it become a springboard for community activity. It has the advantage of flexibility so that depending upon the personnel available, it can vary from being very basic to a well co-ordinated and complex activity. It does not require highly trained personnel or expensive equipment and buildings, and is cost effective.

Ideally, the under-fives' and the antenatal clinic should be housed together and conducted simultaneously to form a proper MCH clinic. But this development has not yet occurred and in most countries the two clinics are conducted separately.

Like all health programmes, the mere setting up of antenatal and under-fives' services does not produce an impact on the health of the community unless certain epidemiologic criteria are met. The most important of these is that of coverage. A minimum of 80 per cent of the pregnant women and children under the age of five should attend on a regular basis before measurable benefits can occur. The other requirements are

(1) The frequency with which the clinic runs. A daily clinic especially for the under-fives' will be more beneficial than a weekly one, which is in turn better than a monthly clinic. For rural areas, the ideal will be to have one antenatal and one under-fives' clinic shared in rotation by a cluster of villages in such a way that no home is a distance of more than two miles from the clinic.

(2) The individual mother or child should attend at least once a month for health supervision but within a day of onset of any illness.

(3) A suitable antenatal card and, for children, a parent-retained growth chart should be available.

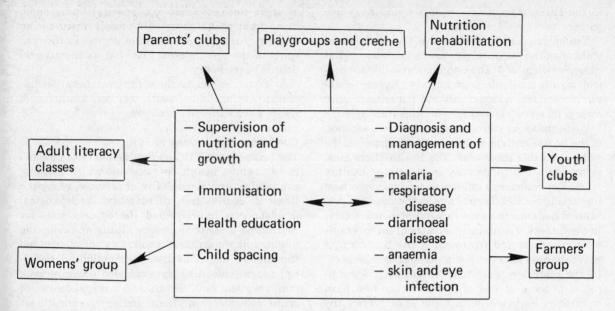

Figure 29.3   Activities of the under-fives' clinics

(4) Those who do not attend regularly are usually the ones with problems. There should be provision for home-visiting and follow-up care of such families.

(5) Criteria should be established for the identification of the pregnant woman, child or family who is 'at risk' of disease.

Community participation, a key factor for success

Success or failure of the community health services is usually decided by community involvement and support. To what extent are the services looked upon as part of their social and cultural life by the people and not something alien imposed from outside? The establishment of a continuing dialogue with the community generating bonds of mutual trust and friendship and involvement of the community in planning, implementation and evaluation of health programmes are some of the factors contributing to popularity of health programmes.

Part of the objective of a rural health programme is to develop local awareness, bring about community organisation through group activities and develop local leadership for self-reliance. Some of the community groups mentioned such as farmers' clubs, youth clubs, women's organisations, play

groups, literacy and handicraft classes in fact act as pegs on which several mutually supportive activities hang together. The village health worker and the trained birth attendant are two examples of the willingness by the village leadership to commit resources to the health effort. In the same way, the village council acting through the health committee or other community groups is often able to contribute resources for other forms of activities.

A conceptual model of a community health programme

On the basis of the above discussion, a conceptual model for a district health programme is suggested in figure 29.4 as follows. At any given time in a district there will be some sick, some ambulatory sick and a large number of healthy people. This is suggested on the left-hand diagram in the figure. Services are required for all these three groups as shown in the middle diagram. In-patient care for the sick and out-patient services for the ambulatory sick are easy to understand. What is not widely appreciated is the fact that services are also necessary for maintaining the healthy in a state of good health. But here there are two important considerations. Firstly, the services should be delivered to the people in their homes, at their places of work, in the schools, in the fields, in the market place, in the places of worship – in fact wherever people gather.

Examples of such services are the mother and child health services as discussed above, but nutrition (chapter 5) and communicable disease control, mainly tuberculosis (chapter 14), leprosy (chapter 15) malaria (chapter 20) and parasitic disease control (chapter 21) also play an important role.

When the above two criteria are met then addition of the *at-risk concept* will make the diagram on the right hand side come true. The health effort aims to maintain the community in the upper healthy layer. Environmental influences tend to push them into the lower sick layer. Here is the need for prevention and cure to merge into comprehensive care. In the context of a minimum of 80 per cent coverage, early diagnosis and treatment is the best form of prevention, as for example in malaria or diarrhoea. In the context of such a coverage, early identification of those at risk of disease is the best form of curative medicine. Within the same service the dichotomy between care and prevention disappears and becomes the concept of comprehensive care.

Primary health care

Many of the concepts discussed in the foregoing sections have been brought together under the heading of Primary Health Care (PHC), first enunciated at an international meeting in Alma Ata in 1978. PHC is not to be misunderstood as first contact care. It stands for health care in its broadest sense, and involves activities and involvement in the following eight elements

(1) Safe and clean water, and sanitation including environmental health.
(2) Adequate nutrition.
(3) Immunisation against common infectious diseases, as well as the control of endemic communicable diseases.
(4) Mother and child health.
(5) Minor treatment facilities, and care of emergencies.
(6) Referral services.
(7) Health education about the prevalent health problems.
(8) Community participation in the planning, implementation, monitoring and evaluation of health activities.

Different countries have interpreted PHC in the light of their existing health infrastructure, as well as their socio-economic and political background. Some countries have carried out major restructuring of their health services, and not always in the true spirit of the principles of PHC but as a matter of political expediency.

As countries make their progress towards universal coverage with health services, a number of issues have surfaced as follows.

Comprehensive or selective PHC

The principles of PHC as first defined are directed more towards health development which includes availability and accessibility of services, along the lines of equity and affordability. Technological developments have created the opportunities for controlling some of the major killing and crippling diseases like diarrhoea, respiratory infections, and the common infectious diseases of childhood. Essential programmes like the expanded programme of immunisation, oral rehydration therapy, control of acute respiratory infections, and so on, cannot wait for the physical, technical and managerial infrastructures of PHC to be in place first. In fact they comprise the cutting edge of PHC. Such programmes are usually listed under the heading of Selective Primary Health Care.

The different terminologies create unnecessary confusion, and tend to draw attention away from the fact that the main objective of PHC is to make essential health care universally available in a society. A rational approach will be to exploit fully all new developments for controlling local health problems whilst working towards the goal of PHC.

Lack of resources

In the 1970s when the elements of PHC were being defined, it was estimated that not more than 20 per cent of the population in the developing world enjoyed regular health coverage. Universal coverage meant expanding the health services four to five fold. This is an impossible task, bearing in mind the triple difficulties of inflation, international debt burden, and the readjustment policies enforced by the international monetary organisations. The economic realities have forced countries to consider a variety of innovative approaches like the use of auxiliaries, community health promoters and traditional healers including birth attendants. More recently attempts have been made to transfer costs of services to the consumers, for example, the Bamako initiative in West Africa.

Rapid urban growth

Most developing countries have experienced mushrooming of their urban populations. Whereas urban growth prior to 1970s was mainly through in-migration, it is now taking place through natural increase. The growth of squatter areas, urban slums, and inner city decay is now universal in all developing countries. Up to 40 per cent of the population of the average city in the Third world are living in such neighbourhoods, mostly below the poverty line (defined as having to spend 80 per cent of the family income to obtain the necessary requirements of calories from common staple foods). Poverty, family disintegration, and lack of traditional social networks present special challenges to PHC in such communities.

The health problems of squatter and inner city populations stem from three main causes as follows

(1) Direct problems of poverty arising from unemployment, limited education, and low income. The physical manifestations are undernutrition, early abandonment of breast feeding so that the mother can work, and involvement with illegal activities.

(2) Environmental problems arising from poor housing, overcrowding, inadequate water and sanitation, lack of waste disposal, and often proximity to industrial hazards. The physical manifestations are infectious and parasitic diseases, accidents and poisoning, and lack of personal hygiene.

(3) Psycho-social problems arising from stress, alienation, insecurity and family instability. These manifest as depression, low self esteem, alcoholism, drug abuse, violence and abandonment of children.

PHC as initially defined in 1978 must evolve further to meet the new challenges of the 1990s.

Seven faces of paediatrics revisited

The inadequacy of present day paediatric care in developing countries is mentioned on page 22. It is pointed out that hospital paediatric care is just one of the seven facets of child care. It has received undue importance at the expense of other aspects of child care. The widespread morbidity in young children has understandably resulted in paediatric sickness assuming a dominant position in health care planning. Yet if the major illnesses of children are preventable, then why are they not prevented?

The conceptual model in figure 29.4 emphasises paediatrics of prevention, of community health and of life-style and habit at home through community involvement and participation. The auxiliary and the village health worker, including the village midwife, are the chief agents, with the district hospital and the health centre providing professional, educational and administrative support. There is potential for expanding the work of the under-fives' clinic to prevent emotional and physical handicap and to diagnose problems early. One additional facet to the under-fives' programme is the 'child-to-child' programme to extend health into the school curriculum and improve the care of the toddler through the older sibling.

Primary care for all by the year 2000! Will it remain a dream, or become reality? The knowledge exists and resources can be mustered if only professional skill can be mobilised.

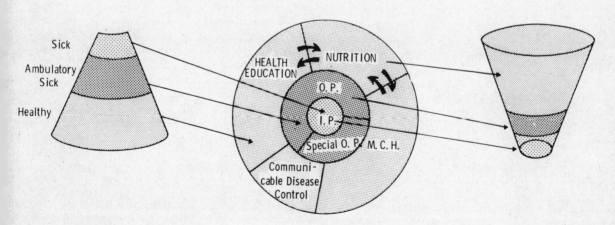

Figure 29.4 Health care model

Further reading

Aarons, A, Hawes H, Gayton J. *Child-to-Child*. Basingstoke and London: Macmillan, 1979.

Amonoo-Larston R, Ebrahim G J, Lovel H J, Ranken J P. *District Health Care. Challenges for planning, organisation and evaluation in developing countries*. Basingstoke and London: Macmillan. 1984.

Ebrahim G J. *Social and community paediatrics in developing countries: caring for the rural and urban poor*. Basingstoke and London: Macmillan. 1985.

Ebrahim G J. *Practical mother and child health in developing countries*. Basingstoke and London: Macmillan 1991.

Ebrahim G J. and Ranken J P. (Eds). *Primary Health Care: reorienting organisational support*. Basingstoke and London: Macmillan. 1988.

Ebrahim G J. Village health workers. *In*: Wallace H, Ebrahim G J, (Eds). *Maternal and child health around the world*. Basingstoke and London: Macmillan, 1981.

World Health Organisation. *Health For All* series No. 1 to 6. Geneva: W.H.O. 1978 (No. 1), 1979, and 1981.

Index